Preventive Mental Heal

Gayle L. Macklem

Preventive Mental Health at School

Evidence-Based Services for Students

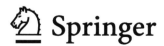 Springer

Gayle L. Macklem
Massachusetts School of Professional Psychology
Newton, MA, USA

ISBN 978-1-4614-8608-4 (Hardcover)   ISBN 978-1-4614-8609-1 (eBook)
ISBN 978-1-4939-2161-4 (Softcover)
DOI 10.1007/978-1-4614-8609-1
Springer New York Heidelberg Dordrecht London

Library of Congress Control Number: 2013945167

Springer is part of Springer Science+Business Media (www.springer.com)

Preface

The National Association of School Psychologists updated its *Model for Comprehensive and Integrated School Psychologist Services* in 2010. The 2010 model includes recognition of the need for systems-level services for school-based mental health professionals. The model broadens the responsibility of school psychologists to include knowledge of systems theory to influence school practices. This text is designed to assist school psychologists, school mental health counselors, social workers, and administrators in preventive work. It is designed to develop a strong working knowledge of prevention science and public health, ecological models so that school-based mental health professionals can collaboratively influence the development of comprehensive services for all children, at all levels in schools.

The text includes a very specific skill set needed for this important work. It teaches the skills of locating and selecting strong evidence-based preventive curricula and programs. It includes strategies to increase student engagement and motivation through active learning as well as strategies to engage families through school and family partnerships. Moving schools toward system change involves challenging shifts in thinking and in how work is accomplished in schools. Critical data collection skills are needed to include measures of organizational readiness and knowledge of theories of change. Much of this work may feel "new" to those who have worked in schools for some time, as many concepts come from the business world rather than from the education field.

In order to become advocates for change, school-based mental health workers will need to use their knowledge of the trajectories of the risky behaviors in which some adolescents engage, as well as of the factors influencing the externalizing disorders and internalizing disorders that students may develop. The critical need for implementation fidelity in preventive programming and skills for making improvements in implementation are addressed. The skills needed to learn to make safe adaptations to evidence-based programming so preventive work can engage diverse populations, and can fit local schools, are addressed in detail. Adapting evidence-based programs for young children is included. The many and various tools needed for preventive work in schools are covered to include resource mapping, needs assessment, universal mental health screening, developing a logic model, choosing a theory of change, process evaluation including monitoring, and outcomes evaluation. Finally, a few examples of practitioners at the school systems level attempting to develop comprehensive mental health programming are described.

As the student populations and our schools are rapidly changing and becoming more diverse, it is critical that school-based mental health professionals become significantly more aware of cultural differences. Professionals must know how ethnicity, culture, gender, and other differences affect mental health issues. Mental health awareness, understandings, and belief systems differ. This affects mental health programming. Instructional practices make a difference for students of different races, ethnicities, and genders. Different strategies are needed at different times, for different situations, and for different students and their families. Schools and school practices must be relevant for all students and families.

Many different evidence-based and promising curricula and programs addressing social-emotional learning and various preventive efforts to change behavior are described. There is much valuable material and resources to access. As each set of skills is addressed, readers are challenged to try out and use some of the specific skills. Completing this work will prepare school-based mental health professionals to make important inroads into efforts to change schools so that they can meet the mental health needs of the populations they serve.

Systems thinking is challenging at first. As practitioners, mental health professionals, and school leaders become more comfortable with systems thinking, they will increase confidence in their ability to effect change. This will have significant benefits for the children and families they serve.

On a personal note, there are several individuals who have contributed to this effort. Andria Amador of the Boston Public Schools and Melissa Pearrow of UMass Boston generously shared their work in developing a comprehensive behavioral health plan in Boston, Massachusetts. Others may learn from their efforts. Bob Lichtenstein of the Massachusetts School of Professional Psychology (MSPP) invited me to teach *Preventive Mental Health in Schools* in the MSPP School Psychology training program in Newton, MA. This opportunity allowed me to solidify and share my thinking in regard to population-based mental health services. Most importantly, Dick Macklem has served as a sounding board for this text. It would be hard to describe how much his unswerving support, patience, and good advice have helped and literally made this work possible. I am exceedingly grateful.

Newton, MA, USA   Gayle L. Macklem

Contents

List of Challenges

List of Tables

Chapter 1
Providing Preventive Services in Schools

A substantial number of school-aged children and adolescents in schools are impacted by problems affecting their mental health (Weissberg, Kumpfer, & Seligman, 2003). Too many adolescents get involved with risky behaviors. Too many children and adolescents have not developed sufficient social–emotional competencies to function at their best. Frequently cited estimates indicate that as many as 20 % of school-aged children have mental health problems affecting their behavior and learning (Duchnowski, Kutash, & Friendman, 2002). In many large urban school districts, as many as half of the total student population have learning, behavior, and/or emotional problems (Center for Mental Health in Schools, 2003).

There are currently strong calls for schools to step up to the challenge of meeting the mental health needs of all school-aged children and adolescents. This presents a tremendous additional burden for schools as well as an enormous opportunity for service. In order to appreciate the challenge and to take steps to move in the direction of comprehensive mental health services for children in schools, it is necessary to appreciate the extent of the problem and to evaluate the current service models used in schools. To move forward, a population-based perspective is needed. This entails knowledge of the public health model of prevention and taking an ecological approach to mental health services in schools. The terminology and "systems thinking" will be new to some school-based professionals, but until we move in this direction, we cannot even begin to address students' needs in the area of mental health.

The Need for Mental Health Services in Schools

Mental health is neither a single state nor is it stable. It is a continuum that changes over time. Mental health also changes across groups of students in additional to whatever is going on within a single student (Murphey, Barry, & Vaughn, 2013). More than half of diagnosable emotional disorders have onsets by age 14 (Kessler, Berglund, et al., 2005). Estimates of the number of adolescents with diagnosable

G.L. Macklem, *Preventive Mental Health at School: Evidence-Based Services for Students*,
DOI 10.1007/978-1-4614-8609-1_1, © Springer Science+Business Media New York 2014

disorders are difficult to determine. Teens are not eager to disclose their problems, definitions vary, and disorders are determined by clinical rather than biological means. Depression is the most common type of emotional difficulty in adolescents, although it often coexists with other diagnosable disorders.

According to a 2011 survey of 12–17 year olds by the Centers for Disease Control and Prevention (CDC, 2012b), 29 % of high school students reported sadness and hopelessness almost every day for 2 weeks or longer during the past year. The group with depression was slightly higher than adolescents with conduct disorders. Ten percent of adolescents reported anxiety and 5 % reported symptoms associated with eating disorders. Substance abuse is strongly associated with emotional disorders. Teens with mental disorders are more vulnerable to risky behaviors, with suicide as the most disturbing consequence. Importantly, the first symptoms of a mental health disorder are seen 2–4 years before a disorder can be diagnosed (Biglan, 2009). This does not necessarily mean that these symptoms would be easily identified, but with training, school staff may be able to identify early symptoms or less obvious symptoms. Teachers and other school personnel can be taught to watch for irritability, anger, social withdrawal, and physiological symptoms. Training all school staff members to be more aware of and to work toward prevention and early intervention could make a huge difference in the lives of school-aged children.

According to Volpe, Briesch, and Chafouleas (2010), the "overwhelming majority" of students who could be helped by preventive efforts, do not receive services (p. 240). In fact, they are not even identified. Of the one in five adolescents with a mental health disorder, most students do not look for, or receive, needed services (Murphey, Vaughn, & Barry, 2013). In a study of 3,042 students aged 8–15 with the goal of building a national database on mental health among youth, researchers found only half of the students with diagnosed mental health disorders had sought treatment (Merikangas et al., 2010). Although proven and promising programs exist, there are many barriers affecting needed services. The most obvious include stigma associated with mental health difficulties, lack of attention to prevention by schools, poorly coordinated systems of care, and shortages of trained service providers.

Barriers also include the traditional model of pullout services in most schools and the negative environments in many poor community schools (Rones & Hoagwood, 2000). Disparities in mental health care have been well documented. Sixteen- and 17-year-old boys are the least likely of all school-aged students to be given help for mental health problems. Lesbian, gay, bisexual, or transgender adolescents; homeless teens; incarcerated teens; children under the child welfare umbrella; uninsured adolescents; and adolescents in rural areas have particular difficulty accessing treatment. Publically funded insurance is available to some students, but even in this case many states have limits on those services.

There is general agreement that the mental health problems of children are "widespread" and begin when children are quite young (Stagman & Cooper, 2010, p. 3). Children and adolescents with problems in the area of mental health do not achieve in school at the same rates or to the same level as their peers. They are more likely to be involved in the criminal justice system. They are more likely to experience problems in school, they may fail in school, or they may drop out. It is important to emphasize again that most students do not receive needed services. Even when students are insured, they may not receive services. For those who do receive services, care is often deficient due to use of interventions which are not evidence-based and do not have empirical support. Problems impeding mental health services are found in regard to both infrastructure and lack of finances in schools. Although evidence-based practices (EBPs) are one of the major preventive strategies, there are many barriers to adopting the best interventions.

Students in poor communities are especially impacted. They tend to have fewer qualified teachers. Parents in these communities are less involved for understandable reasons (Williams & Greenleaf, 2012). Students in these communities have less access to books, computers, and other resources. More generally, there are serious discrepancies in schools in regard to race, ethnicity, gender, class, disability status, and sexual orientation. Racial/ethnic minority students are more often placed in special education. They are more often punished more severely than their White counterparts. They are more often punished for minor disciplinary acts. They are more often suspended and expelled than White students for the same behaviors. They are more likely to be retained and to drop out of school. Children with disabilities are bullied more frequently. They are sexually harassed and isolated. Sexual minority students are harassed, isolated, and more subject to violence than their peers.

Kutash, Duchnowski, and Lynn (2006) published a monograph outlining approaches to school-based mental services. They pointed out that the Individuals with Disabilities Education Act (IDEA) actually added some confusion in regard to which agencies are responsible for mental health services, i.e., community mental health facilities or schools. School-based professionals have not typically taken on the role of social change, yet a student's behavior is a result of interactions between the child and the environment that are not effective. Schools must emphasize social and educational equity and equal opportunities. School mental health professionals are in a position to advocate for equal and fair support for every student. Additionally, it is important for school-based mental health professionals to align with parents who lack skills and knowledge to access resources and to teach parents and students about their rights (Williams & Greenleaf, 2012). Although most children and adolescents who need mental health services do not get services, and because schools are the most likely place that youngsters might receive services, there is now a strong focus on schools as the key or even primary site to provide mental health services for children and adolescents.

Williams and Greenleaf (2012) recommend that school professionals work with groups of students rather than individuals and redefine their roles. Researchers interested in moving mental health services to schools, or in improving the mental health services that are already in place in schools, stress using data to change the roles of school-based mental health workers and add advocacy to their roles. School psychologists, for example, are urged to gather data and factual information to support their own role change and advocate for those changes not only in their own schools but also at the district level (p. 52).

Current Services Models

The issue is not that schools ignore the need for mental health services to students but rather that the current models are insufficient to meet needs. School mental health providers currently provide an estimated 70–80 % of mental health services to the subgroup of students who do receive services for mental health issues (Rones & Hoagwood, 2000). The typical model in school mental health has been individual counseling for children with mental health difficulties and case management (Ringeisen, Henderson, & Hoagwood, 2003).

A majority of schools in the United States provide individual counseling and case management; about half of schools provide some group counseling, but very few provide parent services (Kutash, Duchnowski, & Green, 2011). About one-third of school districts lean solely on school-based mental health workers to provide services and a quarter of schools use only community agencies. A little more than half of schools in the United States have contracts with outside agencies to augment in-school staff services. Weist (2003a) warns however that community providers should never be brought into schools if this might be used to replace school-based mental health workers. Community-based mental health providers should only augment the work already being done in schools. Slightly more than half of schools use some sort of social–emotional curricula, although this may be an underestimate given strong movements to implement curricula in this area and the expanded types of programming considered under the umbrella of social–emotional learning (SEL). Kutash and colleagues argue in favor of preventive efforts that are equally effective in the emotional and academic domains for at-risk populations.

Unfortunately, mental health delivery systems in schools are often designed in a piecemeal fashion, and programs are implemented in a disjointed and fragmented manner (Adelman, 1996). Mental health practitioners, such as school psychologists, work in isolation and are not included in decision-making in many schools. Student mental health services are considered desirable, but not essential. In order to address this, a comprehensive preventive intervention perspective is needed. Mental health services and programs must be comprehensive, overseen and monitored by school-based teams, and be considered essential by school staff members and administrators.

The public wants safe and orderly schools (Billings, 1996, p. 487) and there is strong support at the federal level for the integration of education and mental health in schools as evidenced by the Surgeon General's report (USDHHS, 1999) and The President's New Freedom Commission on Mental Health (2003). More and more there is a growing consensus that mental health programming should be located in schools. At the same time, there has been limited progress to support sustained mental health programming within the ecologies of schools (Atkins, Hoagwood, & Seidman, 2010). Efforts that focus on mental health promotion, prevention, and/or intervention compete with one another for attention in school settings. This competition is exacerbated by reductions in funding for schools. Clearly there is concern around the unmet psychosocial needs of children and their families. Educators, in general, agree that mental health and education should be integrated, but this would require enormous changes in service delivery in schools.

Atkins et al. (2010) propose a new paradigm for mental health services in schools. They recommend that in-school mental health professionals become "educational enhancers" to assist teachers who would become the first-line change agents. Mental health school-based professionals, such as school psychologists, mental health counselors, and school social workers, could help teachers manage their classes and provide effective instruction for students. This would embed mental health staff in the classroom as consultants to improve implementation of preventive programming. There is a critical need to integrate models to enhance academic success and learning and to promote mental health at the same time. School resources need to be reallocated to implement and sustain support for emotional and behavioral health, to improve outcomes for all school-aged children, and to support the active involvement of parents. The mental health needs of the entire school population must be considered.

The goal is a continuum of services in schools from primary prevention to treatment of serious problems (Adelman & Taylor, 2003). Programs need to be coordinated with one another and with educational programming. Instead of a reliance on reactive strategies, schools need to focus on prevention (Schrag, 1996). Instead of a focus on disability and the weaknesses of students and families, schools need to focus on strengths. Coordination must become the goal rather than compartmentalizing issues and concerns. Appreciation that student and family concerns are interconnected must be widespread. Communication must be clear among all stakeholders.

Schools have been providing services in the area or domain of mental health service since the end of the nineteenth century (Kutash et al., 2006). It is not that there have been no efforts to address these issues; there have been a number of efforts to make systems changes in schools such as school-linked services, integrated services, interagency services, and comprehensive systems of care (Schrag, 1996, p. 491). However, these efforts are not standard practice in the majority of schools. Forness (2003) advocated for schools, and school psychologists in particular, to become more aggressive in identifying mental health concerns, given "rarely" has there been "a substantial focus on early detection" (p. 63).

Some progress is being made. The three-tiered model has provided the impetus for recent changes in academic, social–emotional, and behavioral programming in schools (Forness, 2003, p. 111). The three-tiered model represents a different perspective influencing delivery of school services (Meyers, Meyers, Graybill, Proctor, & Huddleston, 2012). Prevention efforts from this perspective focus on the system as a whole or on an identified subsystem or component within the larger system. The three-tiered model includes services for every student in a school population. Tier 1 services support the total school population. Tier 2 provides for students at risk for mental health, behavioral, or academic difficulties. Tier 3 services those students with identified issues in various domains.

Making changes in the way things are done is a "formidable task" (Huang, Hepburn, & Espiritu, 2003). In attempting to change schools, school discipline and turf issues complicate the change process. In order to develop the skills for prevention work in schools and to learn to build comprehensive mental health services in schools, it is necessary to learn the language and theory of prevention science. This may initially be experienced as new and complex. An introduction to the terminology and concepts is provided here, with many individual chapters ahead to explore the concepts in depth. The approach will become more comfortable and familiar as school-based mental health professionals develop expertise in systems thinking.

A Brief History of Prevention Science

"Prevention requires a paradigm shift. Successful prevention is inherently interdisciplinary" (Report of the Committee on the Prevention of Mental Disorders and Substance Abuse, 2009, Slide #7). In general, less attention has been given to prevention than to treatment when considering the mental health problems of students in schools. Prevention research has not caught up with treatment research (Rishel, 2007). According to the American Psychological Association (APA) Task Force on Evidence-Based Practice for Children and Adolescents (2008), prevention programs are important. They reduce rates of social, behavioral, academic, and psychological problems in students.

Prevention is a multidisciplinary science to which many disciplines have contributed (Weissberg et al., 2003). This has resulted in a variety of terms, which can create confusion for school professionals when reading prevention-focused articles in peer-reviewed journals. Gerald Caplan (1964) described prevention as primary (for everyone), secondary (for at-risk groups), and tertiary (to prevent complications or relapses). Gordon (1987) used labels to include universal (for everyone), selective (for at-risk groups), and indicated (for those at the highest risk). Romano and Hage (2000) added health promotion and institutional change, making the three-tiered model into five tiers.

The Institute of Medicine (IOM) later described preventive efforts "universal" when the entire population would be serviced; "selective," when the needs of subgroups considered at-risk were addressed; and "indicated," when the highest risk individuals with symptoms of mental health disorders were targeted (Mrazek & Haggerty, 1994). In the 1990s, the prevention field as a whole adopted the terms universal, selective, and indicated. The three-tiered model commonly used in psychology and in education uses a third set of terms: Tier 1 or universal, Tier 2 or targeted, and Tier 3 or intensive services (Strein & Koehler, 2008). The three-tiered models from various fields explain their tiers in a similar manner. The universal level services all students while the targeted level serves at-risk students. The intensive tier may serve those exhibiting notable symptoms, those identified for special education services under federal/state laws and regulations or those with diagnosed disorders but who do not need educational services (Table 1.1).

Table 1.1 Preventive mental health terminology

Public health model	Institute of Medicine (IOM)	National Institute of Mental Health (NIMH)	Schools using RtI or SW-PBIS	Current service model in schools
Primary	Universal	Universal	Tier 1	General education classroom
Secondary	Targeted	Selective	Tier 2	Small group service
Tertiary	Indicated	Indicated	Tier 3	Individualized or small group services

Note: RtI stands for Response-to-Intervention; SW-PBIS stands for School-Wide Positive Behavior Interventions and Supports

National interest in prevention began with a report by the National Advisory Mental Health Council (1990). This was followed by work of the National Institute of Mental Health (NIMH 1993, 1998) and the IOM (1994). The 1994 IOM report differentiated prevention from treatment and pointed out the importance of prevention. Preventive interventions must be put in place before significant symptoms appear in children and adolescents (Greenberg, Domitrovich, & Bumbarger, 2000).

Prevention science integrates models from public health, sociology, epidemiology, and developmental psychopathology (Greenberg et al., 2000). Complex studies of causation and risk have contributed as well. Mental health risk factors may be constitutional and involve skill deficits or delays. They may involve emotional difficulties, family issues, and complications. They may derive from interpersonal issues or problems in school. Risk factors may be associated with poverty, injustice, and/or neighborhood dangers and disorganization. There are multiple routes to emotional and behavioral difficulties in that different combinations of risk factors might contribute to the same disorder. Search for a single cause of various mental health disorders may be a waste of time and resources. Because risk factors contribute to a number of negative outcomes, it makes sense to target multiple risk factors when locating and selecting preventive strategies and to focus on reducing interacting factors. At the same time, it is important to increase protective factors. Protective factors can decrease risk or buffer their effects, disrupt the progressions, or prevent onset of problems.

As applied to schools, universal prevention addresses all of the students in a school system. Universal prevention is proactive rather than reactive. It does not require risk status. It minimizes stigma. Universal prevention is a broad and positive approach. The advantages of universal prevention include the avoidance of labeling and the possibility of addressing a range of problems, while promoting resilience at the same time. Universal prevention can decrease the risk of students developing mental health disorders. Universal prevention programs tend to engage teachers in implementing the interventions. They can engage parents in reinforcing social–emotional learning skills (SEL) taught in school (Kutash et al., 2006). The disadvantages of universal preventive efforts include spending money and effort on children who may be fine without the intervention. The low dosage of universal programming may be insufficient to help those at significant risk. The greatest impact of universal programming may help only a small group of students. On the other hand, even small positive outcomes may make a significant difference in the lives of children and their families and may prevent mental health difficulties when healthy students later encounter stress or risks.

Current Directions in Prevention Science

When designing or choosing universal prevention programs or preventive interventions, school-based mental health professionals must learn to select interventions that target multiple risk factors. Mental health disorders have multiple risk factors (Domitrovich et al., 2010). The common risk factors to many different disorders include poverty, family conflict (coercion), poor self-regulation, and aggression in social relationships (Biglan, 2009). Students who do not learn to regulate their emotions are at high risk for future behavioral problems and emotional problems. Risk factors predict multiple outcomes and negative behaviors. Health-risk behaviors co-occur, particularly in adolescence. Preventive efforts need to address multiple risk factors in order to affect multiple outcomes. Building protective factors is equally important in decreasing risk. Much of the current prevention research has focused on elementary schools, and this work has resulted in a number of evidence-based universal prevention programs, although most of these focus on preventing behavioral or externalizing disorders.

Nation et al. (2003) proposed coordinated programming to prevent mental health problems. This would involve using a research-based risk and protective factor framework involving all stakeholders and targeting multiple outcomes. Programming over time would be delivered to specific age groups in a culturally appropriate manner. All students would receive training in social–emotional and ethical values. Policies, practices, and environmental supports would be established. Teachers would be trained and supported to implement programming with fidelity. Evidence-based programming would be scientifically adapted to fit to local school communities and would be continuously monitored.

Greenberg et al. (2000) point out that multi-year prevention programs would have longer lasting benefits. Preventive efforts need to start early, and efforts should be aimed at risk and protective factors rather than at specific disorders. Additionally, researchers point out that the targets of prevention must include both the school and the home environments. Interventions need to be at the environmental level. This means promoting nurturing environments, reinforcing prosocial behaviors, monitoring progress, and setting limits for students who need it (Biglan, 2009). School settings for preventive efforts make sense. However, school professionals must realize that prevention efforts are challenging because access to environmental supports and protections are limited for many children (Opler, Sodhi, Zaveri, & Madhusoodanan, 2010).

Preventive programs have demonstrated benefits for all age groups of children and adolescents and for all mental health disorders (Opler et al., 2010). The data to support the effectiveness of primary prevention efforts to prevent psychopathology and to promote healthy development in high-risk students is "ample" (p. 230). Primary preventive efforts can improve the understanding of mental illness. Primary preventive efforts can improve coping skills in all children. Preventive efforts work better when they address children's social environments, include family and peers, and address issues in the surrounding community. Preventive programs are more effective when implemented early and when they include booster lessons later on. Preventive efforts are most effective when targeting risk or protective factors rather than a specific symptom and when they are integrated and coordinated with other efforts.

The Medical Model Versus Population-Based Models

School mental health services have been developed based on the medical model. The medical model ties students' educational and academic problems to the child alone (Gutkin, 2012). This model makes servicing all children in need "nearly impossible" (p. 4). Also of concern is the fact that diagnosing pathology does not necessarily result in strong treatments with empirically validated interventions specific to the diagnosis. The medical model does not feature environmental strategies and interventions that might promote generalization and decrease the likelihood of reoccurrence of problems.

The medical model misses many students who need some sort of support in schools. For example, there are many children in schools who have subclinical symptoms and would not qualify for special education services. Significant numbers of students experience mental health issues that are not defined as "disabling" (Baker, Kamphaus, Horne, & Winsor, 2006). The problem with the medical model is that it is both resource-intensive and the impact on broader problems is limited. School-based mental health professionals need to move beyond individual child treatment to developing and implementing interventions that are "relevant to the contextual needs of a dynamic education system" (Ringeisen et al., 2003, p. 165).

Schools are not going to succeed when they continually take a reactive approach to solving problems. Success is more likely when schools take a comprehensive approach that utilizes prevention science (Burns, 2011). Burns defines prevention science as "the process of identifying potential risk and protective factors" (p. 134).

When the *entire school* setting is the target of preventive efforts, the school mental health professionals or a school prevention team is utilizing a "systems" framework (Strein & Koehler, 2008). Moving beyond servicing individuals to servicing all students, or to servicing systems, requires systems thinking. Systems thinking addresses the systems that affect both the school and the individual student.

Behavior in a system develops in continuous loops or circles (Darnton, 2008). Contrary to the typical school services three-tiered triangle model where as many as 80 % of students would fall in the broadest group at the universal or Tier 1 level, an urban school system may have very high numbers of children needing services. In a study of a small city with four elementary schools with diverse students, almost 56 % of students exhibited behaviors in need for selective or indicated prevention services (Baker et al., 2006). This fact should make it clear that assigning percentages of students serviced to the well-known tiered triangle does not work. The prevention tiered model uses circles that overlap and are integrated to explain what school-based mental health services should look like.

Systems thinking is a point of view that focuses on patterns of interrelationships between components of the whole organization instead of dealing with parts of the whole (Hargreaves, 2010). Systems thinking is interested in how behavior is generated and focuses on what causes the behavior. Systems thinking allows those interested in prevention to connect preventive efforts with contexts and with the diverse perspectives of stakeholders.

In order to move schools to new mental health service delivery systems, there will need to be changes. Mental health workers and other professionals in schools will need to learn new ways of thinking and will need new tools. Change involves multiple individuals and subgroups, and the relationships between subgroups can be complex. All stakeholders' views are important. The dynamics of a system must be understood when change is attempted. The goals of the system change must be clear and agreed upon.

School-based professionals will need competency in systems change and organizational consultation in order to be successful in changing schools (Meyers et al., 2012). In order to help all students, particularly the students who have been bypassed or neglected, and to meet the urgent need for mental health services for students, interventions need to take place at the systems level.

The Public Health Model

The public health model with its emphasis on prevention is becoming more prevalent in the minds of those who want to meet the needs of *all* students. The public health view of school-based service delivery focuses on systems-level interventions. Systems-level interventions may be the "first line of defense against mental health and learning problems" in students (Meyers et al., 2012). Prevention work can involve indirect services such as teacher or parent consultation, staff training, conducting needs assessments, reorganizing school resources, reducing barriers to learning, or assessing systemic readiness to change among other challenges. The public health model places prevention "first" (Hyde, 2012).

The public health model, as applied to schools, comprises a number of components. It features comprehensive services so students receive services according to their needs. It addresses not only the child but also the complex environments surrounding the child including the classroom, friendships, the school, the family, and the community cultures. This is the "ecological developmental approach" to mental health services for students. The approach may also involve mental health and behavioral screening and surveillance of processes. It requires EBPs with a focus on data-based problem solving. This is necessary because behavior is the result of interactions between individual students and the various environments that affect them (Glanz & Rimer, 2008).

Federal policy advocates for the public health model, focusing on populations rather than on individual students (Kutash et al., 2006). The President's New Freedom Commission Report on Mental Health recognized the importance of schools in regard to children's mental health by recommending improving and expanding programs with the goal of increase access to mental health services for students (President's New Freedom Commission on Mental Health, 2003). Schools already provide some degree of prevention services at least in regard to prevention of negative behaviors. However, the quality of the programs being implemented in schools is questionable (Langley, Nadeem, Kataoka, Stein, & Jacox, 2010). The public health model as applied to schools starts with an examination of the risk and protective factors influencing a particular concern. Goals are directed not only to reducing risks but also to strengthening protective factors. The steps of the model involve first identifying problem through data collection (also labeled surveillance) at the population level (all students). Second, causes or antecedents are determined as well as how these might be changed to reduce risks. Third, preventive interventions are researched and evaluated. Fourth, action is taken to prepare for intervention, followed by implementation and monitoring the interventions selected. However, there are considerable concerns around the implementation and evaluation of programming in schools, and yet another challenge involves integrating mental health programming with academics.

Ecological Theory and Models

Changing systems is more likely to result in lasting change as compared to changing individual students who will return to the environments and to the people who supported the original behaviors that the mental health professional may have tried to change in the first place. If health behavior is to be changed, theories are the tools to assist the process (Crosby, Salazar, & DiClemente, 2013). Theories are systematic ways of appreciating concepts and hypotheses that may explain or predict the behaviors that mental health workers may want to change (Rimer & Glanz, 2005). Most of the health behavior theories were borrowed and adapted from the social and behavioral sciences but also draw from sociology, anthropology, consumer behavior, and marketing. Theories can guide planners to develop appropriate preventive interventions. Theories help explain the forces that impact a given behavior, help target what to change, what to monitor, what to measure, and clarify the processes for changing behavior.

The "ecological approach" of focusing on competency and improved functioning as compared to reducing symptoms is helpful in moving toward the integration of education and mental health in schools. The goal is to eliminate the past practice of providing tangential services (Rones & Hoagwood, 2000) while reaching toward integrated mental health services.

Although the ecological approach is described as "new," ecological models have been around for a long time (Crosby et al., 2013). Ecological models have been used in the field of public health and have been considered to be important since the

Table 1.2 Bronfenbrenner's ecological model

The ecological model as described by Bronfenbrenner featured interlocking levels of environmental systems surrounding and interacting with the individual student. Bronfenbrenner's
theory of human development was frequently revised over time. His earlier work described
the well-known ideas of the *microsystem* (immediate settings), the *mesosystem* (interactions
between the individual student and surrounding environments), the *exosystem* (people and
places that influence the student indirectly such as the neighborhood), and the *macrosystem*
(culture, beliefs, social structure of the school system, federal/state/local policies) affecting a
child (Doll, Spies, & Champion, 2012; Swearer, Espelage, Love, & Kingsbury, 2008; Tudge,
Mokrova, Hatfield, & Karnik, 2009)

Bronfenbrenner's later work acknowledged the role the individual child plays in her own
development. In addition, Bronfenbrenner considered proximal processes that have to do with
contexts that interact with the biological and genetic aspects of the developing child on a
regular basis and over time. This is a process–person–context–time model (PPCT). Based on
the most recent version of the theory, mental health workers would assess the types of
interactions relevant to a student's developmental outcomes of interest, investigate the ways
in which students' ages and genders influenced outcomes, and attend to the characteristics
change in response to the interactions. Mental health workers would investigate the proximal
environmental influences such as school, home, socioeconomic status (SES) of the family,
and the family culture. Professionals would consider all of these influences at a particular
time and over (Tudge et al., 2009). This perspective is even more important when considering
groups of children

1980s (Richard, Gauvin, & Raine, 2011). One influential ecological model was that
of Bronfenbrenner (1979) (Table 1.2).

In 2003, the IOM published a study addressing the education of public health
professionals (*Who will keep the public healthy? Educating public health professionals for the 21st century*). This publication focused attention on the ecological
model of public health. The ecological approach is broad and offers a unique perspective (Richard et al., 2011). This approach is expected to lead to more powerful
and effective preventive interventions. The ecological approach emphasizes prevention and early intervention that influences one or more environmental systems surrounding the child and thereby changing those connected to these systems (Gutkin,
2012). The ecological model increases the number of providers in a school system
to include teachers and possibly peers. The approach determines what works in light
of the specific caregivers involved and the relevant environments that influence student behaviors. The ecological approach avoids blaming, misunderstanding, judg-
ing, or discriminating against individuals (Hyde, 2012; Richard et al., 2011). It uses
every influence around a problem behavior to build supports for lasting change. The
ecological approach guides practice (Golden & Earp, 2012).

The concept of ecology includes everything that might influence a student's
mental health to include the classroom environment, time of day various activities
occur, school schedules, school climate, curricula, school organization, teacher perceptions, adult–student relationships, peer relationships, home–school partnerships,
expectancies, parenting styles, and instructional styles (Ysseldyke, Lekwa,
Klingbeil, & Cormier, 2012). Any or all of these could potentially influence students' mental health. An understanding of the ecology of success in school leads

mental health professionals to the early school years where positive behaviors can be shaped and ecological supports established more easily (Doll et al., 2012). Early intervention involves the use of EBPs, universal screening, multiple tiers of supports, progress monitoring, data-based decision-making, and learning to improve these processes over time (Greenwood & Kim, 2012). Intervention at the school level addresses the total school environment (Trickett & Rowe, 2012). Preventive work involves groups and the school community rather than individual students (Williams & Greenleaf, 2012). An ecological view may also include concern about equal opportunities for all students.

School climate, teacher–student relationships, parent–child relationships, and peer relationships each in turn affect the behaviors of students and their functioning. The school climate itself is an important ecological consideration as well as a preventive factor. School climate involves the curricula, the teacher's view of interpersonal relationships within the class, and teacher support. A student's behavior is related to many factors in the external environment. There are a variety of actions that can improve school climate. These include:

- Collaboration around decision-making
- A safe, orderly school with discipline that is consistent and fair
- The involvement of parents
- Student interpersonal relationships
- Staff dedication to learning (Ysseldyke et al., 2012)

Teacher–student relationships can be improved by helping a teacher understand that expressing interest in students' lives beyond school can make a difference. Teacher interest and personal attention can strengthen relationships and may improve engagement. From an ecological point of view, students' peer networks become a key area for examination. School-based mental health workers need to consider multiple settings and interpersonal interactions from a strength-based perspective in order to determine how to improve outcomes for students. The work of prevention and intervention requires collaboration between all of these systems.

The ecological model identifies missing supports for learning rather than identifying deficiencies (Doll et al., 2012). It examines the ecology of the school in interaction with students rather the student alone. Within an ecological model, a student's academic success depends on multiple tiers of influence that extends well beyond the child. Changes in any single system influencing students would affect all of the other systems. Surrounding the student with a caring community comprised of high-quality relationships fosters academic engagement and prevents negative consequences such as dropping out of school. Academic engagement is improved when the social aspect of the school is caring and supportive, when students expect to be successful, and when students have some autonomy so they can direct their own goal-directed behavior. The ecological approach of focusing on competency and improved functioning as compared to reducing symptoms will help schools move toward the integration of education and mental health services.

School Mental Health

School mental health covers a broad range of interventions and diversity of services designed to meet student needs (Franklin, Kim, Ryan, Kelly, & Mongomery, 2012). At best, the focus is the total student population and all of the programs and services in the school system from mental health promotion, to prevention, to intervention. Children spend a large amount of their time in schools, which makes schools a logical place to deliver mental health services (Domitrovich et al., 2010).

Weare and Nind (2011) examined 52 reviews of attempts to meet mental health needs in schools. They determined that the impact of efforts to enhance mental health and to prevent emotional difficulties in schools at the universal level has resulted in small to moderate outcomes. Higher risk students benefit more in regard to prevention of disorders and bullying. When considering efforts to develop social and emotional competencies in students, the impact has been moderate to strong. Universal programs when implemented in isolation are not as effective as universal plus targeted models. Prevention efforts need to begin in the earliest grades, address broad competencies, and be in place over several years.

School-based mental health professionals may be more successful implementing prevention programs initially, but teachers need to take over if programming is going to be sustained and become part of the routine of the school (Weare & Nind, 2011). Information-based preventive approaches are not as effective as active teaching approaches such as games, simulations, and group work. A major deterrent in prevention work in schools has been a lack of attention to fidelity of implementation, which has reduced the impact of programs. The more flexible bottom-up approach of preventive efforts in Europe and Australia contrasts with the top-down approach of work in the United States according to Weare and Nind. Bottom-up may work better in regard to sustainability, although the best answer may be a balance between top-down and bottom-up approaches.

An important component of prevention work in schools is the use of evidence-based programming. The implementation of EBPs is a major prevention strategy that has valid scientific support (Stagman & Cooper, 2010). Unfortunately there are many barriers to overcome in adopting EBPs in schools. Poor implementation fidelity is a major barrier. The challenge of transporting a program from well-funded and conducted university-based studies to the school setting can present huge difficulties. Another barrier is that there may not be an evidence-based program available for a particular problem that a school identifies. Although the number of randomized controlled trials has dramatically increased between the early 1990s and the present, according to Brownson, Colditz, and Proctor (2012), it takes 15–20 years for research studies on programs to be ready for dissemination so that they can be used with strong confidence in schools.

Several principles of prevention have been proposed that may allow researchers to describe the characteristics of effective programs. Principles of prevention assist practitioners in choosing a program that will work (Nation et al., 2003). In developing these principles, researchers examined reviews of prevention programs

Table 1.3 Principles associated with preventive programs that worked

1. Effective programs were comprehensive involving multiple interventions and settings
2. They included some type of active skill building with hands-on experiences and interactive instruction
3. Programs had sufficient dosage; i.e., they were implemented long enough to make a difference
4. They included booster sessions to prevent decay
5. They were theory driven, focusing on risk and protective factors
6. They provided strategies for changing risk factors
7. Building relationships were a critical component of programs that worked
8. Effective programs were attached to critical developmental periods and delivered at times of school transitions
9. The programs were relevant and culturally appropriate
10. Finally, effective programs were evaluated and improved

Source: Nation et al. (2003)

dealing with substance abuse, risky sexual behaviors, school failure, dropout, and prevention of aggressive/antisocial behaviors. Nation and colleagues distilled nine principles associated with programs that worked (see Table 1.3).

School staff members implementing the programs were well trained, received needed supports, and were supervised. These principles can help school teams choose programs that have a good chance of being effective, given school staffs have other expertise in implementing programming.

Once a school team identifies evidence-based programs these programs need to be placed into a comprehensive model. Integrated models of school mental health preventive services are more efficient (Domitrovich et al., 2010). Integrated models retain the critical or core strategies of each intervention and merge the strategies that overlap. An integrated model delivers a group of approaches, all at the same time. Integrated models are expected to have additive effects. Importantly they may reduce overload on school staff members. This is critical because schools are so focused on academic outcomes. Integrated models have the potential of improving effectiveness and increasing sustainability.

A continuum of mental health preventive services would include support for psychosocial development at the preschool-level, preventive early-schooling interventions for at-risk students, and regular ongoing supports for all students, at all school levels. Preventive interventions would be implemented *before* students evidencing symptoms are referred for intensive services (Adelman & Taylor, 2006). Preventive services would include:

- Involving all stakeholders
- Enhancing community partnerships dealing with inequity
- Consideration of diversity issues
- Balancing risk factors and protective assets
- Using evidence-based approaches and strategies

Mental health goals must be connected to the mission of schools and become part of a full range of student learning supports addressing barriers that interfere with learning. Given the restrictions of school resources and the fact that some schools are challenged by the fact that there are more students who are not doing well than those who are doing well, preventive work will require redeploying existing resources. Schools need to do more to provide public health interventions and to enhance children's mental health.

Tools for Preventive Work

One of the tools of preventive work is social marketing. Social marketing is a technique used by government and agencies to encourage people to change their behavior (Darnton, 2008). It uses business-inspired marketing approaches to reach goals. Social marketing involves selecting behaviors to address. It identifies barriers to change and designs approaches to overcome barriers. Approaches are piloted and evaluated after they have been implemented. Knott, Muers, and Aldridge (2008) developed a cultural capital framework. Knott et al. argue that interventions must address social and cultural norms. Cultural capital has to do with attitudes, values, and aspirations of individuals. These determine behavioral intentions. Over time behaviors become social norms. Social norms influence attitudes, values, and aspirations. All of these become a loop. Cultural capital impacts knowledge and skills and is a measure of assets.

Preventive interventions are designed to change the societal context for behavior (Knott et al., 2008). Systems change can be perceived as unfair by some stakeholders, particularly when change is attempted by establishing new policies. Engaging stakeholders in the process is likely to be associated with equity and acceptability. When change is contemplated, it is important to make every effort to reduce risk and increase choice or opportunity.

As school-based mental health professionals begin to address systems change, they may want to start at the classroom level. An example of a preventive tool which can be used at the classroom level is the ClassMaps Survey (Doll, Spies, Champion, et al., 2010; Doll et al., 2012; Doll, Spies, LeClair, Kurien, & Foley, 2010). Using the ClassMaps Survey, teachers would be able to distill a description of the classroom learning ecology, which would lead to problem solving. Teachers and students working together make changes in routines and practices to increase student engagement, improve interpersonal relationships, and strengthen student autonomy. This tool is also a good example of the ecological approach used in a component of school system.

Looking Ahead

Over the past few years, there have been massive cuts that have impacted the mental health care systems in the United States, particularly for youth with the most serious mental illnesses (Honberg, Diehl, Kimball, Gruttadaro, & Fitzpatrick, 2011).

An 11-state survey representing a variety of population sizes and regions of the United States determined that programming has been underfunded. Locally controlled school policies have not made the situation better. In fact, local control appears to have complicated implementation of programming in schools that were funded by their states (Behrens, Learn, & Price, 2013). This has occurred at the same time that both professionals and the general public are more aware of the fact that school systems are not meeting the needs of children and adolescents. The Patient Protection and Affordable Care Act (PPACA, 2010) (January 2014) will cover mental health disorders and substance use disorders as of January 2014. Each state will determine the benefits for children and adolescents in their respective states raising possible equity issues.

The president's plan to protect our children and our communities by reducing gun violence (2013) (http://www.whitehouse.gov) included the improvement of mental health services. The president advocated for making certain that children and adolescents get treatment for mental health issues. Stipends and tuition reimbursement for training additional mental health professionals were presented as a priority. The plan included providing mental health first aid training for teachers through Project AWARE: Advancing Wellness and Resilience in Education (2013). Project AWARE addresses the encouragement of students and families to seek treatment. Mental Health First Aid is a program that teaches adults to identify, understand, and respond to signs of mental illnesses and substance use disorders. It includes skills in assessing risk, listening nonjudgmentally, giving information and reassurance, encouraging students to get help, and supportive strategies (http://www.mentalhealthfirstaid.org). The proposed plan is evidence of a national interest in improving mental health services for children and their families. There is reason to be optimistic. Preventive mental health is important work. It is necessary work. It can be done.

Prevention in Action Challenge: Create a Resource Map

Consider a school system with which you have some familiarity, and look carefully at its mental health services delivery system. Briefly describe the services model. Create a Resource Map (chart) to show the mental health services the school system provides: at each grade level; at Tiers 1, 2, and 3; the professionals in the school system who provide the services; the mental health curricula or programs already in place; whether or not the school system uses a needs assessment tool; how service decisions are made; how students receiving services are monitored; what data is collected; and whether or not there is a team in place for planning, analyzing data, and evaluating mental health programming.

(continued)

(continued)

Resources for maps and charts:

1. Oregon Health Authority. (2008–2009). *Oregon School Mental Health Inventory: A self-assessment and planning tool for addressing mental health within a coordinated school health program* (pp. 7–10). Middle and High School Version. Oregon: Author. Retrieved from https://public.health.oregon.gov

2. Center for Disease Control and Prevention. (2008). *Mental Health and Social Service School Questionnaire.* Atlanta, GA: Author. Retrieved from http://www.cdc.gov

3. National Assembly on School-Based Health Care. (2009). *Assessment tools for school mental health capacity building.* Washington, DC: Author. Retrieved from http://www.cde.state.co.us

4. Price, O. A., & Learn, J. G. (2008). *School mental health services for the 21st century: Lessons from the District of Columbia school mental health program.* Washington, DC: Center for Health and Health Care in Schools. (See A guide for mapping school-based mental health activities, p. 74).

5. Center for Mental Health in Schools at UCLA. (n.d.). *School-community partnerships: A guide.* Los Angeles, CA: Author. (See *Who and what are at the school?*, p. 121). Retrieved from http://smhp.psych.ucla.edu

6. Center for Mental Health in Schools at UCLA. (2007). *A resource aid packet on addressing barriers to learning: A set of surveys to map what a school has and what it needs.* Los Angeles, CA: Author. (See: Survey of learning supports system status, pp. 12–14).

Chapter 2
Locating and Selecting Evidence-Based Preventive Curricula and Programs

McCall (2009) suggests that there is a new appreciation of the importance of research and evidence influencing mental health practice. This is particularly important given interventions often used in schools and in mental health clinics have not been evidence-based in the past (Waddell & Godderis, 2005). When a program is considered evidence-based, it was developed based on scientifically supported theory. The design of the program is described in detail. Outcomes are reported including outcomes over time. The original study to determine whether or not the program works was conducted in a scientific manner, and there is some positive outcome (Sherman, 2010). The requirements to use strong and proven programs have increased. Practitioners want to know what works to help children and adolescents.

The concept of evidence-based practice originated in Ontario, in 1992, in the medical field. Shlonsky and Gibbs (2004) describe evidence-based practice as "a systematic process that blends current best evidence, client preference (wherever possible) and clinical expertise, resulting in services that are both individualized and empirically sound" (p. 137). In school psychology as in other fields, interventions that are considered to be evidence-based, need to provide information about how the intervention can be applied, and whether or not the intervention is efficacious when implemented and evaluated (Kratochwill & Shernoff, 2004). In school psychology, the scientist–practitioner model advocates for evidence-based practice.

Shlonsky and Gibbs (2004) argue that other types of practice such as "best practices" can change quickly. Evidence-based practices are updated on an ongoing basis. Practitioners in all of the mental health fields have access to research and practice data through the Internet so it is much easier to stay current than ever before. Practitioners have responsibility to track down the best evidence for prevention work. Evidence-based practice covers a wide range of practices used in the mental health services (Hoagwood & Johnson, 2003). A variety of agencies and work groups have established lists of interventions that are considered evidence-based. Various groups have developed standards. The primary one in the medical field is the Cochrane Collaborative Group. In psychology, the American Psychological Association (APA) has recommended standards for programs to be considered evidence based.

G.L. Macklem, *Preventive Mental Health at School: Evidence-Based Services for Students*, 19
DOI 10.1007/978-1-4614-8609-1_2, © Springer Science+Business Media New York 2014

Interestingly what qualifies as evidence is debated in the literature (Tseng, 2012). "Evidence" and "research" are terms used for data derived from scientific approaches. In education, the concept of "research" is used very broadly to refer to empirical findings, data, practice guidelines, personal experiences, experiences of others, and feedback from stakeholders. The term "research-based" in education has also been used to describe programs and products that have been studied as part of a research process. This definition is clearly extremely broad. Researchers, on the other hand, consider evidence-based practices as research studies designed using randomized controlled trials (RCTs) and showing positive results.

Research must always be interpreted and acted upon. Those who use research need to be able to determine the quality and credibility of studies based on professional norms, professional training, knowledge they have accumulated over time, personal goals, rules of evidence, and whether or not the research can be used to address a particular problem (Tseng, 2012). Whether or not the research can be used in a local school is critical as well. It is critical that schools determine who among their professionals have the most knowledge about interpreting research data, such as school psychologists working with small teams of stakeholders, and give those individuals time to do the work.

Research-based practice takes place in social systems and can be influenced by these systems (Tseng, 2012). Research-based practice takes place within an organization and is influenced by organizational culture affecting its use. Research can be used to make practice decisions or it can be used tactically or politically to support a position.

Federal policies have strongly affected school systems in regard to use of evidence. Researchers are interested in how school professionals define and interpret research evidence because it appears that educators do not always distinguish between informal communication or unsupported "evidence" and research evidence. Educators tend to focus on what they think works in their own schools, and many do not trust research because they believe that it can be easily manipulated (Tseng, 2012). Individuals, who claim that their comments are supported by research, without providing data to support their arguments, do not help the process. They add to the cynicism of the public about the value of research. Preliminary work by researchers suggest that relationships between administrators at various levels and school staff members influence whether or not research is used in schools (Finnigan, Daly, & Che, 2012). Other researchers have found that opinion leaders in organizations are seen as resources in regard to evidence-based programs. Opinion leaders may or may not have the background and training to determine the strength of a given practice or program.

Criteria to Determine the Evidence Base of Research

According to the Association for Behavioral and Cognitive Therapies (http://www.abct.org), there were no guidelines for schools in regard to which interventions to choose for various child and adolescent problems before the 1990s.

In 1997, the Substance Abuse and Mental Health Services Association's (SAMHSA) Center for Substance Abuse Prevention developed a hierarchy to rate programs. Operational criteria were proposed by the APA in 1998 to describe treatments (Hoagwood, Burns, Kiser, Ringeisen, & Schoenwald, 2001). According to these criteria, "well-established" interventions/treatments would have the support of two or more efficacy studies or nine single-subject case studies, demonstrating that the treatment was better than placebo, another treatment, medication or that it was just as good to another already established treatment. "Probably efficacious" interventions would have two or more studies, or three single-case studies, showing the intervention better than a Wait-list control group condition. An intervention with a single study that would meet the criteria for "well-established" would be considered "probably efficacious" until additional strong studies were available.

Criteria around the participants in efficacy studies were established among several interdisciplinary groups building on the APA work. For interventions to be considered evidence-based, they must meet the following criteria:

> ...at least two between-group design studies with a minimum of 30 subjects must be conducted across studies representing the same age group and receiving the same treatment for the same target problem, at least two within-group or single case design studies with the same parameters must be conducted, or there must be a combination of these (Hoagwood et al., 2001, p. 1180).

In addition, the group determined that most of the studies around a particular intervention must have positive outcomes and be administered with acceptable treatment integrity.

A complication is that interventions validated in efficacy studies may not work well in different settings with heterogeneous populations. Or they may not work well when implemented by busy mental health workers with high caseloads, whose training may be different from the developers or university researchers who implemented the efficacy studies. Or school cultures may or may not support the intervention.

There has been a major change in how prevention takes place, fostered by federal agencies efforts to identify programs that have sufficient evidence to support their use (Botvin, 2004). The several federal agencies generated lists of strong programs and provided funding to support their use. However, not only were there different definitions of what constituted as "evidence" but a lot of the research available was actually efficacy research of clinical treatments (Hoagwood et al., 2001). Additional agencies developed lists of evidence-based programs, but again, each used their own criteria. Some quickly became out of date, others did not share their criteria, and still others listed programs that were determined to be evidence-based from data that consisted of only one efficacy trial.

The agencies or organizations reviewing and listing programs that they consider to be evidence-based tend to differ in how they determine which program to include. They differ in their focus on "types" of programs to consider. Some are interested in social–emotional learning, others in reducing dropping out of school or violence prevention, etc. (Kutash, Duchnowski, & Lynn, 2006) (Table 2.1).

Table 2.1 Evidence-based registries

There are a number of registries to help school teams determine where to begin when searching for evidence-based programs that may fit a particular school
California Evidence-Based Clearinghouse for Child Welfare (http://www.cebc4cw.org/search/)
Center for the Study and Prevention of Violence, Blueprints for Violence Prevention (http://www.colorado.edu/cspv/blueprints/ratings.html)
Cochrane Summaries (http://summaries.cochrane.org/search/)
Collaborative for Academic, Social, and Emotional Learning (CASEL) (http://casel.org/in-schools/selecting-programs/)
Helping America's Youth (http://helpingamericasyouth.org)
Lifecourse Interventions That Work: A Matrix of Evidence-Based Programs Compiled from Various Registries (http://www.childtrends.org/Files/Child_Trends-Lifecourse_Interventions.pdf)
Matrix of Children's Evidence-Based Interventions (http://www.nri-inc.org/reports_pubs/2006/EBPChildrensMatrix2006.pdf)
National Registry of Evidence-Based Programs and Practices (NREPP) (http://www.nrepp.samhsa.gov)
Office of Juvenile Justice and Delinquency Prevention (OJJDP) (http://www.ojjdp.gov/programs/index.html)
Preventing Drug Abuse Among Children and Adolescents: Examples of Research-Based Drug Abuse Prevention Programs: see Chapter 4: Examples of research-based drug abuse prevention programs (http://www.drugabuse.gov)
Promising Practices Network on Children, Families and Communities: Programs That Work (http://www.promisingpractices.net/programs.asp)
What Works Wisconsin: Evidence-Based Parenting Program Directory (http://whatworks.uwex.edu/Pages/2parentsinprogrameb.html)

There is a range of criteria used to consider whether or not a practice is evidence-based although there is some consistency around the basic considerations. For example, an RCT or a very rigorous quasi-experimental design (QED) is considered by most rating agencies to be the highest level of evidence for mental health practices. Empirical data indicating the presence of effectiveness has been required by many of the various agencies to list a program or practice on their respective list. Kutash et al. (2006) feel that there is sufficient evidence to indicate that many school-based mental health interventions to prevent mental health problems, or to improve the functioning of students, are effective.

Today, practitioners need to find and use the most effective interventions due to lack of time and concerns around the ethics of using programs without an evidence base. In 2001, the federal No Child Left Behind Act (NCLB, 2001) adopted the concept of using practices that have strong support. Tilly (2008) noted that the phrase "scientific research-based practice" in some form can be found in the NCLB statute 111 times. Unfortunately, we do not as yet have scientific research-based interventions for all behaviors that children may exhibit. Available data is still often qualified in spite of enormous progress developing and examining programs and practice. The mandate to use scientific research-based practices does not specify how programs, or interventions, should be delivered.

The term "scientifically based research" was taken from the NCLB statute and incorporated into the IDEA 2004 amendments (Tilly, 2008). Next, California's Safe and Drug-Free Schools and Communities joined the movement (Sherman, 2010). The 2004 amendments to the Individuals with Disabilities Education Act (IDEA) indicated that a local education agency could use a process to identify specific learning disabilities that measures whether or not a child responds positively or negatively to "research-based" interventions (Burns, Jacob, & Wagner, 2008). The Bush initiative to improve education in the United States established the Institute for Education Sciences (IES) as the source of federal funding, making it clear that there would be an emphasis on scientific rigor in research in the field of education (Reeves, 2011).

Concerns Around the Mandate to Use Evidence-Based Programs and Practices

Practitioners at the school level are interested in how well evidence-based interventions can be implemented in the school setting (The Evidence-Based Intervention Work Group, 2005). There has been concern about defining "evidence" when it has been used too strictly. Schools are more interested in whether or not a program is effective and funding may be limited by a particular definition of evidence-based (Waddell & Godderis, 2005). A preventive intervention may work with one age group but not another. A program may not address needs of the family or the school context. Because fragmentation of services is so prevalent in schools, it may be difficult to get agreement on the role of evidence-based practice in schools.

There is a range of degrees of rigor in research studies, ranging from work that is evidence-based to evidence-informed, to evidence suggested, or to work based on opinion and consensus (Huang, Hepburn, & Espiritu, 2003). Even when data is strong, an intervention that would fit one disorder would not affect or might negatively affect a second disorder evident in the same student. And, even when strong data to support a program is available, parents may choose not to allow it, funding may not be available, and staff may not have had training in the strongest approach. According to Weisz (2006) most evidence-based treatments are for single specific disorders when school-aged children are dealing with more complex problems. Children and adolescents may present problems that are manageable 1 day and reach crisis proportions the next day. What is needed are simplified treatments focused on a few critical skills that can be taught, practiced to mastery, and work well.

The adoption of evidence-based practice is still problematic. As recently as 2007, Kratochwill, Volpiansky, Clements, and Ball claimed that school psychologists were not prepared to conduct evidence-based prevention and intervention. Teachers for the most part have not been trained in evidence-based practices.

Combine these concerns with what is described as the antiscientific stand of educators; use of evidence-based practice may be an uphill battle. Kratochwill et al. (2007) reported that only 19 % of schools implemented a research-based curriculum in response to a Department of Education policy requiring schools to abide by principles of effectiveness.

Efficacy and Effectiveness

There are a number of things to consider when determining the evidence base of a prevention program. For example, when examining a research study, it is important to look for elements of "rigor." The elements of methodological rigor include the design of the research study, how constructs are conceptualized, the measurement strategies, the integrity of the program, and the duration of the study (Braverman & Arnold, 2008). When conducting a literature search or evaluating a program, it is important to determine whether or not the research is convincing in regard to a program's ability to get the intended results under ideal conditions (efficacy), and this is determined by examining the methodology of studies (McCall, 2009).

Efficacy has to do with positive outcomes of a program under ideal conditions, whereas *effectiveness* has to do with the effects of a program when it is implemented in the field under naturalistic conditions. Efficacy trials have strict and highly controlled research designs. They are implemented with strict researcher control by highly trained staff. An effectiveness trial of a program might be run in a school with a typical school population and implemented by general education teachers. In effectiveness studies, quality of implementation is critical, or outcomes may be negatively affected. For a program to be considered "effective," it must meet all of the criteria for "efficacy." For a program to be considered "ready for dissemination," it must meet the criteria for efficacy as well as the criteria for effectiveness (Flay et al., 2005, p. 3).

In an efficacy study, the study is generally well controlled with a homogenous population with no comorbid problems (two disorders occurring together) (Flay, 2007). The interventions are highly standardized when delivered, with the goal of getting strong effect sizes. Effect sizes are an estimate of the size of an outcome or of an association between two variables (Ferguson, 2009). They offer a better measure of the size of effect between the variables in the study because the number of participants in the several studies is not relevant. An effectiveness study is conducted in one setting, typically with resources and experts to implement the intervention. A specific implementation protocol is used and carefully monitored. An effectiveness study generally deals with a heterogeneous population that constitutes a representative sample. The interventions in the study tend to be brief, not overwhelming to implement, not requiring experts to implement the intervention, and are adapted to the setting. An effectiveness study works in various settings and can be implemented by a variety of staff with competing stresses (academic demands). Protocols tend to be adapted in schools because the setting is as important as the population.

The outcomes of effectiveness trials may not be impressive because participants may not be very motivated, participants may have several mental health issues, implementation may not be as well controlled, and the setting may be varied or challenging.

Efficacy trials are likely to produce significant effect sizes because interventions are more intensive and are delivered with a high level of expertise, yet the impact is limited because of the selectivity of those who participate and those who implement the interventions (Prochaska, Evers, Prochaska, Van Marter, & Johnson, 2007). The outcomes may be impressive but this is not a "real-world" condition. Efficacy trials are difficult to generalize because the number of settings, times populations, times problem combinations, is so huge (Flay, 2007). However, as studies are repeated with many trials and the whole body of research at a particular point is reviewed and a meta-analysis is conducted, the likelihood of generalization is greatly improved.

Once both efficacy and effectiveness trials are completed and outcomes are positive, there is data to say that the program is practical. Program designers next write a manual. They offer technical support, develop and make available tools for data collection, and provide cost information for implementers. At this point the program can be considered ready for dissemination (Flay, 2007). Of the many prevention programs available, the best programs have moderate positive effects. Large effect sizes have been determined for cognitive-behavioral approaches, for programs evaluated using RCTs, and for interactive programs. Effect sizes at the indicated or selective levels are about three times that for universal programs *because* the participants in these programs are already showing symptoms or are at high risk. When students are mentally healthy, it is more difficult to show effects of programming.

Process for Locating Evidence-Based Programs, Interventions, and Strategies

Locating a program to fit a local school or school district takes time, expertise, and an organized approach. SAMHSA's Strategic Prevention Framework (SPF) (2009) was designed to help school professionals and local communities identify and select evidence-based interventions that would address local needs and reduce substance abuse problems. The SPF identifies evidence-based interventions as those interventions or programs included in federal registries of evidence-based interventions, those published in peer-reviewed journals with positive effects, or those with documented effectiveness supported by other sources of information and the consensus judgment of informed experts. The Wilder Foundation (http://www.wilder.org) published a brief on evidence-based interventions and practices (2009, August) offering suggestions for this process. Sherman (2010) also described this process. It is easy to access federal registries online.

The National Registry of Evidence-Based Programs and Practices (NREPP) (http://www.nrepp.samhsa.gov) is an excellent source for evidence-based interventions and programs that are relevant for schools, especially because one of the focuses of the registry is on preventing and treating mental health issues. Federal registries provide brief descriptions of various interventions and the strength of those interventions. The list of programs is limited to those that meet the criteria of the site. Some federal sites focus on specific problems. The Office of Adolescent Health, U.S. Department of Health & Human Services, (http://www.hhs.gov) lists evidence-based programs associated with teen pregnancy prevention. NREPP lists evidence-based programs for substance abuse prevention. Blueprints for Violence Prevention, the Center for the Study and Prevention of Violence at the University of Colorado (CSPV) (http://www.colorado.edu), provides lists of violence prevention programs. The U.S. Department of Education, What Works Clearinghouse (WWC), has a search site to locate studies that are of very high quality. This site rates programs against the WWC standards, and research studies are determined to meet the standards without or with reservations (http://ies.ed.gov) (Table 2.1).

According to the WWC: Procedures and Standards Handbook (Version 2.1) (2011), WWC looks at each study once it is screened in and determines if it provides strong evidence (meets evidence standards), weaker evidence (reservations), or insufficient evidence (does not meet standards). Only well-designed and well-implemented randomly controlled trials are considered strong evidence. QEDs with equating (the control group is determined to be as similar as possible to the experimental group) meet standards with reservations. The QED studies must show that the experimental and comparison group are equivalent in regard to observable characteristics to meet standards "with reservations." In addition, the WWC specifies the *extent of evidence* available for the programs it has reviewed. For example, as of 2013, the extent of evidence to support the *Positive Action* program (Li et al., 2009), *Coping Power* (Lochman & Wells, 2002), and *Early Risers* (August, Realmuto, Hektner, & Bloomquist, 2001) was medium to large, whereas the extent of the evidence for *Too Good for Violence* (Bacon, 2001), *First Steps to Success* (Walker et al., 1998), and *The Incredible Years* (Webster-Stratton, 1982) was small as of the time the WWC evaluated the data.

There are many other nongovernment agencies that list evidence-based programs including university groups and groups advocating for a particular disorder. Huser, Cooney, Small, O'Connor, and Mather (2009) at the University of Wisconsin–Madison publish a resource list of registries with lists of evidence-based programs. The list includes both government and nongovernment agencies, a description of what each agency evaluates, and how to access the lists. Importantly, the list is updated periodically. The Center for School Mental Health at the University of Maryland School of Medicine provides summaries of evidence-based program registries (http://csmh.umaryland.edu). Heartland Area Education Agency (http://www.aea11.k12.ia.us) offers a compilation of reviews for social–emotional programs. Terzian, Moore, Williams-Taylor, and Nguyen (2009) provide a "research-to-results" brief that presents issues to consider when searching for evidence-based programs. Additionally, the brief lists online agencies and the information that each provides as well as appropriate search terms. This resource is very helpful.

A second source of evidence-based programs for practitioners is peer-reviewed journals. These can be challenging to access. Local colleges with relevant majors may provide access to their databases for guests. Schools need at least one person on their teams who have the technical expertise to interpret research studies and judge the quality of the studies that are located. School psychologists have this level of expertise. It is important for school-based teams searching for programs to realize that one study is insufficient to provide evidence in support of a program or preventive intervention. Reviewing several studies or a small group of studies for consistency of findings is important (Sherman, 2010). Each study needs to be examined further for its underlying theory or conceptual model, whether or not it meets the needs of the local school population, whether or not it explains the mechanism of change, whether or not the study group matches the local school, whether or not competing explanations were ruled out, if the findings are clearly specified, and if the conclusions come from the data. Sherman provides some additional questions for consideration.

If agency and government lists do not provide the program to match the community and a literature search is not helpful, selecting interventions based on other sources of information that may support a particular intervention must be done with caution. Sherman (2010) provides some guidelines for this situation. It is important to make sure that the intervention:

- Has a documented theory of change
- If it looks very much like the interventions described in registries or in the peer-reviewed journals in regard to content and structure
- If it has been implemented successfully multiple times, with a pattern of positive effects
- If it has been reviewed by external experts and representative of the local culture

This places a considerable burden on the local school team for decisions and requires extensive documentation.

Given the financial strains on schools, the time constraints, and insufficient training, some schools lean toward packaged curricula, which *claim* to be evidence-based (McCall, 2009). The research literature often has limited information describing the program or preventive intervention making it difficult to implement the program in a school system. Selecting programs that may not work is a waste of time and resources. The complexity of locating and selecting a program, strategy, or intervention that is most likely to work requires research. This is necessary to prevent school personnel from buying-in to a program that will not produce results. Selecting an evidence-based prevention program is not an easy task.

Literature Search

Unfortunately, the term "evidence-based practice" has been used too freely. The phrase has been connected to practices that are loosely connected to a study, without determining the quality of the evidence, whether or not there are critical limiting factors, or whether or not there may be contrary data. Evidence-based practice is a process that is empirically sound, combining the most current and strongest data with needs and practitioner expertise. Shlonsky and Gibbs (2004) argue that from the time it was first introduced, evidence-based practice has been misunderstood and misused. They describe a helpful process of decision-making as follows:

- Formulate an answerable question about the prevention of a specific problem.
- Find the best evidence to answer the questions.
- Determine the validity, impact, and practicality of the preventive interventions.
- Match the preventive intervention to the needs of the local population taking backgrounds, conditions, preferences, and values of the local population into consideration.
- Evaluate the effectiveness and efficiency of the process (Shlonsky & Gibbs, 2004, pp. 139–140, 147).

A literature search of research can be overwhelming as information is increasing exponentially. One source, MEDLINE, adds 10–20,000 new citations each week.

Practitioners need to learn how to search efficiently. They need to learn how to evaluate the evidence that they find critically. Once these skills have been mastered, searches will take considerably less time.

The Rigor of Research Studies

Today there is a strong emphasis on evidence-based decision-making (Puddy & Wilkins, 2011). In order to determine the best available research evidence, both the strength of the evidence and also the effectiveness of the intervention must be determined. In examining the strength of the evidence, it is important to look at how rigorously a program has been evaluated along a continuum. A prevention practice may be rigorously evaluated but not independently replicated and therefore fall into a different category, somewhat less rigorous. The continuum of evidence of effectiveness involves the effect of the studies (short-term, long-term, or both), internal validity, research design, independent replication, implementation guidance, and both external and ecological validity. The effectiveness continuum in more detail ranges from effective, some evidence of effectiveness, undetermined effectiveness, and finally, ineffective. Validity is determined by use of a control group, multiple measurement points, and gathering information on whatsoever might influence outcomes. The range in regard to internal validity runs from true experiment, quasi-experimental, nonexperimental, sound theory only, to no research and no sound theory.

There are real challenges to convincing practitioners to use evidence-based practices, one of which is the fact that not all practitioners agree whether or not some interventions should be considered evidence-based (Rubin & Parrish, 2007). When evidence-based practice is expanded to include the integration of the very best evidence, with clinical expertise, and the desires of those who will participate in the intervention, there is an opening to use interventions, which were not determined to be efficacious.

As powerful as RCTs may be, they may not be possible due to ethical concerns and costs (Sibbald & Roland, 1998). Clinical judgment does not take priority over research studies using RCTs. However, there are reasons that practitioners might accept other sources of evidence. We do not as yet have RCTs for all aspects of mental health practice. RCTs when available might not fit the local population, and when fidelity of intervention is rigid, outcomes may not be as good (Rubin & Parrish, 2007). Although RCTs, systematic reviews, and meta-analyses of RCTs may represent the strongest evidence, other research designs may provide provisional support for an intervention. In some cases, these may actually be the best evidence available. This does not excuse practitioners from searching for RCTs when selecting interventions. The more recent softening of standards has made it even more difficult for practitioners to carefully read journal articles and evaluate the research designs, read study limitations, and avoid misconstruing statements made as conclusions.

Once a prevention program that initially appears relevant is located on a list of evidence-based programs, it is important to locate the efficacy study or studies and examine the study carefully. Reading and understanding the research methodology of a study is extremely important because it allows the reader to understand the value and limitations of the results of the study (Vitiello, 2010). It is possible to judge the quality of a research study by studying the details provided (Lohr, 2004). Strength of evidence of a program depends on the size of studies and how robust the group of studies on the topics may be. The task is to look for the same findings across studies with different populations. Strength of evidence is different from the size of the effect or impact. Results that are dramatic in one small isolated study are not as strong as small effects in a group of studies reporting the same outcomes. Each study in turn needs to be judged for quality and strength before making conclusions about a body of studies or aggregated data.

The ability to evaluate the methodological structure of a research study requires some basic expertise. Evidence based practices offer evidence based on research that involves randomized trials with control groups, studies that match groups of participants in control and experimental groups, studies in which those implementing the preventive intervention do not know which participants are in each group, statistical analysis, and carefully considered and correct conclusions based on the data collected (McCay, 2007). The advantages connected with evidence-based practices include the ability to choose preventive interventions based on data rather than on subjective decision-making, support of the program from a broader base, and the provision of guidelines or manuals to help implement the program with fidelity.

Evaluating evidence is complex. The quality of evidence refers to the degree to which someone can be sure that an estimate of effect of a research study is correct.

When searching through studies for preventive interventions, the quality of the study must be determined, consistency of results across studies must be determined, and appropriateness of the study design must be considered (Kropski, Keckley, & Jensen, 2008). The *quality* of a study is gleaned from the methodology as well as the execution of the study. *Consistency* refers to whether or not the effects of an intervention are similar across studies. In reviewing the methodology of a study, RCTs provide "high" quality of evidence, quasi-experimental trials provide "moderate" evidence, observational studies provide "low" evidence, and all other evidence would be considered "very low." Characteristics of studies that would weaken the quality the study might otherwise provide include baseline differences, high level of attrition, questionable validity of the instruments or the techniques used, sparse data, reporting bias, uncertainty of external validity, serious design limitation, and uncertainty of directness. Factors that would increase or strengthen the evidence would be lack of confounders, consistent and direct evidence (GRADE Working Group, 2004; Kropski et al., 2008).

The Canadian Task Force on the Periodic Health Examination introduced the idea of a hierarchy of evidence to rank interventions (Evans, 2003). The order of hierarchy depends on the question asked by a school team in that different research questions are answered by different types of study and study designs (Petticrew & Roberts, 2003).

Research Types and Study Designs

School teams conducting a search need to appreciate that not all evidence is equal. Research designs fall on a continuum ranging from RCT, to QED, to single-group design, to exploratory studies, and finally to a needs assessment (Puddy & Wilkins, 2011). Hierarchies are about effectiveness.

Meta-analyses aggregate data from multiple studies and thus provide considerable information to answer questions asked (Ho, Peterson, & Masoudi, 2008). They are often used to summarize data from experimental studies. As long as the studies in the meta-analysis are strong and as long as the outcomes of those studies are not tremendously different, the data will be strong. A meta-analysis of similar, well-run, randomized and controlled trials is considered by many to be one the best if not the best level of evidence (Garg, Hackam, & Tonelli, 2008). Possible deterrents to the quality of the meta-analysis include the issue that studies comprising the meta-analysis may be confined to published studies, and results may be biased in that publications are biased themselves toward positive outcomes. Given the strengths and weaknesses, practitioners must carefully read meta-analyses.

Locating a meta-analysis of studies in the literature around a particular mental health concern is very helpful. Most evidence-based practices, according to Kratochwill and Shernoff (2004), come from reviews of the literature, around a particular student problem, involving a meta-analysis. A meta-analysis is one of the most used approaches to synthesizing research results in the social sciences, combining numbers of studies and determining an overall effect size (Reeves, 2011). A meta-analysis of studies RCTs that have been implemented well and a similar is considered one of the highest levels of evidence (Garg et al., 2008; Hadorn, Baker, Hodges, & Hicks, 1996). Meta-analyses are limited in that there is a bias against the publication of negative results and sometimes small studies are included (Walker, 2008b), and they are only as reliable as the methods that the researchers used to estimate the effects in each of the original studies (Garg et al., 2008); but, meta-analyses can help guide practitioners decide whether or not implementing a given program is even feasible in their school district. Meta-analyses combine studies to increase sample size, summarize the results of multiple studies, analyze differences among studies, increase precision in estimating effects, and supplement experimental research. Sources such as government reports, book chapters, and conference proceedings provide useful data, but these are considered "gray" literature (not peer reviewed). Decision-making is complicated by the fact that there is so much information to synthesize and the fact that decisions may be made by a group.

Systematic reviews have been considered critical for implementing evidence-based practice and considering a set of questions (Schlosser, 2007). They save practitioners time in that many consider them excellent sources of information on a given disorder or behavior. Unfortunately they differ in quality. Systematic reviews evaluate available studies with the same goal as meta-analyses, but do not always use quantitative methods to summarize results and so are not as strong as meta-analyses (Ho et al., 2008). Schlosser's online brief (http://www.ncddr.org) provides help in evaluating systematic reviews.

The so-called *gold standard* of research studies has to do with interventions determined to be effective in studies using random assignment of participants to the experimental group and control group. In this way those participants in each group are as similar as possible before the intervention is implemented (Schaeller, 2002). Gold standard studies comprise the highest level of evidence (Jacobs, Jones, Gabella, Spring, & Brownson, 2012). The most reliable data on the efficacy of preventive interventions is found in well-designed *randomized controlled trials* (RCTs) (Moher et al., 2010). RCTs are the strongest method of demonstrating effects of prevention studies (Walker, 2008a). An RCT places individuals randomly into each of the experimental and control groups to make sure that there are *no systematic differences* between the groups (Sibbald & Roland, 1998). RCTs are the most rigorous way of determining cause and effect and provide the best evidence in the absence of systematic reviews (Glanville, Lefebvre, Miles, & Camosso-Stefinovic, 2006; Sibbald & Roland, 1998). RCTs allow practitioners to say that the preventive intervention is the cause of an effect (Flay, 2007).

In order to have high validity, the research study must distinguish the outcomes from any other influences (Weisburd, Lum, & Petrosino, 2001). This is accomplished through randomization. Groups will not be exactly the same in every possible manner, but differences will be distributed randomly. Well-designed and conducted RCTs often form the most reliable input to systematic reviews and meta-analyses of health care interventions and, where practical and ethical, can provide the best evidence in the absence of systematic reviews (Glanville et al., 2006).

Randomization avoids making errors when studies are interpreted (Walker, 2008a, 2008b). Focusing simply on the study design, the highest level of support for a prevention program would consist of at least *two* successful RCTs with follow-up, successfully replicated at least *twice* by researchers other than the program developers. Good support might be two successful RCTs using a wait-list control group, while one RCT study showing results equal to an established treatment would constitute moderate support.

Although some researchers have strongly advocated for RCTs (the medical standard) in education, others claim that double-blind experiments are impossible (Reeves, 2011). For example, the establishment of the WWC proved to be controversial with its rigid criteria for a determination of scientifically supported educational methods and the fact that programs cannot reach its standards for experimental studies. Currently the *rigor* versus *relevance* debate is moving toward relevance although the advocacy for RCTs is still very strong. Even in the medical world, RCTs are challenging to apply to individuals.

The *cluster-randomized trial design* randomizes schools rather than individuals. In this way all of the students in the study from each school receive the same preventive intervention, and contamination between groups does not occur (Jaycox et al., 2006). A complication of this design is that a larger number of participants is needed (sample size) to obtain equal power as compared to study designs that randomize participants. In addition to needing more schools in the study, matching must be very careful. Even within a randomized trial, there can be variation depending on the quality of the study and transfer among groups can occur if students in the same school receive different interventions. Scheduling in schools can negate randomization of individual students. For example, students from separate classes may have the same recess, which would contaminate the study.

Quasi-experimental studies involve a wide range of nonrandomized prevention studies. QEDs are used when randomization is not possible. They are used when a control group is not available or when there are ethical concerns (Ho et al., 2008; Jaycox et al., 2006). Ethical considerations typically prevent withholding of an intervention that is known to work (Harris et al., 2006). This is a particular concern in studies conducted with school populations. In quasi-experimental studies, care must be taken to make sure that results reflect treatments rather than any differences between groups that existed before the program was implemented (Jaycox et al., 2006). Nonrandomized studies may overestimate or in some cases underestimate the outcomes for a prevention program if the study is not well designed (Weisburd et al., 2001).

The major weakness of a quasi-experimental study design is the lack of random assignment. QEDs use *matching* to try to make groups equivalent, but this is challenging. One possibility is to lean on statistics to increase equivalence of groups (Weisburd et al., 2001). Statistical association is helpful but cannot determine causality. Alternative explanations of the data are possible in this design. Confounding variables particularly if they are not measured can threaten results. The quasi-experimental pre–post intervention is used to determine the benefits of a particular preventive intervention (Harris et al., 2006). There are four QED groups for studies in the social sciences and in prevention work, each of which have subtypes. The four categories include:

- A QED with no control group
- A QED with a control group but no pretest
- A QED with a control group that includes a pretest
- Interrupted time-series designs (using several waves of observation of both the intervention and comparison groups before and after the intervention) (http://www.csulb.edu)

Another way to describe common designs of this group would be a pretest/posttest study without controls, an interrupted time-series design, and a pretest/posttest study with a contemporaneous control. In a pretest/posttest design, observations are made before and after implementing the intervention (Ho et al., 2008). The *time-series design* employs multiple observations or involves collecting multiple data points before and after the intervention. The goal involves establishing that changes occur in outcomes after the intervention and that changes are most likely to come from the intervention rather than from other variables. A control group strengthens the QED, but because the control group is not randomized, outcomes may be confounded or biased. There is also risk of regression to the mean with multiple measurements in the case of the time-series design.

Huey and Polo (2008) point out that when evaluating studies that would be appropriate for ethnic minority students, additional considerations are needed to include the following:

- At least 75 % of students in the study must be from ethnic minority groups.
- A separate analysis is needed, to determine significant outcomes for ethnic minority students as compared to controls.
- Ethnicity must not moderate outcomes, or the program must be effective with ethnic minority students in spite of moderator effects (p. 264).

Nonexperimental designs do not use randomization, and there is no control or comparison group (Steinberg, Bringle, & Williams, 2010). Nonexperimental research is more varied than experimental research (Muijs, 2004). The most common methods in educational research include the use of surveys, observational research, and analyzing data sets that are already available. The most popular involves surveys using standard questionnaires. When the researcher does not get involved in selecting participants but simply observes them, the design of the study is nonexperimental or observational (Ho et al., 2008). When nonexperimental designs are used to answer descriptive research questions using a survey, this would be a posttest only, single-group design (Steinberg et al., 2010). A cohort study is a study in which groups are followed over time to determine the impact of an intervention in a school. A cohort study can be retrospective or prospective. In cohort studies, statistical methods attempt to control for confounding variables, but they can't explain unmeasured confounders. In cross-sectional studies, measurement takes place at one point in time and groups may be compared. Case studies generally result in the weakest data as far as causality is determined. Different research designs answer different questions (Cook & Cook, 2008). Whereas nonexperimental designs cannot answer questions about causation, they can at times serve as the only or the best available data to guide decision-making (Table 2.2).

When effectiveness of a prevention program is the question, the RCT provides the highest level of evidence (Evans, 2003). But, RCTs answer only the question of effectiveness (Evans, 2003). Evidence on the effectiveness (does it work?), appropriateness (do school staff feel the outcomes are important or will be beneficial?), and feasibility (how should it be implemented?) of preventive intervention are important given factors that can have an impact on the success or failure of a

Table 2.2 Levels of evidence

Preventive interventions range from well supported by empirical evidence to unsupported by evidence (Puddy & Wilkins, 2011). Research studies may not fit neatly into a particular category. Determining the strength of the evidence of a research study is only one step in evaluating a curriculum or program. School teams must also determine if implementing a preventive intervention is feasible, if it would be acceptable, and if it is appropriate for the school setting

Experimental designs

1. Experimental design with participants randomly assigned to an experimental and a control group (another treatment). At least two randomized controlled trials with independent evaluators demonstrating efficacy. At least 30 participants per group. Published in peer-reviewed journals

   (a) Participants randomly assigned to both an experimental group and to a waiting list control group

   (b) Random assignment of communities, schools, or classrooms

2. Experimental design with two or more randomized controlled trials and at least 30 participants per group. Outcomes superior to wait-list or no-treatment control group

3. Experimental design with one randomized controlled trial and at least 30 participants per group. Outcomes superior to wait-list or no-treatment control group, or equal to established treatment in other experiments

Quasi-experimental designs

1. Quasi-experimental design with matched controls on important characteristics but not randomly assigned. Multiple studies with well-matched comparison groups published in peer-reviewed journals. At least 30 participants per group

2. Quasi-experimental design with equated groups compared using statistical controls. At least 30 participants per group

3. Quasi-experimental time-series design with a comparison group using multiple data observation points over a long period

4. Quasi-experimental time-series design without a comparison group using multiple data observation points over a long period

5. Quasi-experimental with comparison group not well matched

6. Pre–post studies with matched but not equivalent groups with follow-up measures

7. Pre–post studies without a control or comparison group

Nonexperimental designs

1. Nonexperimental, sound theory only. Program participants are studied over several years

2. No research, no sound theory

3. Risk of harm

Sources: Chorpita and Daleiden (2009a, 2009b), Paulson and Dailey (2002), Perez-Johnson et al. (2011), Puddy and Wilkins (2011), Saxena and Maulik (2002), and Williams-Taylor (2010)

program. If the program can't be implemented with fidelity, or participants don't want or like it, its value is questionable. Therefore, in addition to the study design, additional considerations include replication, external validity, ecological validity, implementation guidance, and evidence of effectiveness. Independent replication can vary from partial to full, with or without evaluation (Puddy & Wilkins, 2011). External validity refers to whether or not a program can still have effects when implemented with different populations, and in different contexts. Ecological validity has to do with whether or not a program simulates real life condition of a particular setting such as a school. On a continuum, this factor can range from two or more applied studies in different settings, two or more applied studies in the same settings, real world-informed, somewhat real world-informed, not real world-informed, to possible applied studies in similar or different settings. Implementation guidance can be comprehensive, partial, or none.

Additional Considerations in Program Selection

Evidence of outcomes comes from RCTs, but information about process, such as how outcomes were achieved, the quality of the implementation, and the context, comes from different data. Petticrew and Roberts (2003) suggest that typologies as described by Gray (1996), rather than hierarchies, may be more useful in conceptualizing the strengths and weaknesses of different methodological approaches. In a typology, the value of various research methodologies would be evaluated on three variables: effectiveness, appropriateness, and feasibility. School teams must determine the extent to which a program meets criteria for effectiveness. Did the program "work" in the efficacy study with the population, staff, and budgets similar to the local school or school system? Appropriateness may refer to school and community values or goals. Feasibility needs to be determined by checking to see whether the school or district has the services, personnel, and financial potential to implement the program.

Identifying and selecting an evidence-based intervention or program requires an understanding of the basic psychological processes involved in student problems, the associated risk and protective factors, and the theoretical framework that supports the intervention (Kratochwill & Shernoff, 2004). In addition, knowledge is needed around how to get behavioral change when implementing a prevention program. In order to make decisions scientifically, practitioners need to determine the best available research evidence for the specific identified problem they want to address, they need to determine availability of local resources, and they need to assess the needs, values, and preferences of stakeholders who will be affected by the prevention effort (Jacobs et al., 2012).

Programs must have a strong theory of change and evidence of *how* or *why* the programs produce effects (McCall, 2009). Cost-benefit analyses need to be determined. This would indicate whether or not the program would benefit enough students to justify the expense of implementing the program. The effect size needs to be determined as well. Some researchers feel that an effect size below 0.40 is not acceptable for educational programming (Reeves, 2011).

Even after locating a program or programs that have sufficient research evidence to determine effectiveness and some data to indicate that the program might be effective in a particular community or school district, it is important for school teams to reflect on the characteristics of effective programs or, more specifically, determine which elements of the evidence-based program are critical. Schools need to know what really matters in practice, and studies or program evaluations may not include this information.

The next level of precision in practice may be the "common elements" approach (Stephan, 2012). Common elements outperform treatments with a manual partly because they are more acceptable to providers (Borntrager et al., 2009) and also because outcomes are better and faster (Weisz et al., 2012). School teams need to consider the crucial elements of the program that would be critical in order to implement a particular program and whether or not these could be tweaked or scientifically adapted (McCall, 2009). "Core components," also called the "active ingredients" or "essential functions" of a program, are those that have been found to affect outcomes. Identifying these and focusing on them make a difference in implementation. They also allow for accurate interpretation of outcomes, making adaptations, and are critical in preventing "program drift," which occurs when those implementing programs make spontaneous changes in the program as they implement it (Greenwood, Welsh, & Rocque, 2012). When evaluating programs under consideration for adoption, school staff members can look for clear descriptions of the core components and also look for the dosage needed and the strength of the core components. They can review the activities that define the core components to determine if they can be implemented in a local school and if they are able to find assessments that can measure them. If not evident, program developers can be contacted to ask about core components and fidelity measures.

If school leaders do not understand the value of evidence-based programming, less well-trained local staff will make the decisions. Unfortunately, decisions made by local "experts" can be biased by their own experience, which may not include use of evidence from research (O'Connor & Freeman, 2012). Andrews and Buettner (2012 update), at the Center for Learning Excellence at the Ohio State University, urge school teams to locate the original article describing the particular program and determine if it is an evidence-based, promising, or untested program. Next, search for additional studies to determine if outcomes hold over time. Determine if the team feels that the program could be implemented in the school, if it is based on effective principles, if participants found it helpful, and if the program has been replicated at multiple sites. The team needs to determine how much of the program must be implemented to get acceptable results (dosage) or if the program has been part of a meta-analysis or review of programs article.

Determining the Appropriateness of Preventive Strategies and Programs

Although there is an ever-increasing body of literature on evidence-based programs available for practitioners, an additional task before selecting the evidence-based program of interests is to determine if the program is the best "fit" for the local school, school system, or district. A compendium of program choices is helpful, but this does not substitute for examining each possible program to determine if meets identified local needs (Kutash et al., 2006). The program must be available. The program must fit into the total school schedule of programming or at least complement programs already in place (McCall, 2009). Of critical importance is whether or not the program is acceptable to the intended stakeholders, as most programs require changes in roles for school workers (Flay, 2007).

By 2007, there was a shift to thinking of a continuum of evidence such that the degree of evidence was important, but the *context* was important as well. Instead of simply choosing a program on a list, school teams must determine what they need, think about whether or not a program fits their local population, and consider the local context (Sherman, 2010). The CDC Division of Violence Prevention, Evidence Project Overview (http://www.cdc.gov) provides a framework for thinking about evidence. This framework includes the best available research evidence, experiential evidence, and contextual evidence. All of these help determine whether or not a prevention program can result in intended outcomes. Contextual evidence includes factors such as whether or not a strategy is useful feasible to implement and accepted by all stakeholders in the community. Although this is considerably more work than simply choosing a program on a list, it may increase the likelihood that the program once implemented will actually work as it was designed to do.

Using an Evidence-Based Prevention Program

Jacobs (2008), known for expertise in ethical practice, urges school psychologists to recommend intervention techniques "that the profession considers… responsible, research-based practice" (NASP-PPE, IV, C, #4). Also, when selecting interventions, preference should be given to strategies and interventions described in the peer-reviewed professional journals and are determined to be effective (Jacob, 2008, BP V Chapter 121, p. 1928).

As of 2002, fewer than 30 % of schools in the United States were implementing evidence-based programs (Ringwalt et al., 2002). This may not have changed to a significant degree today. Barriers to use of evidence-based practice in schools are associated with confusion around use of the term "evidence-based." Even when some professionals in schools are aware of the empirical evidence to support a given practice, they do not have time to complete the work associated with the practice. There may be some individuals in schools more influenced by clinical judgment than empirical data. Many school professionals do not have the training to implement evidence-based practices in their schools (Kratochwill & Shernoff, 2004). Cost may be another factor.

Crosse et al. (2011) examined research-based programs used in schools during the 2004–2005 school year. The program data they collected involved prevention of alcohol, tobacco, and other drug use and school crime prevention. They found that only 7.8 % of schools implemented strongly supported programs: and of those, less than half implemented the programs with fidelity. They estimated that only 3.5 % of all prevention programs that met the criteria to be considered research based were implemented in schools during that period. The mean number of prevention programs implemented in schools during the study year was 9; 14.8 % of schools did not use any prevention programs, whereas 11.1 % of schools used more than 20 different prevention programs. Middle schools implemented more programs than elementary or high schools. There is a lot more work to do in schools.

Prevention in Action Challenge: Identify the Strength of Study Designs

Read the following descriptions of several studies' research designs (methodologies) and determine the level of evidence that the studies represent. Evaluate the rigor of the several research designs. Use Table 2.2 to make your determination.

1. Fonagy et al. (2009) studied 1,345 third to fifth grade students in nine elementary schools in a Midwestern city to determine the efficacy of a manualized psychodynamic social systems approach to prevention of bullying called *Creating a Peaceful School Learning Environment* (CAPSLE). Schools served as clusters and were randomly assigned to intervention conditions. The unit of inference remained at the individual level. Three schools participated in the CAPSLE condition and three in an individually tailored intervention service condition as a control. Baseline data was collected and additional data was collected twice a year for 2 years during implementation. Effectiveness data was collected twice a year for the following year. Over 3 years 74 % of eligible students participated.

2. A nationally representative sample of 7,313 students in grades 6–10 completed the bullying and depression items in the Health Behavior in School-Aged Children 2005 Survey. Wag, Nansel, and Iannotti (2011) determined that more than half of students reported that they had bullied someone or had been verbally bullied themselves at least once in the past several months. More than half were involved in relational bullying. Cyberbullying was less common than other types of bullying, but victims were more depressed by this form of bullying.

3. A group of 106 third and fourth grade students participated in a study of a social–emotional curriculum. They were assigned by classroom to either a treatment or to a wait-list. Students completed two questionnaires pre-intervention. Harlacher (2008) asked teachers to complete a scale for each student at each assessment period. Students completed questionnaires immediately post-intervention and at 2-month follow-up.

4. One hundred and forty-four kindergarten children from ten classrooms participated in the study. Harrist and Bradley (2003) worked with three schools randomly assigning classrooms to experimental or control groups to evaluate the intervention *You can't say, you can't play*. Classrooms that were team-taught, or shared the same recess time, were excluded. Ratings were collected from teachers, children, and observers in regard to students' social acceptance at baseline. Data was collected again 12 months post-intervention.

5. Students from two equivalent school cohorts were compared at two time points. The data collected from the first cohort in grade 7 (Time 1) provided the data for pre-intervention, and the second cohort when they were in grade 7 (Time 2) provided the data for post-intervention, 1 year

(continued)

(continued)

    later (Olweus & Limber, 2010). The two sets of data were compared. The students in both cohorts had been in the same schools for several years and therefore differed only in a minor way from their adjacent cohort with which it was compared at Time 2. As new cohorts entered the program, each in turn was assessed. Several cohorts served as both baseline (Time 1) on one set of data and as the intervention (Time 2) group in another set of data to protect against selection bias.

6. In one area, six schools implemented a program and five schools served as the control group. Eight hundred and thirty first, second, and third grade students participated (Leadbetter & Sukhawathanakul, 2011). Schools were recruited from adjacent school districts, and groups were matched on household income, children's living situation, sex, and number of schools attended since kindergarten. The levels of parents' education were higher in intervention schools. Self-report data was collected from students, and data from parents was collected in regard to children's victimization. Three sets of data were collected for 18 months.

7. Taub (2001) conducted a longitudinal study with students in grades 3 through 6 to determine the effectiveness of an intervention. The target school was chosen due to behavior problems at the school; there were no reported behavior problems at the comparison school. Teachers in the control school were reluctant to be involved in the study because their students would not benefit from the program.

8. Fifty-nine African-American girl in two urban middle schools participated in a cultural program (Belgrave et al., 2004). Pre- and post-intervention data was collected. Two students moved and five did not attend very well. The final sample was limited to 35 girls. There was no baseline difference between the two groups. The intervention group showed significant differences on measures.

9. Twenty-eight elementary schools were randomly assigned to a group which received a social skills training curriculum or a group which received no treatment (Jenson, Dieterich, Brisson, Bender, & Powell, 2010). Five groups of self-report data were collected over 3 years. One thousand, one hundred and twenty-six students participated in the study. The curriculum was delivered in four 10-week modules over 2 years time.

10. Intervention and control classrooms from five schools participated in a study of sixth, seventh, and eighth grade students (van Schoiack-Edstrom, Frey, & Beland, 2002). Only two classrooms were randomized because teachers were not cooperative and one middle school had all intervention classrooms and no control classrooms. Because both intervention and control students came from four of the five schools, the schools were considered to be equivalent in ethnicity and in students receiving free or reduced lunch. Students completed confidential surveys at pre-intervention. At post-intervention, the data was collected between 1 and 5 weeks across classrooms.

Chapter 3
Student Engagement, Motivation, and Active Learning

Data from the 2008 to 2009 school year indicated there were 607,789 students who dropped out of school, grades 9–12 (U.S. Department of Education, 2011). Dropout rates increased with grade level. Of particular concern was the fact that only 64 % of African American students completed public schooling as compared to 82 % of White students. The decision not to complete schooling is a process that is drawn out over many years. School dropout is a complex problem involving school experiences, and both family and community factors. One of the first indicators is poor attendance or academic problems beginning as early as elementary school (Christenson & Thurlow, 2004). Importantly the dropout issue can be prevented.

As educators and researchers examined the possibility of preventing school dropout, additional concerns such as the issue of disengagement become relevant. For example, a Canadian study determined that up to one-third of 13,330 students in Quebec schools reported decreases in interest in school, along with an unwillingness to learn, and lessening compliance with school rules (Archambault, Janosz, Morizot, & Pagani, 2009).

Because more students than one might think are bored, unmotivated, or uninvolved in schools, researchers and educators have become interested in how to engage students in learning (Appleton, Christenson, & Furlong, 2008). Student engagement is a complex, multifaceted concept involving cognitive, behavioral, and affective engagement (Estell & Perdue, 2013). Student engagement is strongly tied to positive outcomes for school-aged children (Mahatmya, Lohman, Matjasko, & Farb, 2012). The positive outcomes include academic achievement and importantly, school completion. Student engagement has been studied in connection with school dropout and school completion but taking a broader view, every school has some students who are disengaged. Less-engaged students tend to be male, from a non-White or Asian group, of lower SES, or students who are receiving special education services. Student disengagement becomes a serious concern by middle school. By the time students are in high school, estimates indicate that from 40 to 60 % of adolescents can be considered disengaged (Klem & Connell, 2004).

The negative outcomes of disengagement are serious. There is a relationship between school disengagement, negative behavior, and use of substances. The aspect of engagement that is involved in these behaviors has to do with emotional engagement. When emotional engagement to school is strong, risky or delinquent behaviors are less likely (Li et al., 2011). Emotional engagement, but not behavioral engagement, is associated with peer support (Estell & Perdue, 2013). Students' positive interactions with peers in less-structured times of the school day, and also in clubs and sports after school, have been found to influence affective school engagement. Parent educational support predicts behavioral engagement while teacher emotional support is connected to academic achievement. A longitudinal study of 6,864 students in grades 5 through 11 (predominantly European American) determined that both behavioral and emotional positive engagement were protective and reduced the odds of starting to use substances or engaging in delinquent behaviors. If teens attend classes regularly, feel close with school staff members, and feel that school is important to them, this data indicates that they will have support to avoid trouble. Active participation in school activities, solid student–teacher relationships, involved parents who support their children and monitor them, and supportive communities can make a difference.

Educators and researchers are interested in increasing achievement, improving behavior, and developing a stronger sense of belonging in students to counter school dropout (Taylor & Parsons, 2011). A focus on student engagement is one approach to deal with low achievement, school boredom, feelings of alienation, and school dropout (Fredricks & McColskey, 2011). Student engagement has been used as an outcome measure for preventive efforts in schools. When children are engaged they tend to perform better. Engagement typically decreases unfortunately as students progress in schools reaching a critical level when students reach high school increasing risk of dropping out of school.

Student Engagement

The focus on the issue of school dropout has forced schools to attend to school engagement (Yazzie-Mintz, 2009). In examining the relationship between student engagement and student achievement, researchers have explored self-regulation, motivation, class size, school attendance, and other factors. The goal of studies in student engagement has been to prevent losing socioeconomically disadvantaged minority students from school (Taylor & Parsons, 2011). More recently, student engagement has been a focus of classroom management strategies. Student engagement is considered an outcome measure and a process for learning in and of itself. Disengagement is a serious concern of educators as completing education has become necessary in the contemporary USA. As a result, student engagement has become a goal of school reform. Reengaging students has become central to the effort of preventing dropping out of school (Reschly & Christenson, 2012b).

Engagement is a recent concept and concern of researchers and school personnel. Student engagement is difficult to conceptualize because there is lack of agreement around the definition of student engagement and in regard to the number of subtypes of engagement (Reschly & Christenson, 2012b). Student engagement has been used to refer to different things in research studies and different terms have been used to describe the core dimensions of the concept.

Fredricks, Blumenfeld, and Paris (2004) proposed a three-part conceptualization of engagement to include cognitive, behavioral, and emotional/affective components. Reschly and Christenson (2006) added "academic" as a component. Reeve (2012) adds "agentic" engagement, which refers to a student's active and intentional contribution to the *flow* of learning rather than passively receiving content (p. 151). Agentic engagement recognizes the effort of individual students to personalize what they are learning and may be seen as a high level of motivation. "Reaction to challenge" has been proposed as another aspect of engagement, although it is not a major subcategory (Klem & Connell, 2004). This behavior relates to whether or not a student engages or withdraws when the possibility of failure is present.

Student engagement is important because it facilitates learning; it can predict how successful students will be, and it gives teachers' feedback so that they can make adaptations necessary for student learning (Reeve, 2012). Strong engagement predicts academic performance and attendance in both elementary and also in middle school (Klem & Connell, 2004). Teacher support facilitates engagement for students particularly in elementary school. Student engagement can be influenced and changed. It can be improved through changes in relationships and through support from teachers, peers, and parents. It can be improved through changes in instruction.

Most of the literature focuses on three core aspects of engagement. According to Fredricks and McColskey (2011), the *emotional* aspects of engagement include identification, feelings of belonging, whether or not students like and enjoy their classes, and how attached they may be to others in school. The *cognitive* aspects of engagement include investment in learning, willingness to work, exertion of effort, whether or not students persist, and how self-regulated students may be. *Behaviors* associated with engagement may relate to participation in learning or in social interactions, participation in the associated activities of school such as extracurricular activities and sports, and time on task. Connectedness to school is a component of engagement (Li et al., 2011).

Other researchers have expanded factors associated with the three core subtypes of engagement. For example, emotional or affective reactions of students in school include not only whether or not students are bored or interested but also emotions such as happiness, sadness, and anxiety (Mahatmya et al., 2012). Emotional engagement includes attitudes toward schoolwork and relationships (Bingham & Okagaki, 2012). The cognitive aspect of engagement includes the willingness to master difficult tasks. This aspect also includes intrinsic motivation, and use of metacognitive strategies. Behavioral engagement can be seen in whether or not students ask questions or if they contribute to discussions in class.

Researchers make a distinction between "indicators" of engagement and "facilitators" of engagement (Appleton et al., 2008). The former would refer to attendance or behavior while the latter might refer to peer attitudes toward school or achievement, or parent attitudes and support.

An interesting small study was presented at the National Association of School Psychologists Annual Conference in 2012 (Saeki & Quirk, 2012). The goal was to develop a model to explain the relationship between school engagement and social-emotional functioning among primarily Hispanic/Latino students. Researchers felt that motivation must first influence engagement before outcomes can be influenced. This preliminary finding suggested that addressing motivation first would have the greater effect on behavioral functioning and social-emotional functioning. Both motivation and engagement contribute to functioning but for this group of students, motivation mediated the relationship between engagement and social-emotional and behavioral outcomes.

Age and Grade Differences in Engagement

There are developmental considerations of engagement. In early childhood, engagement of young children can be observed when children play together helping one another and sharing; when they can complete tasks with effort and focus; and when children follow the rules and directions given by teachers (Mahatmya et al., 2012). Engagement peaks in middle childhood during elementary school. Engagement at this level can be observed as students *actively* participate in tasks and activities. Also at this developmental period positive events, relationships, and situations beyond the school affect engagement in the classroom. Students who are cognitively engaged are more successful when interacting with others and this in turn encourages school engagement. Student perceptions of school characteristics in seventh grade influences their participation in school activities, their identification with school, and their use of self-regulation strategies in eighth grade, which in turn affects achievement (Wang & Holcombe, 2010). On the other hand, social-psychological and behavioral disengagement from middle school can result eventually in dropping out of school (Orthner et al., 2010).

Archambault, Janosz, Fallu, and Pagani (2009) studied 118,727 high school students and found that global engagement, and in particular behavioral engagement, predicted school dropout. Unfortunately, negative relationships with classmates and teachers can also affect engagement in the opposite direction (Mahatmya et al., 2012). Engagement decreases as students move to middle school. Some of the factors that affect this decline include an emphasis on extrinsic motivation, competition, lectures versus discussion, new and expanded numbers of peers, and an increased emphasis on evaluation. Protective factors include parent participation in and assistance with homework, home stimulation, and enthusiastic teachers. Strong connectedness pays off in higher grades and is related to better outcomes in adulthood (Bond et al., 2007). Student engagement predicts school completion for students with disabilities as well as for those without disabilities even when family factors and personal variables are controlled (Sharkey, You, & Schnoebelen, 2008).

Bond et al. (2007) conducted a longitudinal study of 2,678 students in grade 8, grade 10, and 1 year after completing high school. They examined both social connectedness and school connectedness. Social connection in this study was determined by whether or not a student had someone they could trust and confide in, and who knew them well. School connectedness was determined by whether or not students were committed to school, and believed that school was important. Researchers found that low school connectedness in early high school predicted risky behavior and poor academics. Students with the best outcomes had good social and school connectedness in grade 8 and were less likely to experience later mental health problems, or to get involved in risky behaviors. Additionally, they were more likely to have good academic outcomes. This group experienced the lowest depressive symptoms. Students strongly connected to school in tenth grade were less likely to smoke. On the other hand, students with low social and school connectedness were more likely to use alcohol later on. Students in this group were at risk of not completing school. School completion was associated with either poor social connectedness, or low school connectedness or both.

The real complexity of the relationship between social and school connectedness was seen when connectedness of the two variables were discordant (Bond et al., 2007). Adolescents with good social connections and poor school connectedness were the most likely to use marijuana, to smoke, and to get involved in regular use of alcohol. School connectedness was a protective factor for substance use for this group. This group was at heightened risk for anxiety and depressive symptoms. One possible explanation was that students who do not find school relationships rewarding would find positive relationships elsewhere. School professionals must appreciate that the school experience is social as well as academic. School connectedness is associated with student–teacher relationships, peer relationships, and feelings of belonging. Student–teacher relationships are more influential that student–student relationships for learning and for continued school engagement, suggesting that teachers need to build positive relationships with students who are at risk of disengaging or who are experiencing interpersonal conflict. School-based mental health staff members need to help students deal with conflict and offer opportunities for increasing a sense of belonging.

Diversity and School Engagement

The meaning of "achievement" depends on culture (Trumbull & Rothstein-Fisch, 2011). Social goals can be motivating for students and can be more motivating for students of some cultures than others. For example, good relationships with parents, classmates, and teachers are very important for immigrant Latino children, with the teacher–student relationship strongly affecting engagement. Latino students' goals may be to please others, to be with others, or to be successful "for the group."

Social support is a somewhat different concept. Asians and Asian Americans use social support less than European Americans (Kim, Sherman, & Taylor, 2008). Students may be cautious about sharing or asking for help in order to avoid creating stress for others and to maintain harmony. The tendency not to look for social support is found in Chinese, Japanese, Korean, and Vietnamese cultures although this may not be the case for students who have considerable exposure to American culture. Asian Americans are more likely to seek and accept social support when it is offered emotionally, without the accompanying demand to share or *discuss* details of difficulties. When social support is offered, it must be culturally appropriate to meet needs. For Asian Americans this means "being there" rather than talking about problems. Talking about an issue could exacerbate the distress for some students.

Immigrant adolescents who speak their native language at home have been found to have good attitudes toward school in general. Yet, they do not have as strong a sense of belonging as native American students. This difference reflects stronger cognitive and weaker emotional engagement (Chiu, Pong, Mori, & Chow, 2012). Immigrant students have the challenge of cultural barriers, decreased educational and cultural resources, and must learn their new school's norms quickly in order to adapt. Their parents may be more optimistic around the connection between school and upward mobility, which can be very helpful to their children. This group of students is often placed in schools with fewer resources and they tend to experience more safety issues. They may have relationships with teachers that are less strong because of cultural differences. Many factors affect the engagement of immigrant students. Some may be supportive, and other factors may be barriers, to school and interpersonal engagement.

Ethnic minority students are quite diverse but are increasing in numbers in American schools. For these students, engagement and motivation are both important (Bingham & Okagaki, 2012). Some studies support the idea that racial and ethnic minority students with strong identities tend to be more engaged. Although the idea that minority students need to give up their ethnic identify in order to engage in American schools is not supported.

The belief that doing well in school fits with one's racial or ethnic identity can be protective against negative effects of discrimination as it affects engagement. Discrimination or the perception of discrimination interferes with engagement, especially in the case of elementary aged Mexican American children (Bingham & Okagaki, 2012). Researchers have found that when academic achievement is considered a value of one's group, this is particularly helpful for African American girls. Parent involvement predicts engagement of both boys and girls in African American families. In fact, the expectations of parents that their children will do well, supports engagement in general for minority students. Native American students who are strongly identified with their community and who actively take part in their community have more interest in school. The value of hard work and effort is related to engagement for Asian American students. Asian American children spend more time on schoolwork and are more involved in the activities associated with school than other student groups.

When differences between home and school exist for racial and ethnic minority students, engaged peers can make a difference. Friends can provide social connections and support. Although the research is sparse, access to similar peers can support emotional engagement with school and schoolwork (Bingham & Okagaki, 2012). Some studies suggest that same-race or same-ethic group peers who are friends can make a difference in both emotional and behavioral engagement, although this has not been found consistently among all minority groups. Same-race peers help Asian and African American students in regard to emotional engagement; whereas for Latino and White students, simply having a best friend was more important. A negative peer factor for Mexican American children is being around classmates who drop out of school.

School climate can be protective for all students, as can strong positive relationships with teachers, especially when the teacher is of the same race and the class size is not too large (Bingham & Okagaki, 2012). This effect is stronger for disadvantaged children and is stronger for behavioral adjustment for low-income Hispanic students.

Student Motivation

A concept related to student engagement is student motivation (Appleton et al., 2008). Motivation has to do with psychological processes, while engagement refers to active involvement in an activity. Reschly and Christenson (2012b) suggest that it may not be particularly important to differentiate between the two terms when the goal is prevention. Context affects both, and both are linked to the important outcomes of prevention work. One aspect of engagement, cognitive engagement, is quite similar to the concept of motivation. For some researchers, the two terms represent different concepts but the concepts are related. Reschly and Christenson (2012b) write "…motivation is necessary but not sufficient for engagement" (p. 14). Mahatmya et al. (2012) feel that motivation is a "precursor" to student engagement. Motivation is private, difficult to observe, and is subjectively experienced. Engagement is observable and can be seen by others (Reeve, 2012). Both motivation and engagement require teacher support.

It is evident that when children and adolescents are engaged in learning, they will most likely learn, but often teachers and mental health workers are taught to engage students by reinforcing them (Center for Mental Health in Schools at UCLA, 2012a). Public praise can stress some students because it makes them stand out from the group. Critical feedback may motivate those students whose goal is to meet expectations (Trumbull & Rothstein-Fisch, 2011). Being aware that their group is stigmatized by having low status is connected to anxiety around academic achievement and decreased intrinsic motivation (Gillen-O'Neel, Ruble, & Fuligni, 2011). African American, Chinese, and Dominican students, as young as second grade, say that their ethnic group has less status than other groups. The association between being aware of stigma toward one's ethnic group, and decreased motivation along with increased anxiety, has also been found among fourth graders. Possible contributions to this association include school factors, acculturation stress, and/or high-stakes testing.

There is considerable interest in teaching approaches that may engage students. There is a great deal of theory around teaching approaches but the research in this regard is not extensive. It is critical to enhance intrinsic motivation in order to engage students. Engagement can be increased by giving students choices, involving them in cooperative activities, working on projects, and inviting students to participate in school management and policy (Center for Mental Health in Schools at UCLA, 2012a). Additionally, it is important to match instruction to student differences in motivation. School tasks must be challenging, interesting, emotionally positive, and supported by teachers and the school climate. Learning must be challenging but also attractive (Taylor & Parsons, 2011). Teachers must talk about the process of learning and how to improve learning, They must discuss both content and process. Projects that make a difference are important and students need input or control in evaluating their own learning. Ownership and responsibility for their own learning must be fostered in students.

School Dropout and Noncompletion of Schooling

The very strong focus an academic achievement in education policy has brought the issue of "dropout" front and center (Yazzie-Mintz, 2009). The National Center for Education Statistics (Stillwell, 2009) report indicated that only 75 % of students who began high school completed high school in 2008; i.e., one-quarter did not graduate on time. Accurate school dropout data is difficult to compile due to the different ways in which data is collected and reported (Garrison, Jeung, & Inclan-Rodriguez, 2009). The numbers of dropouts reported may not be realistic in some cases. The U.S. Department of Education now requires schools to use a 4-year adjusted cohort graduation rate when reporting data, which may provide for better estimates of the problem (Dianda, 2008). No matter how data is collected, urban schools have a serious problem with students not graduating. Problems begin very early in schools, as early as when students are not ready to begin formal schooling. This is followed by complications of social promotion and general student attitudes about school not really "counting" until ninth grade. Many educators and researchers feel that schools have a serious problem with "in-school" dropping out due to boredom and loss of support and extracurricular programs due to; cut-backs, lack of after-school supervision, and lack of relevance. No Child Left Behind (NCLB) has created its own pressures with intensely focused attention to basic skills and losses of opportunities for students to take classes that interest them. Add to this the added stress of high-stakes testing. Economic issues, poor communities and neighborhoods, and family issues contribute to the problem of school dropout as well as limiting resources to deal with the problem.

There is no single risk factor to predict dropping out of school. Hammond (2007) identified 25 risk factors, 60 % student centered, and 40 % family factors, all of which were considered significant. Individual factors included background characteristics, immigration status, limited English proficiency, disability, early adult responsibilities, high-risk attitudes and values, poor behavior, poor school achievement, educational mobility, and disengagement. Family issues included a high level of stress, family dynamics, family attitudes/beliefs/values around education and schooling, monitoring of homework, and parental expectations. School risks included ineffective school structure, limited resources, the student body itself (characteristics and performance), school policies around discipline and retention, high-stakes testing, and high standards without support. Community risks included a school's location, school type, poverty, unemployment, other demographic variables, crime rates, and community stability. Interactions among the various risk factors are very complex and effect students differently according to the presence or absence of protective factors and a student's developmental level.

Given school disengagement occurs over time, school professionals need to identify the risk factors that are relevant in their local school. Hammond (2007) lists a number of programs that a school team can examine. They are organized depending on which risk factors the program addresses, as well as whether the program would be considered a primary, selected, or indicated prevention intervention. Schools can improve education and engagement of students with disabilities can address and improve issues for minority children, and can work harder to engage families. The most successful programs identify multiple risk factors across several domains (Hammond, 2007). Effective programs include teaching skills, providing support, reaching out to parents, and addressing the school environment. The programs, once identified, must be implemented in the same manner in which they were designed. Although a large number of programs have been designed, many have not been evaluated rigorously in regard to their effectiveness. Many have not collected long-term data or used a control group. School teams investigating preventive interventions must use their expertise, or involve a mental health professional with expertise in selecting an appropriate program that fits a particular school.

Dropout rates are worrisome in both huge city secondary schools and in poor rural schools. Schools in the largest 50 American cities are having particular challenges where only half of students are completing secondary school. The situation is *more serious* than has been previously understood. Recent data indicates that more than two out of five students in high schools do not feel that they are an important part of their school communities (Yazzie-Mintz, 2009).

Students drop out of school for a variety of reasons, both personal and institutional. Mac Iver and Mac Iver (2009) report that school disengagement can be seen in four behaviors that are developing as students move through school: frequent absenteeism, work incompletion, failing courses, and suspensions. Poor attendance during early schooling is a predictor of later dropping out of schools and absenteeism in ninth grade is a very strong predictor of dropping out of school. Missing more than 2 days per month over time requires attention and intervention. When a student fails math or language arts courses, subsequent motivation is negatively affected. Dropout rates are decreased in schools in which students can form positive relationships with staff members, but strategies such as gathering at-risk students together in schools do not help. Monitoring and reviewing student progress in regard to academics, behavior, and attendance; and, developing an early warning system with early intervention planning school-wide are very important.

Using both observational and self-reported data from the NICHD Study of Early Child Care and Youth Development, researchers found that improving classroom quality was not enough to change student engagement from poor to adequate in students with prior difficulties (Dotterer & Lowe, 2011). The problem is bigger than this for students who are *already* disengaged. This fact argues for a tiered approach to prevention of dropping out of school. Prevention of school dropout requires a variety of approaches including community and school level approaches as well as individual approaches (Kerka, 2006). Systems thinking is needed when addressing the dropout problem.

Preventing Dropping Out of School

Dianda (2008) advocated for the implementation of strategies from preschool, though and beyond high school. She stressed the point that the school dropout problem contributes to crime, the costs of welfare and public assistance, and lack of positive participation in communities. The problem perpetuates disproportionality, and increases health costs making it a national problem. When considering universal prevention, many evidence-based programs are available to deal with academic, social-emotional, and behavioral difficulties of students that need to be implemented scientifically across all school levels. It critical to identify risk factors by tracking and analyzing data showing early signs that students may drop out of school, beginning in the middle grades or earlier (Kerka, 2006) (Table 3.1).

Schools need a tiered prevention and intervention system to provide assistance at the *first sign* of school difficulty.

When considering secondary or targeted prevention, students at risk can be identified as early as sixth grade and in some cases even earlier. The indicators include poor grades, poor attendance, grade retentions, behavior problems, and disengagement. Prevention of school dropout requires school level approaches (Kerka, 2006). Kennelly and Monrad (2007) identified some of the prevention efforts that have the "best bet" for preventing dropping out of school. These include monitoring all students' academic progress, attendance, and behavior; providing tutoring and counseling; using a homerooms system; providing transition programs at critical points; offering catch-up courses; redesigning smaller learning communities; and tiered interventions. Community engagement helps as well, as does high expectations on the part of teachers and parents. Studies show that school level factors are more important than trying to focus on variables such as poverty or race. Schools need to address what they have in their power to change.

Table 3.1 Key issues to address at the universal level of prevention

- Advocating for social justice for students and families
- Helping homeless children transition from school district to school district
- Improving education for English Language Learners
- Working to retain minority boys in school
- Working on disproportionate placement in social education programs
- Connecting with families to provide options for students so that they can attend school
- Providing alternatives to retention
- Increasing time on task in basic skills
- Reducing class size
- Providing tutoring for at-risk students

Source: Dianda (2008)

Dounay (2008) argues that schools should receive funding for students who are older, who want to return and earn their high school diplomas. Schools also need to have alternative ways to demonstrate competency in content areas and have *credit recovery* choices and options. Schools need more flexible options for students who already have children, or who need to work. Additionally, it is important to prepare students who need real-world learning environments to be able to get credit so they can later apply for jobs with career options. Schools need to find ways for students to earn both high school and college credits for some of their work.

Klima, Miller, and Nunlist (2009) identified alternative educational programs and mentoring as having a modest but statistically significant effect on preventing dropping out of school. Academic remediation alone was not successful. The alternative intervention that has had some success is a model called *Career Academies* involving both academics and work-based learning in the community. *Career Academies* was initially designed in 1969 in Philadelphia at the Thomas Edison High School for lower income students in grades 10–12. The program spans 3 years and the model is a school-within-a-school (Lehrt, Johnson, Bremer, Cosio, & Thompson, 2004). A manual is available for implementation. Alternative schools have not had an effect on graduate rates although they have had a negative effect on dropping out.

Salvador (2012) took a very broad view of dropout prevention, and searched for programs that impacted high school graduation as well as programs with outcomes involving school engagement. In order to be determined "well supported" programs, Salvador required two or more studies involving randomized controlled trials, publication in peer reviewed journals, implementation in the community, and significant effect sizes. Included were high quality child-care programs, home visit and home intervention programs, high quality preschool programs, child parent centers, literacy support, community-based programs such as *Big Brothers Big Sisters*, and multifamily group interventions. Unfortunately, only a few programs that fit easily into schools were listed:

- *ALAS* (Rumberger & Larson, 1994)
- *Early Risers Skills for Success* (http://www.psychiatry.umn.edu)
- *Positive Action* (http://www.positiveaction.net)
- *Families and Schools Together* (FAST) (http://www.familiesandschools.org)
- *Strengthening Families Program* (http://www.strengtheningfamiliesprogram.org)
- *Check and Connect* (http://checkandconnect.umn.edu)
- *New Hope Project* (http://www.mdrc.org)

The National Dropout Prevention Center for Students with Disabilities (http://www.ndpc-sd.org/dissemination/model_programs.php) listed six dropout prevention programs:

- *New Hampshire's Achievement for Dropout Prevention and Excellence* (APEX) *Program* (http://www.ndpc-sd.org)
- *The Achievement for Latinos through Academic Success* (ALAS) Model
- *The Advancement Via Individual Determination* (AVID) Model (http://www.ksde.org)
- *Check and Connect* (Lehrt et al., 2004)
- *The Coca-Cola Valued Youth Program* (http://www.idra.org)
- *The Iowa Behavioral Alliance* (http://www.ksde.org/)

These programs may not be equally well supported by research studies (Thurlow, Sinclari, & Johnson, 2002).

WWC provides a dropout prevention section with a *Practice Guide and Recommendations* along with the level of evidence to support each recommendation (Dynarski et al., 2008). Recommendations with *moderate* evidence include personalizing learning to develop a sense of belonging and to foster a learning climate, and engaging students by providing skills needed for graduation and for life. At the targeted level, adult advocates and academic support were recommended. Multilevel issues for three levels of intervention were included in this report because dropout prevention is complex and must include multiple components. The authors warn that preventive efforts take time, even years, to result in outcomes that can be measured.

Dynarki and colleagues listed seven programs as showing potentially positive impact on students. *ALAS* and *Check and Connect* had positive effects on staying in school and progressing in school with *Check and Connect* showing actual positive effects and *ALAS* showing *potentially* positive effects at the time they were evaluated. The *Check and Connect* model was developed in 1990, originally for students with behavioral difficulties in urban middle schools. The approach is comprehensive (Lehrt et al., 2004). The *Check and Connect* program has two components, a monitor/mentor, and individualized attention (Sinclair & Kaibel, 2002). The program can be coordinated by a school psychologist and is a targeted intervention for at-risk students. The *ALAS* program was designed for at-risk middle and high school Latino students, includes mentors or advocates, student training, and parent training.

At the tertiary prevention level, more individualized interventions are needed or interventions for specific subgroups might be appropriate. Cobb, Sample, Alwell, and Johns (2005) looked at studies that combined the use of a cognitive-behavioral intervention with high school students with disabilities (behavioral, emotional, or learning disabilities) and measured a dropout prevention outcome. They were particularly interested in social alienation and lack of social skills as well as how to use the social skills students had learned under stressful social pressures. Sixteen studies were identified, five of which were single-subject designs, and three specifically addressed retention or dropping out. They concluded that cognitive-behavioral interventions were *moderately effective* in reducing dropout and aggressive behavior in both younger and older students with disabilities in schools. Particularly recommended were cognitive strategies that used self-management or self-control procedures.

In an interesting study, Spielvogle (2011) conducted a randomized controlled study of engagement. This was a pilot study of fifty-one 13–19 year olds to determine if an engagement strategy could motivate them to participate in treatment. The engagement strategy was motivational interviewing (which identifies the student's past coping methods, explores what the student chooses to share, and what the student anticipates in treatment). An ethnographic approach was used to learn how a child of a different culture perceives what happens to him/her. The process was designed to build trust and encourage sharing feelings about barriers to treatment and feelings for treatment itself. Teens who participated in the engagement intervention had better initial treatment attendance although the effect was medium.

Instructional Practices

Many factors involved in student disengagement have to do with student perceptions of ineffective instruction (Yazzie-Mintz, 2009). The educational literature stresses that teaching techniques matter. Teaching approaches are critical to improving and enhancing engagement (Griffiths, Lilles, Furlong, & Sidhwa, 2012). Teachers are encouraged to move from didactic to constructivist pedagogy. They are encouraged to use peer-based collaborative learning with multiple forms of feedback, along with assignment choices (Taylor & Parsons, 2011). Teachers are urged to encourage students to become co-designers of their learning. When students were asked about types of class work that engaged them on the High School Survey of Student Engagement (HSSSE), 61 % rated discussion and debate as engaging, and 60 % rated group projects engaging. Students positively rated student presentations (46 %), role-plays (43 %), art and drama (49 %), and projects involving technology (55 %).

In the general classroom, a number of strategies have been suggested to help students connect to activities. Some of these include collaboration between students, intensifying how work is presented and acted upon, providing activity options, engaging students in lessons, and establishing a working relationship with students

(Center for Mental Health in Schools at UCLA, 2012b). Project-based learning has recently become popular again. Project-based learning requires students to conduct in-depth research and share it. Patton (2012) documented a process of project-based learning that is useful along with resources for planning and critiquing projects in the form of a teacher's guide. Project-based learning is featured in high school reform efforts (Davis & McPartland, 2012).

Instructional practices can make a difference for minority students (Bingham & Okagaki, 2012). Instructional practices that reflect the values of various groups can positively affect engagement. Many African American students prefer higher levels of movement and auditory input/stimulation. Incorporation of sharing, working together, and attending to group needs, is important for American Indian students. Sadly there seems to be more information available on practices that do not work than on practices that work.

Given the focus on prevention, it is critical that researchers and practitioners determine ways to prevent students from becoming excessively bored, from losing interest, and from feeling alienated from the group or the content. Schools must provide more personal connections with teachers and opportunities for active participation in the classroom to promote engagement in class, such as hands-on activities in small groups (Anderson, Christenson, & Lehr, 2004).

Practices to improve engagement have emerged from the literature to include social interaction, fostering relationships, and dialogue; exploration through problem-based learning; relevancy using real-life scenarios multimedia and technology; learning from experts in the field; learning to communicate with others; challenging instruction; and authentic assessment which includes sharing conversations with students to talk about how they are learning (Taylor & Parsons, 2011). It is also helpful to require student interactions and to make sure that discipline policies are reasonable (Finn & Zimmer, 2012). Novel topics, universally relevant themes, physical activity, and opportunities for exploration increase student interest (Ainley, 2012). It is important that teachers attend to the initial reaction of students to content or method of presentation. Students who react with moderate to high interest tend to hold on to that level of interest. Lam, Wong, Yang, and Liu (2012) urge teachers to make sure that tasks have real-life significance as this has a particularly high correlation with student engagement. Tasks need to be relevant to students' lives. Practical application of tasks needs to be explained.

Emotional engagement may drive other dimensions of engagement (Lam et al., 2012). Emotional engagement has the highest positive connection to instructional contexts. Boredom is a fairly common experience in life in general and also in schools. It can be problematic in that there is an association between boredom and depression, impulse control, and risky behavior. Eastwood, Frischen, Fenske, and Smilek (2012) consider boredom in terms of attention. A student feels bored when he or she cannot engage attention in order to participate in an activity. The student attributes the problem to the environment rather than to an internal ability. Boredom is a form of disengagement from school (Yazzie-Mintz, 2009).

Yazzie-Mintz (2009) used the HSSSE, a tool developed by the Center for Evaluation and Education Policy (CEEP) to examine student beliefs.

This study involved 103 schools from 27 states, representing urban, suburban, and rural areas. The HSSSE measures cognitive engagement, social/behavioral engagement, and emotional engagement. Students reported that education was their primary reason for going to school, but social and family reasons were also important to them. Sixty-six percent of high school students reported that they were bored every day in class. One out of six students said they were bored in every class (17 %) and only 2 % said they were never bored. Eighty-one percent of students who reported boredom, felt that the class material wasn't interesting, 42 % reported the work wasn't relevant, 33 % felt work wasn't challenging, and 26 % found work too difficult. More than a third of students reported they were bored because they had no interaction with their teacher(s). Boredom is a problem for students who may drop out, but it is also a problem for students who stay in school.

Active Learning

There is a large literature available around active learning. A good deal of the literature is theoretical, although there have been a number of studies on the effects of active learning using college student populations, in science classes in particular. There is empirical evidence to suggest that interactive teaching strategies are better than didactic methods (Khan & Coomarasamy, 2006; Miller & Cloverdale, 2010; Scime, Cook-Cottone, Kane, & Watson, 2006). Data at the university and professional training levels suggest that nondidactic teaching works well (Deslauriers, Schelew, & Wieman, 2011; Lo & Prohaska, 2011; Lorenzo, Crouch, & Mazur, 2006; Michael, 2006). Interactive teaching styles are rated highly by students in undergraduate education and some evidence has been found to suggest that retention is better when teachers use this style (Costa, van Rensburg, & Rushton, 2007). At the high school level, Johnes (2006) found that an interactive approach led to better performance.

There is a strong emphasis on active learning in the prevention literature, particularly in the dropout prevention and drug abuse literature. Important for prevention work, meta-analytic studies of prevention efforts that involved prevention of drug and alcohol abuse, and were implemented in schools, were more effective when they included interactive teaching strategies (Ennet et al., 2003). Tobler et al. (2000) conducted a meta-analysis of prevention programs in schools. The synthesis of 207 universal drug-use prevention programs indicated that interactive programs had better effects. Lectures that focused on communicating knowledge were not as effective. Interactive approaches worked when the goals were delaying drug use, preventing initiation of drug use, and/or were focused on reducing drug use. Interactive approaches worked for tobacco, alcohol, and marijuana use. The programs that were noninteractive were only "marginally" effective. More intensive programs that were interactive worked particularly well. Prince (2004) conducted a meta-analysis of 57 studies and found support for active, collaborative, cooperative, and problem-based learning. Student resistance skills are higher in active-learning programs that provide multiple opportunities for students to practice the new behaviors.

There is also data to support the use of an active-learning approach with younger students. Active-learning techniques such as role-play improved skills for children in sexual abuse prevention training (Blumberg, Chadwick, Fogarty, Speth, & Chadwick, 1991). Wurtlele, Marrs, and Miller-Perrin (1987) worked with kindergarten students and found that modeling and active rehearsal skills were more effective than watching films designed to train the same skills. When children became active in child sexual abuse prevention programs, they benefitted more, and the effect size was greater (Davis & Gidycz, 2000). Active long-term programs were more effective for students at every age.

Activity-based learning, especially discussions in small groups, helps students develop a deeper understanding of scientific concepts and helps students apply that knowledge (Hussain, Anwar, & Majoka, 2011). Teachers play a critical role in facilitating intrinsic motivation (Skinner & Pitzer, 2012). They do this by including interesting and challenging activities that are fun. They encourage children to identify their interests and goals. Teachers need to find ways to help students complete tasks that are not so much fun. Students in classrooms need to be protected from public criticism and negative feedback. These safety issues protect engagement from decreasing. School psychologists and other mental health workers need to work with teachers around these issues.

In the academic area, studies indicate that active information processing enhances learning (Catrambone & Yuasa, 2006). Active learning is considered important for mastering both facts and also procedures. Active learning takes more time but is helpful when attacking new tasks. Mahatmya et al. (2012) concludes that children in middle childhood must actively participate in order to achieve and engage in school tasks, arguing that active interactions with the environment drive development. In reviews of universal and after-school social-emotional learning programs, interventions that included active learning were found to be more effective (Payton et al., 2008).

Sequenced training requires active learning and sufficient time in order to master learning goals (Durlack, Weissberg, Dymnicki, Taylor, & Schellinger, 2011). Active-learning strategies are important for skill acquisition. More successful prevention efforts are interactive. They use coaching, role-play, and structured activities. Nation et al. (2003) describe varied teaching methods as one of the principles of effective prevention programs. They argue for hands-on experiences to include role-play, more than one teaching method, active practice of skills and new behaviors and activities. A text by Ratiani et al. (2011) for teachers on disaster risk reduction supported by UNICEF, lists a variety of interactive teaching approaches to include learning by doing, role-play, and case study. In a meta-analytic review of drug prevention programs, most of which were conducted in schools, Cuijpers (2003) found that interactive drug prevention programs resulted in significantly less tobacco, alcohol, and illegal drug use. Noninteractive programs did not have the same success. Also important, most of the successful programs were universal programs. Winters, Fawkes, Fahnhorst, Botzet, and August (2007) recommended school administrators or a prevention team overseeing implementation of a prevention program, monitor student engagement as well as whether or not implementers use interactive strategies. In a yearlong program, quarterly collection of engagement data would be most useful.

Increasing Engagement Through Active Learning

School mental health workers have various roles in prevention activities. At the targeted level, school psychologists and other mental health workers may work with small groups of at-risk students. Thinking about student engagement, it is important to be able to generate active-learning opportunities for at-risk students at the Tier 2 and Tier 3 levels. There are several reasons that this skill may be valuable.

1. A subset of students participating in a Tier 1 prevention program may need more practice mastering a skill or concept and may not be highly motivated to master the skills. In this case an active-learning lesson may motivate students.
2. A school may select a prevention program or prevention intervention that does not include the degree of active learning that some students require in order to remain engaged. Small group active lessons may support learning in this case.
3. It may be difficult to locate a targeted intervention that fits well with the universal level prevention program; yet, the issues need to be addressed comprehensively. The mental health staff; i.e., school psychologist, counselors, or social workers may need to develop Tier 2 activities to accompany the lessons in the universal program. This addition would constitute an adaptation to the universal program. Keep in mind it is necessary to monitor and evaluate all changes or additions to universal programs at every step of the way.
4. As Tier 2 interventions are implemented, students may begin to lose focus and engagement. The insertion of an active or interactive lesson may be able to address this problem and re-engage students.
5. As a Tier 2 intervention is implemented, students may not be mastering or using a new skill. The insertion of an active or interactive lesson to practice, generalize, or master a concept or skill may be able to address this problem.

In developing an interactive lesson, recording it in a form that is easy to use is very helpful. It makes the lesson available in the future and once the lesson is in a useable format it can be shared with colleagues. A suggested format would include the following: title of activity, the name of the universal curriculum to which the lesson attached, the age group for whom the lesson would be most appropriate, the objectives for the lesson, the step-by-step directions for implementing the lesson, the materials needed, post-activity questions to help students reflect on and evaluate their learning, adjustments that fit the lesson for students of different ages, extension activities to further learning and generalization, references, cautions, and additional information that may be helpful. A few examples will make the idea clear (Tables 3.2 and 3.3).

Table 3.2 Active-learning lesson: predicting the weather

Active Learning Lesson: Predicting the Weather

Title of Activity: Predicting the Weather

Age Group: Can be adapted for all age groups.

Universal Curricula: This lesson would fit curricula dealing with identifying
feelings (Open Circle), expressing feelings (Al's Pals), identifying others
feelings (Second Step), communicating feelings (Second Step), accurate
awareness of feelings (Coping Power), emotional understanding (PATHS),
and others.

Objectives:

1. Students will enlarge their 'emotions' or 'feelings' vocabulary.
2. Students will learn several words for a basic emotion so they can express
   the particular emotion with varying intensities.
3. Students will be encouraged to continue to practice 'emotions' vocabulary
   words in order to facilitate generalization.

Preparation/Materials:

Copy a map of the United States (or other country) on a large piece of poster board
or use an actual map. Divide the map into five sections. Each of the five sections can
be labeled as follows: 'Overcast,' 'Drizzle,' 'Rain Storm,' 'Wild Thunderstorm,' and
'Dangerous Hurricane.' Prepare cloud cards. The size of each card will depend on the
size of the map. On each card, draw an irregular oval to look like a cloud. Inside or
below this oval print a 'feeling' or 'emotion' vocabulary word. Each student
participating will need a set of cards with 'emotion' words of varying intensity.
Prepare a set of cards for each student in the group. Each set should contain
'emotion' words of varying intensity for the emotion on which you are focusing.

Each set of cloud cards can contain one or more words representing each of several
intensities. For example, one set might contain five cloud cards with the following
words, one on each card: grumpy, cross, vexed, incensed, and raging. If the cards in
each set are given a number and laminated, the materials can be used again and
again.

Below find a list of words to fit the category 'angry words.' For each set of cards,
select words from the several lists so that the set will have a variety of 'anger' words
of varying intensities.

(continued)

Table 3.2 (continued)

1	2	3	4	5
annoyed	smoldering	mad	irate	livid
crabby	huffy	maddened	furious	raging
cranky	aggravated	angered	enraged	raving mad
displeased	sore	angry	infuriated	boiling
grouchy	irritated	indignant	incensed	wild
sulky	cross	irascible	seething	ferocious
grumpy	testy	vexed	burned up	crazed
huffy	agitated	worked up	fuming	fierce
displeased	offended	offended	fiery	violent
uptight	peeved	ireful	outraged	rabid
sullen	petulant	rankled	belligerent	hatred
umbrage	vexed	stormy	bristling	outrage
splenetic	chafed	galled	riled	vengeful
	provoked	chafed	wrathful	inflamed
	nettled	affronted	exasperated	fierce
	frustrated	antagonized	hostile	foaming
	heated	riled	ireful	
	irritable	turbulent	hateful	
	piqued	roiled	inflamed	
	simmering	galled	convulsed	
	fretted	acrimonious	ballistic	
	exasperated	piqued	apoplectic	
	ill-tempered		exacerbated	
	antagonized		impassioned	
			choleric	

Make a large chart to which students can refer in determining where to put their cloud cards on the map.

Overcast	Mild emotion
Drizzle	**Upset**
Rain Storm	**Strong emotion**
Wild Thunderstorm	**Extremely stressed**
Dangerous Hurricane	**Out of control**

Directions:

Explain to students:

You are the weatherperson. Your task is to read the word on one of your cloud cards and explain what the word means. You do not need to give a definition, just explain what the word means, in your own words.

(continued)

Table 3.2 (continued)

Next you need to place the card on the map in the section of the map that matches the degree of emotion that the word conveys. The weather labels in the five sections of the country represent different storm intensities and in the same way, different degrees or intensities of emotion.

Post-Activity Questions:

After all students have explained (not defined) each of the words on their cloud cards and placed the cards on the weather map, discuss the following.

1. Did you find the job of a weatherman/weatherperson easy or difficult? How easy or difficult was it to match the word with weather?
2. Why is it important to know a lot of words to express how you feel? *(If we have more words for our emotions, we will be better able to communicate how we feel. More words for emotions can help us understand ourselves better, help us improve self-control, and allow us to identify strong emotions in others.)*
3. What are some of the things we can do to make sure that we learn more words to express our emotions?
4. Describe some situations or events in which can we could use the new words we learn?

Extension Activities:

1. Repeat the game often using different categories of emotion words (positive emotions and various negative emotions).
2. Post the new words that are being learned.
3. Record the new words in a journal along with the explanation of the word in students' own words.
4. Write stories about the emotion words.
5. Ask students to keep a record of how many times they hear or read the new words they are learning.
6. Ask students to keep a record of how often they use a new emotion word (or words) for a given category of emotions.

Category of Emotion Words	Word	Number of times used

(continued)

Table 3.2 (continued)

1. Make flash cards of the new words and ask student to take them home and place them on the refrigerator in the kitchen.
2. Ask parents to use the new word(s) frequently at home.
3. Ask teachers to use the new word(s) in their conversations with students and to use the new words in their daily lessons.
4. Make 'feelings' thermometers with the words that student want to learn. The thermometer can represent different degrees of emotion. Place these on students' desks so they can communicate quietly to teachers about how they are feeling.

Adjustments:

The major adjustment is to change the emotion vocabulary to fit the age, developmental level, and language ability of the student group with which you are working.

Evaluation/Assessment:

Collect the self-recordings students complete listing how often they use the words, or hear the word(s) outside of class.

Additional Related Articles:

Huyen, N. & Nga, K. (2003). Learning vocabulary through games: The effectiveness of learning vocabulary through games. *Asian ESL Journal.* Retrieved from http://www.asian-efljournal.com/dec_03_sub.Vn.php

Joseph, G. E. & Strain, P. S. (2010). Enhancing emotional vocabulary in young children. Module2. Handout 2.6: Social Emotional Teaching Strategies. Nashville TN: The Center on the Social and Emotional Foundations for Early Learning. Retrieved from http://csefel.vanderbilt.edu/modules/module2/handout6.pdf

Sommer, R, M. (2003). Emotions, anger & emotional honesty. Retrieved from http://www.therapyideas.net/emotional.htm

Suveg, C., Southam-Gerow, M. A., Goodman, K. L., & Kendall, P. C. (2007). The role of emotion theory and research in child therapy. *Emotion and Child Treatment, 14*(4), 358-371. doi:10.1111/j.1468-2850.2007.00096.x

Vano, A. M. & Pennebaker, J. W. (1997). Emotion vocabulary in bilingual Hispanic children: Adjustments and behavioral effects. *Journal of Language and Social Psychology, 16* (2), 191-200. doi: 10.1177/0261927X970162004

To locate word lists for cloud cards:
http://www.sba.pdx.edu/faculty/mblake/448/FeelingsList.pdf
http://www.enchantedlearning.com/wordlist/emotions.shtml
http://www.vocabulary.com/lists/12827
http://www.sengifted.org/articles_social/Lind_DevelopingAFeelingVocabulary.shtml

When students are comfortable with a set of words of varying intensity for a given emotion, create a wordle or **word cloud** at http://www.wordle.net/

Table 3.3 Active-learning lesson: on the other hand

Active Learning Lesson: On the Other Hand

Title of Activity: On the Other Hand

Skill: Alternative thinking

Age Group: This activity is appropriate for elementary and middle school students. It can be adapted for younger and older students.

Universal Curricula: Ability to think of another way of looking at events or situations is a skill taught in all curricula that include social problem-solving, in curricula that teach flexible thinking, in attribution training, and in curricula that teach decision making. Most SEL curricula require this skill to include: PATHS, Open Circle, Strong Kids, Strong Teens, and many others. Additionally cognitive behavioral therapy requires the ability to generate an alternative idea (Coping Cat, etc.).

Preparation/Materials: Trace students' hands, or use a generic hand pattern. Glue the hand patterns to sticks so that each student in the group will have two paper hands on sticks to use.

Objectives:

    1) To practice positive thinking
    2) To learn to generate alternatives to negative statements/situations
    3) To use a concrete exemplar to cue changes in thinking (self-talk)
    4) To change negative self-talk

Directions for Activity: (step-by-step)

Explain to students:

An *'idiom'* is a group of words that have meaning that does not fit the individual words. They are used for a different purpose. An example of an idiom is the phrase, *It's raining cats and dogs* . Cats and dog do not rain from the sky. The phrase simply means that it is raining hard. More examples of idioms include: tongue-in-cheek, smell a rat, bend over backwards, cat got your tongue, for the birds, wet blanket, caught up, make ends meet, let the cat out of the bag and building mountains out of molehills.

(continued)

Table 3.3 (continued)

(Ask students to share which idioms they understand and which are new to them or are confusing. Talk with students about what some of these idioms mean).

Say: There are many idioms that have to do with hands. What might these idioms mean?

have your hands full	to be extremely busy with a difficult job
at hand	close to you and easy to reach
have a hand in something	to help to make something happen
have time on your hands	to have more time available than you need
out of your hands	if something is out of your hands, someone else is now in charge of it
keep your hand in	to do something that you used to do regularly, so that you do not lose the ability to do it well
on the other hand	another point of view; from another standpoint

Say: *'On the other hand'* is something that you say when you are talking about two different facts or two opposite ways of thinking about a situation. This phrase or idiom is used when you are comparing two different facts, ideas, or opposite ways of thinking about a situation.

We can use this idiom when thinking about the way we understand situations. Some people tend to look at the negative side of a situation. On the other hand, some people tend to look at a situation from the positive point of view.

Ask students:

Why might it be helpful to have a positive point of view?
> (Many people who think positively handle stress better, they get more exercise, they eat healthier foods, they feel better and believe it or not, they catch fewer colds.)

Explain: We can learn to think more positively. One way to think more positively is to be nice to yourself. Don't say anything to yourself that you wouldn't say to someone else. Positive thinking takes practice. One way to practice positive thinking is to change negative thoughts so that they become more positive.

Give students the paper hands so that each student has two hands.

Say: We are going to practice using the phrase 'on the other hand' to practice positive thinking. As each situation is described or a statement is made, hold up one hand and if called upon, say how bad you might feel in this situation. Then, if you can

(continued)

Table 3.3 (continued)

think of another way to look at the situation that is more positive, hold up your other hand.

(Call on students who volunteer to share how each student might feel in regard to one or more situation. Next, call on students who volunteer to give students practice in expressing how the situation might be viewed positively).

(Offer students as much practice as needed. Ask students to generate statements from their own experience that can be viewed from more than one perspective. Place students in pairs and have them practice changing negative statements to positive statements; i.e., looking at situations in another way. Students can use the situations below once again with the additional situations they generate themselves).

Practice situations:

Situation	On one hand... Negative Statement	On the other hand... Positive Statement
1. You trip over your feet in front of a girl/boy you like.		
2. You are told that the principal wants to see you in his office.		
3. The teacher moves your seat because you were talking with your best friend.		
4. There is a big party scheduled for the weekend but you have to visit your grandmother.		
5. The exam on Friday is expected to be extremely difficult. You don't think you can pass it.		
6. The team has scheduled an important game on an afternoon when you have to work. Teammates are insisting you show up and play but you are afraid you will loose your job.		
7. You reported a bully to the principal but the kids accuse you of tattling.		
8. You have been chosen to take an advanced math class. You are afraid that you will be the dumbest kid in the class.		

(continued)

Table 3.3 (continued)

9. Your dad is out of work so you have to bring your lunch to school. When you open it up all of the kids laugh because it is not what most kids are eating.		
10. You forgot your homework for the third time this week. The teacher is really angry and tells you to meet her after school. You are really worried that she will call your parents.		

Post-Activity Questions:

1. How easy or difficult was it to think of positive alternatives to the situations described.
2. Are you usually able to look on the bright side or to think of something positive or is this a skill you need to work on?
3. Do you think that being able to think of positive alternatives would help you during stressful situations?
4. What kinds of cues could you use to remind yourself to think of positive alternatives?
5. When might it *not help you* to try to think of a positive way to look at a situation?
6. When trying to think of alternatives what strategies do you use?

Extension Activities:

1. Work with students to create a cue card to remind them to think of another way to look at situations. Agree on a signal to use to remind one another to change negative thinking to positive thinking.

2. If students have difficulty thinking of alternatives, teach this series of strategies:

   a. think of the problem as an opportunity to learn,
   b. think of a weakness as if it were a strength,
   c. instead of thinking that something is impossible, think of it as a possibility,
   d. think of 'meanness' as a lack of understanding,
   e. think of 'against me' as lack of understanding,
   f. look for another purpose for what has happened,
   g. think of a positive value in the situation,

(continued)

Table 3.3 (continued)

---

    h. look for something good in what happened,

    i. identify skills which could be learned from the experience, and
        think of the event as temporary, tell yourself it can change.

3. For students having academic difficulty and are discouraged, have them
    interview very successful students asking the following questions:

        a. What do you do to get ready?
        b. What do you do first?
        c. What do you do next?
        d. What do you see inside your head?
        e. What do you tell yourself?
        f. How do you feel?
        g. How do you do it, step by step?

4. Share the goals of the lesson with parents. Ask parents to remind students to
    think of alternative ways of looking at difficult or discouraging situations.

Adjustments:

If students have difficulty, make a chart with the suggestions found in extension
activity #2. Students can use these suggestions to help them think of ways to
respond to *'on the other hand.'*

The statements/situations can be made easier or more difficult. The discussion
around idioms can be deleted for younger students along with the many examples.
Teach only the single idiom *on the other hand,* and increase practice.

Translating the statements/situations can be practiced without the use of the
concrete hands for high school students, substitute a cue card with a hand or ask
students to use their own hands. A concrete cue may still be useful at the secondary
level. When working with older students, discuss 'context reframing' and 'content
reframing' (Pesut, 1991). *Context reframing* is taking an experience or situation that
feels negative or distressing and showing how the same behavior or experience can
be useful in another context. *Content reframing* is simply changing the meaning of a
situation - that is, the situation or behavior stays the same, but the meaning or the
way you interpret it to yourself is changed. Practice using these two different ways
of reframing.

Caution:

If Asian American students are participating in the group, do some research before
emphasizing positive thinking or positive self-talk.

(continued)

Table 3.3 (continued)

Peters, J.,& Williams, J. (2006). Moving cultural background to the foreground. An investigation of self-talk, performance, and persistence following feedback. *Journal of Applied Sport Psychology, 18* (3), 240-253. doi:10.1080/10413200600830315

References:

Fredrickson, B. L. (2001). The role of positive emotions in positive psychology: The broaden-and-build theory of positive emotions. *American Psychologist, 56* (3), 218-226. doi:10.1037/0003-066X.56.3.218

Fredrikson, B. L., & Joiner, T. (2002). Positive emotions trigger upward spirals toward emotional well-being. *Psychological Science, 13* (2), 172-175. doi: 10.1111/1467-9280.00431

Pesut, D. J. (1991). The art, science, and techniques of reframing in psychiatric mental health nursing. *Issues in Mental Health Nursing, 12*(1), 9-18. Retrieved from http://informahealthcare.com/loi/mhn/

Stoeber, J.,& Janssen, D. P. (2011). Perfectionism and coping with daily failures: positive reframing helps achieve satisfaction at the end of the day. *Anxiety, Stress & Coping, 24* (5),477-497. doi:10.1080/10615806.2011.562977

Treadwell, K. R., & Kendall, P. C. (1996). Self-talk in youth with anxiety disorders: States of mind, content specificity, and treatment outcome. *Journal of Consulting and Clinical Psychology, 64(* 5), 941-950. doi:10.1037/0022-006X.64.5.941

Prevention in Action Challenge: Create a SEL Lesson Using Active Learning

Use the following template to create an active-learning lesson to supplement and support a SEL curriculum. An example of a SEL curriculum is the Strong Kids curriculum (Merrell, Carrizales, Feuerborn, Gueldner, & Tran, 2007a). Some of the concepts included are understanding feelings, dealing with anger, understanding other's feelings, identifying negative thinking, positive thinking, solving people problems, and goal setting. (For additional curricula see http://casel.org.)

Title of activity:
Title of curriculum or program this activity supports:
Preventive curriculum/program concept:
Age group:
Objectives:
Directions for activities (step-by-step):
Materials needed:
Debriefing discussion questions:
Adaptations needed:
Extension activities:
Evaluation/assessment:
References/adapted from:
Additional information:

Chapter 4
Engaging Families Through School/Family Partnerships

Collaborating with families is a critical component of population-based or systems-based strategies to enhance positive social/emotional outcomes for students (Christenson, Whitehouse, & VanGetson, 2007). Family process variables predict student achievement better than family status (Christenson, 2002). Building trust with families, responding to parents' need for information, and providing resources are essential for meeting the mental health needs of students. Student/family systems and school systems must interact together as partners to get the outcomes that everyone wants for the children they serve. Christenson and Sheridan (2001) coined the ideal as "partnering" with parents. The concept is also referred to as home–school collaboration or parent–school engagement. The goal is that schools will reach out to parents bringing them into a partnership with schools to work together for children. In the case of mental health, the mutual goals involve to support and facilitate social, emotional, and behavioral development of students.

There is increased awareness today of the role of the family in their child's education (Christenson, 2004). Educators have a greater appreciation for the importance of shared goals. There is more research available on ways to engage families. The literature is ever increasing in recognition of the need for a partnership between families and schools in order to reach positive outcomes for students.

The goals of partnering, or collaborating, with parents are to create constructive relationships and sustained connections while addressing the obstacles that might interfere with these goals (Christenson et al., 2007). The quality of the parent–school interface is critical (Christenson, 2004). Parent support has more impact on children's and adolescents' school success than income or other demographic variables. Family and schools working together are critical for altering the disparities that exist in outcomes associated with schooling as well as in addressing the mental health needs of all students (Reschly & Christenson, 2012a). Shared goals and two-way communication are critical in this partnership, as is continuity between home and school, because this is protective for students. A need that families have that schools can meet easily has to do with

G.L. Macklem, *Preventive Mental Health at School: Evidence-Based Services for Students*,   69
DOI 10.1007/978-1-4614-8609-1_4, © Springer Science+Business Media New York 2014

information needs. A need for information is considered one of the primary concerns of parents from studies attempting to determine what it is that parents want. Sending information from school to home is *one-way* communication and not the ultimate goal of a partnership. Engaging parents is central to advancing social and emotional learning (SEL) outcomes as well as to academic outcomes. When students see their family members involved in their schooling, they learn the value of education to their family (Anfara, 2008). For schools to reach their goals, family involvement must be increased. Families have rights to be involved in schools as is dictated by NCLB and IDEA (Reschly & Christenson, 2012b). The question is how to make this happen?

There are multiple ecological influences on students. Making a change in the family affects the child and the school. Making a change in the school affects the child and the family. This is an example of "circular causality" from ecological theory, i.e., a change in one system or context affecting a child affects all other systems (Christenson, 2004). Different influences such as family configuration or school climate can result in the same outcome. Two children attending the same school or two children from the same family can have very different outcomes. When all components of a child's success or failure are considered together, the whole may be more important than the several components providing input. The relationships between the adults who are involved with a given student are very important. The dosage and intensity of family–school partnerships determines student outcomes. A child's problems or positive health is hard to explain by citing one aspect of this complex relationship. The responsibility for establishing this partnership and engaging parents falls on the school initially, because parents often wait for the school to make the first move (Reschly & Christenson, 2012b).

There is data to support home–school collaboration and partnering to enhance social–emotional and behavioral skills of students. A meta-analysis of 213 school-based, universal SEL programs showed that participating in SEL significantly improved student's social and emotional skills, attitudes, behavior, and academic performance. In a third of the programs reviewed, parents helped children complete skill-related homework assignments or attended discussion and training groups (Albright, Weissberg, & Dusenbury, 2011; Durlack, Weissberg, Dymnicki, Taylor, & Schellinger, 2011). Albright and colleagues point out that when parents support and reinforce SEL skills using similar strategies, the transition between the two environments is easier and there is consistency in expectations. The consistency improves skills and enhances relationships.

A parental engagement intervention was implemented with parents of children in a Head Start program (Sheridan, Knoche, Edwards, Bovaird, & Kupzyk, 2010). Less than one-third of students were White non-Hispanic. The intervention targeted parent engagement. Children whose parents received the intervention showed gains in interpersonal competence as compared to the control group. The social–emotional gains included stronger attachment behaviors, improved initiating behavior, and reduced anxiety or withdrawal. Aggressive and challenging behaviors did not change.

Barriers to Engagement

Most of the time family involvement activities are designed and implemented on the school's terms. They reflect the school's goals rather than the parents' goals (Reschly & Christenson, 2012a). Communication tends to be mostly from the school to the home in spite of the partnership literature. There are huge social differences between educators and parents in some communities and neighborhood schools (Christenson, 2002). Educators feel it is very difficult to reach some families and they may dismiss some families as "hard-to-reach." These families live in high-risk communities with few resources. They may have less education, be poor, and lack much knowledge about American schools. They may not understand the values of educators or may not have the experience they need to help their children and adolescents. It is challenging for educators to partner with non-English speaking families. School policies do not always match the goal of a shared partnership.

Barriers to good family engagement and family–school partnerships exist at multiple levels, from the family system, to school policy, to state and federal legislation (Reschly & Christenson, 2012a). Parents are mentioned more than 300 times in various parts of the No Child Left Behind Act of 2002 (Anfara, 2008, p. 58). Because the NCLB legislation has not resolved educational problems in the United States, there are currently increased efforts to involve parents and the community into partnerships in children's education (Weiss & Stephen, 2010). However, efforts to involve disadvantaged families have been underfunded, periodic, not sustained, not monitored, or have not worked. The parent involvement that does exist tends to be connected to programs that are funded such as special education. The good news is that interest in family–school partnerships is growing. Schools must take the first step. An excellent place to start is at the kindergarten transition. Another key transition is entry to middle school. First, however, attitudinal barriers must be overcome and needed skills taught well to make real progress in forming strong partnerships.

Obstacles to schools and families working together may be environmental, economic, attitudinal, cultural, etc. Families may not understand that their direct involvement makes a difference or that schools want them to be involved (Weiss & Stephen, 2010). Barriers to family involvement include parents' beliefs about involvement, life contexts, perceptions of invitations for getting involved, as well as class and ethnicity issues (Hornby & Lafaele, 2011). Parents and teachers may have differing concepts of "involvement" (Anfara, 2008). Two family variables have changed over time and these have complicated this process: families headed by unmarried partners and homelessness (Christenson, 2002). School staff members' tendencies to label families are not helpful (single-parent family). Family differences are not deficits. Barriers to parent–teacher interactions include different attitudes, different agendas, and problems around language (Table 4.1).

Schools tend not to reach out to parents who are interested, but not directly involved in the day-to-day activities of the school (Christenson, 2002). Teachers say that working with families is their greatest problem, and point out they have no training to work with families (Weiss & Stephen, 2010). Some teachers feel that

Table 4.1 A few barriers to family–school collaboration

Barriers from teacher's viewpoint	Barriers from parents' viewpoint	Suggested ways to resolve differences
Lack of resources for family outreach and limited time	Limited financial resources	Work toward informal conversations and frequent short contact
Hold stereotypes about families or cultures	Negative past experiences with schools	Block blame, focus on problem solving, reframe positively
Poor communication strategies	Linguistic/cultural differences	Communicate respect, communicate welcome in the family's language
Focus on problems versus solutions	School do not respond to parents' needs	Focus on specific information, give specific examples
Don't recognize parent's constraints	Don't recognize teacher's constraints	Listen and validate other's views

Source: Christenson, Palan, and Scullin (2009)
Additional resource: Rutgers Safe and Drug-Free Schools and Communities Project. (2009). *Strategies for effective collaboration with parents, schools, and community members*. Newark, NJ: Rutgers, The State University of New Jersey, Center for Applied Psychology. Author

their job is difficult because families aren't doing their part. Some school staff members feel that they can't be responsible for that which they can't control. Teachers need experiential and interactive professional development experiences to learn ways of involving families. Teachers also worry about the time commitment involved when they try to reach out to parents, or when the payoff is perceived as too low for their efforts (Anfara, 2008).

Patterns of attitudes of teachers, and other school staff, around invitations to parents to join together in supporting students are related to many parents' decisions to get involved in their child's education (Hoover-Dempsey & Sandler, 1997). Both parents and teachers need to think that parent involvement is important in order for parents to be strongly involved. There must be a belief in shared responsibility (Christenson, 2004). The psychological factors involved include:

- Parents' perception of their roles
- Whether or not parents believe that they have the skills to help their children with schoolwork
- Parents' attitude toward education
- Parents' expectations for their children's performance
- How parents feel about the invitations, demands, and opportunities from the school

Parents' beliefs that they *should* be involved and that they are *capable* of helping are stronger variables, but invitations from the school increase chances of parents' initial decision to get involved.

Communication between groups of different cultures can be problematic due to different ways in which people structure information in a discussion (quickly coming to the point versus inserting a friendly interaction to get to know the other person a bit). Different ways of using tone of voice to emphasize points and a tendency to make assumptions contribute to communication difficulties as well (del Rosario & Webster, 2007). Parents must deal with limited financial resources, negative past interactions with schools, linguistic and cultural differences, and their feelings that schools will not address their needs or listen to them (Christenson et al., 2009). Parent–teacher interactions are even more challenging when teachers focus on problems versus solutions or when they have stereotyped ideas about various cultures and the families with which they must interact. School staff members, teachers, and specialists can work to identify families who are not being reached, make personal contact with them, ask families what resources they may need, and hold conferences at times when parents are actually able to meet.

Teachers and other school staff members require training in involving families as well as in the importance of home–school collaboration. They need help to overcome personal barriers such as the challenge in interacting with resistant, reluctant, or non-English speaking parents. School staff members need strategies for communicating and connecting with families, for involving parents in decision-making, in helping families to support their child's learning, and in recruiting families to strengthen the school. School psychologists and other mental health school workers can ask family members to share their troublesome perceptions of the school and help reframe those perceptions. The goal in this case is to renegotiate and reestablish a collaborative relationship. Cultural sharing conversations are helpful for involving parents of various cultures especially when they are completed early in the year, when meetings are scheduled at times when parents can get to the meeting, and when meetings occur in non-rushed settings (Miller, Arthur-Stanley, & Lines, 2012).

Unfortunately, many observers feel that although we have good ideas about what barriers exist, educational practices have not overcome the various barriers. Reschly and Christenson (2012a) describe disconnects between legislation, policy, attitudes, intentions, and practices (p. 69). They suggest that there is a lack of professional development around the topic for family–school partnerships. "Trust" is difficult to legislate. Developing trust takes time and effort. An additional complication is that school–family interaction and supports change with the developmental level of students and school level. Early on, working toward student readiness, developing basic skills, and facilitating motivation to learn are important. Later, transitions, autonomy, career planning, preventing risky behaviors, and graduation are important. In addition, different families require different supports, more or less time from educators, and more or less effort on the part of schools to become fully engaged.

In a small study, researchers interviewed parents who had elected not to participate in a culturally sensitive parent component of a prevention program (Garcia-Dominic et al., 2010). Using focus group techniques, the barriers identified included competing family demands, social role norms, perceived cost, and perceived value. Maximizing parent involvement requires identification of barriers and alleviating them.

Engaging Parents

Parent engagement can be viewed as a complex activity, which involves parents becoming active in learning activities at home, to include:

- Helping and supervising homework
- Monitoring how children spend their time away from school
- Expressing interest and expectations about school, such as talking about school and what is being learned
- Interacting with school staff and attending events (Henderson & Mapp, 2002)

The literature on parent engagement is complex rather than simple. Some studies show that there is little effect of parent engagement on academic achievement, especially of high school students, for parent communication with schools, for parents volunteering, for parents attending school events, and for parents becoming involved with other school parents. These variables may be mediated by student behavior in that parents may be giving a lot of help to students who are not doing well and this would confound the data. When parents of younger children are engaged in supporting learning at home, the result is higher achievement. Workshops for preschool and kindergarten children that teach parents how to help their children at home seem to work (Henderson & Mapp, 2002). When homework involves parents, students benefit. Families with more income and at higher social class levels tend to be more involved with schools although families of all incomes and social classes are involved at home. Families with more income and education are more comfortable interacting with school staff members and feel entitled to treat teachers as equals. They additionally have easy transportation to schools.

Schools can play an important role in how families are involved in children's learning in schools (Raferty, Grolnick, & Flamm, 2012). There are many strategies and activities that schools could use to increase family involvement in school, but many schools are not trying even the fundamental strategies to affect involvement (Michael, Dittus, & Epstein, 2007). Teachers' attitudes influence parent behaviors. Teachers may or may not encourage parents to visit the school, give parents feedback on how to help, make them feel comfortable, or even believe that it is part of their job responsibilities to solicit family help. Of course some parents' beliefs may clash with teachers' beliefs, making progress difficult. Attitudes may clash as well. In some cases, the school's efforts to involve parents of children who are not doing well may backfire. This might happen because parents have had unrewarding experiences with schools in the past themselves (Center for Mental Health in Schools at UCLA, 2012b). However, when both parents and schools are focused on student learning, when there is a mutual belief that the work of education is shared between home and school, when there are efforts to facilitate parents and schools working together, and when prevention is front and center, parents and schools can say they have a working partnership.

School staff members must embrace the attitude that all parents are involved in their children's learning and all desire that their children are academically successful in school. The literature is clear. School-initiated programs that invite involvement,

Table 4.2 Strategies to help engage parents

Provide childcare during meetings
Arrange carpools
Provide lending libraries
Provide materials for home use
Offer parenting and informational workshops
Provide increased help and communication at times of transitions
Telephone routinely
Require homework that involves parents
Hold focus groups with parents
Ask parents to write comments on homework
Honor the contributions and accomplishment of families and community members
Use a cultural broker when needed

Source: Henderson and Mapp (2002)

are welcoming, and that address parent/family concerns tend to be more successful at engaging parents. When school staff communicate that they consider parents partners, engagement is higher. School staff members need to appreciate that helping children at home is a valuable contribution on the part of parents even if parents cannot get to school to meet with staff (Henderson & Mapp, 2002). There are a number of strategies that can help parents engage (Table 4.2).

Finally, helping families build connections with other parents and with teachers builds social capital. Soliciting parents' input about what would make the school better and asking what kinds of events parents would enjoy may make a difference. School professionals need to determine how they can engage parents in school mental health activities and programs, provide training for school staff in engagement strategies, and find out parents' wishes, interests, and needs.

The Centers for Disease Control and Prevention (CDC) (2012a) recently released a publication on parent engagement. Parent engagement was defined as "parents and schools working together to enhance and improve the development of children and adolescents" (p. 6). "Parent" was defined as the adult primary caregiver or any adults who play an important role in the child's life (Anfara, 2008). The publication offered ways to increase parent engagement. Recommendations included making positive connections with parents, offering frequent and varied choices of activities to involve parents, and working hard to sustain involvement. Schools of course must decide what resources they have available to reach the goals of involving and maintaining parent engagement, but every school can use some of the strategies recommended. Strategies included surveying parents to determine their needs and interests, reviewing ways that the school communicates with parents, educating staff, and planning engagement strategies in detail.

It is important to emphasize that the majority of parents want more information about their children's *progress* (Christenson, 2002). Information needs to be provided systematically. Information about children's progress can include information about how schools function. It is important to keep in mind that family–school

Table 4.3 Strategies for encouraging parent involvement

- Parenting support
  - Assist parents with parenting skills, child development, child management and supervision, modeling healthy behavior, and setting expectations
  - Teach parents how to set up a resource center in the home
- Communicating with parents
  - Design and conduct a variety of effective forms of two-way communications about school programs and children's progress using different media, send many messages home in a variety of ways
  - Establish different ways to get input from parents, use community groups to get information to parents, and provide bilingual interpreters
- Volunteering
  - Recruit and organize help for students, involve parents as volunteers and audiences, determine what expertise is available among the parent population, and find ways to use it
- Learning at home
  - Provide information and ideas about how to help students with homework, activities, and decisions
  - Invite family members to participate in school and community physical activities
  - Encourage children to share with parents what they learn about healthy behaviors in school
- Decision-making
  - Make sure that parents from all backgrounds serve as representatives on school committees, represent all subgroups of parents in the parent–teacher organization, and obtain input from all parents on school decisions
  - Involve parents in setting health-related priorities
- Collaborating with the community
  - Identify and integrate resources and services from the community to strengthen and support schools, students, and their families
  - Link families to community services, ask organizations and business to offer gifts to parent volunteers, and sponsor service learning opportunities

interventions are contextualized, i.e., different strategies are needed at different times, for different situations, and for different families.

Research has identified different types of parent involvement and ways to encourage each type. These are reported in detail in the publication by The Centers for Disease Control and Prevention (CDC) (2012a). Some of the activities in regard to support for parents, communication, parent volunteering, helping parents support their child at home, collaborative decision-making, and community collaboration are found in Table 4.3.

Finally, an important approach is to develop a committee of school professionals to oversee parent engagement. This committee can determine what the school is already doing that is working well at each grade level and school level (http://www.projectappleseed.org). The committee can determine which practices should continue and which should change, how to improve communication to and from families, and how efforts on the part of the school could be evaluated. The Title 1 Parent Involvement section of NCLB requires that every school receiving funds must have a written parent involvement policy, evaluate the content and effectiveness of parent involvement programs annually, identify barriers to increased participation in activities provided for parents, and design more effective strategies to get better results. Parent Involvement Checklists to determine if schools are meeting the requirements can be used more broadly around whole school efforts to involve parents (http://www.ncpie.org). Many checklists can be found online (http://titleone. dpi.wi.gov; http://www.education.ne.gov; http://outreach.msu.edu).

One support that schools can provide to parents is illustrated by the project *Teachers Involve Parents in Schoolwork* (TIPS) (Epstein & Van Voorhis, 2001). The goal of this project was to involve parents in students' homework. When this program was in effect, more families became involved in their child's homework than previously. Van Voorhis (2011) worked with students and families from four urban elementary schools in a study using a quasi-experimental design over 2 years. A majority of students were African American, and 70 % of them received free or reduced price lunch. The students and families participating in the TIPS program became more involved with homework as a family. Additional positive outcomes were reported in regard to math achievement scores and positive attitudes toward math.

Parent Training

Schools can help families by providing parent/family interventions. There are various categories of parent interventions:

1. Those that support parenting practices and skills, support family literacy, and connect families of preschoolers and elementary-aged students with services
2. Short-term interventions to target homework support, preventing behavior problems, or college preparation when children are in middle childhood and adolescence (Weiss, Bouffard, Bridglall, & Gordon, 2009)

Parent training is a very important intervention that school professionals can provide in areas where this is needed. Through parent training, parents learn skills through completing homework, learning from models, and practicing skills (Centers for Disease Control and Prevention (CDC), 2009). A meta-analysis of parent training programs identified three components related to improved outcomes of parent training: focusing on emotional communication skills, teaching parents how to interact positively with their children, and requiring parents to practice with their child during training. Emotional communication skills help parents become closer to their children and help parents have better success at getting their child to do what the parent requests. When parents interact positively with their child, they are in a better position to improve their child's attentional skills and to reinforce their child in a manner that strengthens self-esteem. When practice using parenting skills takes place in a training session, the mental health practitioner can give immediate corrective feedback and encouragement to facilitate mastery of the several parenting skills.

Parent management training has solid support in the literature due to extensive studies to help children with behavior disorders (Lochman, 2000). Ineffective parent interaction with their child is one of the important precursors of poor outcomes for challenging children. Use of harsh discipline, lack of monitoring, lower levels of involvement, and decreased warmth when interacting with their children make a significant contribution to increased aggressive behaviors. Typically as children's behavior becomes more troublesome, parents' behavior becomes more negative. Parents can be trained to remove privileges, to use time-out correctly, and to add work chores rather than responding harshly to negative child behaviors. Parent training for students at risk results in lower rates of aggression, lower rates of delinquent behaviors, and decreased severity of negative behaviors. Parents can learn to reduce their own aversive behaviors, use less physical punishments, and become more effective in the management strategies that they use. When successful, parents feel better themselves, are more positive, and family functioning improves.

Research indicates that parent training has small but significant effects especially on the families most at risk. Meta-analyses show that programs that teach parents to help students with learning activities at home (such as getting involved in student's homework) have moderate to highly significant effects on student achievement (Weiss et al., 2009). Programs targeting family–school relationships have a positive effect on social outcomes. Programs designed to prevent behavior problems that include parent training and family involvement affect cognitive, social, and behavioral skills, although the family component of these programs has not been evaluated separately from the total effects. Data indicates that parents who participate for longer periods of time in programs, and are more actively engaged, benefit more. Family involvement must be systemic and sustained in programs if they are going to be successful.

Parent training is not a panacea however. Lundahl, Risser, and Lovejoy (2006) conducted a meta-analysis of 63 studies involving parent training. They were interested in whether or not parent training could change children's negative behaviors and, additionally, whether or not training changed parents' perceptions and behavior. They concluded that immediate effects were small to moderate. In the case of behavioral parent training programs, follow-up effects were small. Parent training actually worked less well for disadvantaged parents. Parents did better with individually designed training. When child behavior is severe, individually designed parent training may be necessary and schools may need to refer parents to services outside the school.

In schools, school psychologists and other mental health workers can provide training in the use of behavior modification strategies. There is considerable research to indicate that parent training works to prevent behavior disorders when implemented with urban parents of preschool-aged children (Cladwell et al., 2005). Studies indicate that behavioral training for parents of children with ADHD decreases both behavior problems and also has an effect on reducing internalizing problems, although some studies indicate that it has not been as successful in reducing parent stress (Van den Hoofdakker et al., 2007).

As part of behavioral training, parents typically receive 10–12 weeks of training in techniques such as the use of time-out and the use of praise. Carefully examining 79 studies, researchers determined that training parents in behavioral techniques is effective, although many studies lacked detailed information about specific target behaviors or treatment techniques (Maughan, Christiansen, Jenson, Olympia, & Clark, 2005). If behavioral training is implemented in schools, data collection on effectiveness is necessary. Mental health workers need to collect multiple forms of data (teacher reports and student observations) as studies using only parent-reported outcomes can inflate results of effectiveness. There is particular interest in parent training for the treatment of students already identified with conduct problems. A systematic analysis of randomized controlled trials of parent training for this population showed that, in general, parent training is effective for parents of youngsters with conduct problems. However, studies tended to be small so it was not possible to determine which approaches were more effective than others.

It is also important to plan around potential problems when considering parent training. Lochman (2000) points out that a given training approach may not work for all children. Children with particular temperaments may need a different management style than other children. For example, parents may inadvertently encourage inhibition in children who have fearful temperaments by being overprotective. Inhibited children need to learn to overcome their feelings of uncertainty through parental support for independence. Harsh punishment on the other hand may result in increased aggressiveness for boys who have fearful temperaments (Colder, Lochman, & Wells, 1997). Easygoing but encouraging parental management fits children with inhibited temperaments better. Putnam, Samson, and Rothbart (2002) suggest that when children are resistant to control, but not emotionally negative, they do better with parents who intervene and teach them to manage angry impulses.

Examples of Parent Training Programs

An example of a program for aggressive children that involves parent training is the *Coping Power Program.* This program utilizes both parent and child training (Lochman, 2000). The program is typically implemented as students enter middle school. The component of the program targeting students focuses on anger coping. The long-term goal is the prevention of substance use (Lochman & Wells, 2002). Jurecska, Hamilton, and Peterson (2011) randomized two groups of students in four rural public schools. Teacher ratings indicated that there was a positive effect on student behavior in class. Lochman and Wells (2004) found that the *Coping Power Program* with both student and parent components was effective in preventing antisocial behaviors when implemented at the middle school level, and the effects were sustained for 12 months after the program ended. The parent component in this study was not implemented alone without the student component. The students who participated had improved behavior as rated by their teachers. Implementers reported that the parent component was the most critical aspect of the program in regard to sustaining gains. Interestingly the program was less effective for African American students in regard to self-reported delinquency.

It is important that school mental health workers appreciate the fact that parent training that teaches management strategies that do not fit culturally supported beliefs will most likely fail. Cultural norms around the practices of parents play an important role in the ways in which children are raised and which behaviors are considered appropriate. Cultural norms can influence parental acceptance of parent training programs. Cultural norms can interfere with the delivery of programs and can decrease the effectiveness of healthy parenting programs or interventions (Kumpfer, Alvarado, Smith, & Bellamy, 2002; Lubell, Lofton, & Singer, 2008).

Cultural/Diversity Issues in Parent Involvement

The Latino population comprises more than 20 different backgrounds, as well as many different languages, beliefs, and customs (Peña, Silvan, Claro, Gamarra, & Parra, 2008). Acculturation makes a difference in whether or not families may be willing to engage in preventive services. Acculturation is a process. It refers to the process of becoming influenced by the wider society. More acculturated families may be more like the wider society in their attitudes about mental health and services when students have difficulties. Latino families are respectful of authority and rely on the broader family for support. Personal contact and telephone calls help include Latino parents who have limited English. Interventions such as home visits, parent liaisons, workshops, and information provided by the school in the parents' own language are helpful in engaging Latino parents.

The African American community has a variety of different origins as well including Africa, the more than 50 islands of the Caribbean, the Cape Verde Islands, Bermuda, or the United States. These differing backgrounds contribute to differences in families. Spirituality and interactive communication are important for many of the families in these groups (Chandler, A'Vant, & Graves, 2008). It is common for these families to obtain support from extended networks. Some families feel school resources are withheld from their children, so developing trusting relations is critically important. School staff members who openly talk with parents about their concerns can be very helpful in this regard.

Asian families can be very different one from another as countries in Asia have *very* different traditions and preferences (Leung, Wu, Questin, Staresnick, & Le, 2008). School staff members are likely to be working with families whose origins include China, Korea, Vietnam, Singapore, Taiwan, or the Philippines. For many of these families, obedience and respect for elders is a strong value. When communicating with Asian American families, it is important to remember that Asian American parents may not openly disagree or challenge school staff. However, social and economic status (SES) makes a difference in the case of Asian American families. If parents are middle class and were born in the United States, they may not need as formal a relationship with school staffs. Parents from lower SES groups need nonverbal support and extra time when asked to participate in discussions about their child. Note that Asian families also include families from India, Indonesia, Sri Lanka, and other countries whose cultures, beliefs, and traditions may be quite different from mainstream US culture, but whose cultures are very rich.

Indigenous Americans have striking differences in values, beliefs, languages, behaviors, and ways of interacting (Dauphinais, Charely, Robinson-Zañartu, Melrose,

& Bassa, 2009). There are over 500 official tribal groups as well as additional groups not officially recognized in the United States. There is a history of discrimination surrounding these families as well as high rates of poverty, substance use, violence, physical health, and mental health issues. These groups of families have extended kin-ships, practice spirituality, and demonstrate important differences in communication. Generally, their communication styles require additional time in meetings. Meetings may need to be rescheduled after the family discusses issues with others. Asking for the family's perspective and listening to families when there is a concern is critical. Dauphinais and colleagues suggest that when communicating with families from these various cultures, it is important to summarize what has been discussed at the end of meetings to make sure that there is a common understanding.

Parent involvement has been strongly considered as a way to narrow the gap between the success of advantaged and minority students (Raferty et al., 2012). Studies show that parent expectations are stronger than other variables in regard to student success in school because of the attitudes and values students need to work hard. There are some differences among families. For Asian American families and White families, communication, high expectations, and parent participation predicted student achievement. For African American families, parental supervision was particularly effective. For Hispanic parents, communication was a critical vari-able. Parental attitudes and behaviors affect their children's motivation, which helps them engage in schooling. Parental structure in many cases helps students channel effort to achieve.

Colombo (2006) reminds us that forming partnerships with parents who have different languages and cultures takes more effort than establishing relationships with parents who are much like the school staff. The various ways in which parents become involved with schools also depend on parents' cultural orientations (Ryan, Casas, Kelly-Vance, & Ryalls, 2010). Sometimes school personnel try to increase parent involvement with the assumption that lack of involvement is the parents' fault and it is parent attitudes and effort needs to be changed. This attitude on the part of the school does not predict easy success in involving minority parents. School staff must be careful that they don't structure interactions with parents in ways that make parents powerless (Hendricks, 2005). They must keep in mind that minority and linguistically diverse parents may be overburdened and experience limited English. School personnel may not be culturally competent, or they may talk with parents in educational jargon. This needs to be monitored and changed through professional development for teachers and other school staffs.

The challenges of working with parents of various cultures are complex. Not all families from the same background are alike (Guerrero & Leung, 2008). Parents may have individual likes and concerns that have nothing to do with culture or back-ground. At the same time, some parents of various cultural backgrounds have preset ideas about their roles in relation to the school. There are racial differences in beliefs about child problems. Parents may not perceive that some of the services schools may offer are acceptable (Lau, 2006). Parents may trust teachers, consider them experts, and therefore find it difficult to talk with them (Colombo, 2006). Linguistically diverse parents may not question what teachers do because they do not communicate easily. Training parent coordinators is an approach that has been helpful when working with families. Parent coordinators network with families, determine what is needed, and share this with schools who can then try to meet needs. This service model needs to be managed well in that parent coordinators must not have access to confidential information and must be well trained.

Low-income parents are another group that have their own needs as far as schools are concerned. Basically, low-income parents have the same attitudes about education as other parents (Guerrero & Leung, 2008). However, low-income parents have difficulties with transportation, childcare, limited financial resources, and working hours that may interfere with meetings at school held during the workday (Raferty et al., 2012). Furthermore, they may not believe that they have the education needed to help their children. They may not have access to parent networks to help them deal with schools. They may be suspicious of school personnel in the same way that they are suspicious of government. School personnel need to listen to this group of parents and ask parents what they consider to be "normal" behavior for their children and what they need from the school (Ryan et al., 2010). School professionals must keep in mind that should the child's problems be looked at as the family's problem, this would interfere with the comfort level of parents communicating with the school and also with mutual problem solving.

There are many subgroups of families that interact with schools. Gay, lesbian, bisexual, and transgender (GLBT) parents and their children deal with considerable challenges. The children of GLBT parents contend with real and subtle threats and insensitivities. Students report that teachers typically do not intervene to address the subtle indignities. GLBT parents may feel ignored or not acknowledged by schools (Frazier & Chester, 2009). Teachers and other school professionals may benefit from extensive data to indicate that children raised by gay and lesbian parents develop resilience in spite of economic and legal disparities and stigma (Perrin, Siegel, & The Committee on Psychosocial Aspects of Child and Family Health, 2013). The well-being of children is determined by their relationships with their parents rather than whether they are raised by parents of the same or different genders.

Kosciw and Diaz (2008) surveyed national samples of 588 parents and 154 students of LGBT parents in middle or high school. LGBT parents reported being highly involved in schools, contacted schools readily, and were often proactive in bringing up and addressing concerns. Almost half of this group of parents had shared information about their families and two-thirds had talked with teachers about being an LGBT parent. Whereas many LGBT parents did not report negative interactions with school personnel, a fifth of parents in the sample reported that teachers did not acknowledge their type of family. This subgroup indicated that they felt that they could not fully participate in school functions, and quarter of the sample reported mistreatment by other parents at their school. Although this is a national sample, individuals chose to participate in the study so results must be viewed with some caution.

Schools need to create an atmosphere where all views are respected through antibias training for school staff members (Ryan & Martin, 2000). Teachers and other school professionals need information about the complicated concerns of GLBT parents such as custody, daily prejudice, and information about the strengths of families that are not traditional. It is important to ask parents whom they would like to include in planning for students. It is important to review privacy regulations when meeting with families due to possible legal complications. Teachers may need help from school-based mental health professionals in how to talk about family constellations with students in their classes, and what language should be used. Parents should be addressed by the terms they want to be called. Professional staff members need to help families know that they will respect requests for confidentiality once they understand and have talked about the reasons that confidentiality was requested. School professionals must also share with parents the possible loss of feeling fully part of the community when families attempt to hide information. School professionals must keep in mind that there may be some environments, and communities, which are not accepting of all families and children, and children need to feel safe. Steps that schools can take to keep students safe must be taken.

Prevention Programs with Parent Components

In planning preventive activities in schools, there are several representative programs of interest. The *Seattle Social Development Project* (SSDP) is a 6-year multicomponent school-based program focused on preventing delinquency in elementary-aged multiethnic, urban, low-income students (Hawkins, Kosterman, Catalano, Hill, & Abbott, 2008; O'Donnell, Hawkins, Catalano, Abbott, & Day, 1997). In addition to training teachers in classroom management and instruction, parents are offered seven sessions in child management skills when their children are in grades 1–3, with an additional four sessions in skills for supporting academics. When their children are in grades 5 and 6, parents are offered additional sessions focused on reducing risk of problem behaviors. A nonrandomized controlled trial of the program, 9 years post-intervention (in Seattle), resulted in significant positive effects on emotional and mental health in relation to dose, with the strongest effects for groups receiving the full intervention. Long-term effects were studied as well (Hawkins et al., 2008). Quasi-experimental research demonstrated that those students who received the full intervention had significantly better outcomes 12 and 15 years after the intervention ended. Parenting practices improved along with children's social competence. Greater engagement in school, work, and community and fewer mental health problems were identified as outcomes.

The *Incredible Years* (IY) program series has three components:

- A teacher training group format for teachers, counselors, and psychologists
- Two child training programs consisting of 60 social–emotional classroom lessons and activities for children in preschool, kindergarten, and first and second grades, with a targeted intervention for small groups
- Parent training components (Webster-Stratton & Herman, 2010)

The IY parent training program consists of a group and video approach to delivery designed to reduce behavioral problems and, at the same time, promote social–emotional development in children aged 3–8 years. Currently there are three curricula for parents.

The *BASIC* parent component has four levels: parents of baby, toddler, preschool, and school-aged children. These have been recently updated to be appropriate for culturally diverse families and for children of varying temperaments. Other additional features include teaching parents positive interactions with their children and coaching parents to use the skills. Parents are taught how to develop routines, to use proactive discipline techniques, to support children's academic success, and how to collaborate with teachers (Webster-Stratton & Herman, 2010, p. 41). There are additional supplementary programs. One supplement addresses parents' interpersonal risk factors, and the other addresses school readiness. Seven randomized control group trials by the developer indicated that the *BASIC* program improves parent attitudes, reduces harsh discipline, and reduces child behavior problems as compared to wait-listed control groups. Five independently replicated studies in mental health settings or schools supported program effectiveness. One hundred and fifty-nine families with children ages 4–8 years old were randomly assigned to parent training, parent plus teacher training, child training, child plus teacher training, parent and child plus teacher training, or a waiting list control group (Herman, Borden, Reinke, & Webster-Stratton, 2011). Children who received any one of the intervention components were more likely to have lower mother-rated internalizing symptoms at posttreatment compared to children in a wait-list control group.

Webster-Stratton (2009) offered a number of recommendations when implementing the parent programs for minority parents. Holding the parent group in a school can be a non-stigmatizing environment as compared to a clinic. It is important to orient parents in regard to program content and schedule and to encourage questions. Group rules need to be negotiated with members of the group. There must be an agreement around confidentiality. All ideas offered by parents need to be accepted. Asking parents to share their goals in detail will facilitate a collaborative atmosphere. This is also helpful in ascertaining parent expectations and knowledge about child development. The group leader needs to get an idea about what is important for each family, make culture visible, and help parents avoid making assumptions. Culturally relevant images and metaphors to teach concepts are very helpful as are group leaders who match the parents' cultures. The program videos that group leaders select should match the cultures of the parents in the group (video vignettes are available for Vietnamese, Chinese, Ethiopian, Eritrean, Latino, African American, Japanese, and Caucasian adults modeling each parenting skill). Because there may be cultural objections to some of the program skills, leaders will need to be prepared to share the benefits of the various strategies for child management. Interpreters can be trained as coaches. Helping parents feel that they are not alone, forming parent buddies, and inviting extended family members to join the group are part of the many additional recommendations made in this article which can be generalized to other preventive work in schools.

Reid, Webster-Stratton, and Hammond (2007) implemented the IY parent program combined with the universal elementary-level program for students known as the *Dinosaur Social Skills Program*. The classroom component outcomes showed that teachers were more positive and less critical of students, the students demonstrated more social–emotional competence, and they decreased disruptive behaviors. The most at-risk children showed the greatest benefit as is typically found in prevention programs. Parents of moderately at-risk children were randomly assigned to three groups. Outcomes were determined by observations of student and parent behavior at home and in addition by parent and teacher reports. Parents received both the *BASIC* program and *ADVANCE* training with videotape vignettes that included families of different cultural backgrounds. This study is important because research studies up to this point involving comprehensive school-based prevention work had not evaluated the individual components of their programs. In addition, the parent program had not previously been evaluated when used as a prevention program in elementary schools (prior program evaluations were at Head Start). Mothers who received the parent component in addition to their children receiving the classroom component reduced harsh discipline, decreased permissive strategies, evidenced more bonding, used more praise and incentives, and increased in attentiveness and nurturing (Reid et al., 2007). A subsample of students with identified behavior problems showed significant improvement. Teachers reported that mothers in the combined programs were significantly more involved in their children's education. The combined programs were most effective as compared to a group that involved only the *Dinosaur Social Skills* classroom prevention or a control group. The greatest challenge was parent attendance. In spite of intensive efforts to remove barriers by providing childcare, meals, parent buddies reminder calls, gift certificates for attendance, and transportation, 50 % or less of parents attended. Mothers who attended more sessions said they used praise and incentives and decreased harsh punishments.

The *Strengthening Families Program* (SFP) is an evidence-based family skills training program that has been shown to be an effective deterrent for substance abuse (Kumpfer, Pinyuchon, de Melo, & Whiteside, 2008). It was originally developed in the 1980s. There are two versions of the program, one for elementary school families and one for parents and students aged 10–14 years of age (Kumpfer & Tait, 2000). There are three components to include parent training, child training, and family skills training. All components have trainer's manuals. The parents meet for an hour and the children meet separately for the first hour. In the second hour, families meet together. Parents learn developmental expectancies and stress management, how to reward children's behavior, setting goals, making positive statements to children, communication strategies, problem solving, and limit setting. Children learn social skills, communication skills, problem solving, and coping skills. Families practice the various skills through playing games. Implementing the program in schools increased involvement of teachers and improved parent–teacher communication. Teachers and/or school-based mental health professionals can deliver this program with 2 days of training possibly after the school day.

A 5-year quasi-experimental study of the SFP with high-risk families, using four different age versions of the program, determined that all outcome variables were statistically significant, except for reductions in criminal behavior and hyperactivity in 10–16 year olds (Kumpfer, Whiteside, Greene, & Allen, 2010). The largest effect sizes were for improvements in family communication, organization, resilience, and positive parenting in the 6–11 year version. Parent substance use was reduced to the greatest degree in the 12–16 year version.

Since 2003, the SFP has been adapted for African American families, Hispanic families, Asian families, Pacific Islander families, and for Native American families. It has been used in 17 countries. Although some argue that family interventions should be a strong component of prevention programs if they are going to be comprehensive, there is still much more to do to make family interventions appropriate for various cultural or ethnic groups. Because of limited research, whether adapting preventive programs for families is more effective than implementing original programming remains unresolved (Kumpfer, Alvarado, Smith, & Bellamy, 2002). Five studies have been completed to compare the effectiveness of the generic version of the SFP compared to culturally adapted versions for African American, Hispanic, Asian/Pacific Islander, and American Indian families. The data indicated that cultural adaptations reducing dosage or disturbing critical core content increased retention of parents in program. In fact, retention was increased by 40 %. The unfortunate downside was that positive outcomes were reduced when the core components of proven programs were not implemented as they were designed. The research on the SFP has demonstrated this fact clearly.

Prevention in Action Challenge: Complete a Progress Checklist Evaluating Family–School Partnerships

Use one of the parent involvement checklists available online to determine how well a school or school district you know well is doing in this regard, or use the checklist below (see: *A checklist for schools making your Family–School Partnership work* found at http://titleone.dpi.wi.gov/files/titleone/pdf/checklist-for-schools.pdf).

Indicator	Yes	In process	No
There is a written parent involvement policy updated periodically			
Parenting skills are promoted			
Parents are assisted in monitoring their child's progress			
Parents are encouraged to work with teachers to improve their child's achievement			
Parents are provided training in parenting			
The school evaluates barriers to participation by parents of diverse backgrounds			
The school provides resources for parents in languages the parents can understand			
There are efforts to educate parents about shared responsibility for their child's learning			
Parents have reasonable access to teachers and support personnel			
Parents have access to materials (loaned) needed to help their children			
School professionals have some training in communicating with and engaging parents			
Information is sent routinely to parents about programs, meetings, and activities in a format and language that parents can understand			
Parents are encouraged to be actively engaged in their child's education at schools and at home			
Parents serve on committees in this school			
Family learning workshops are held periodically			
There is a family resource center available			
Families are invited to participate in school activities			
Direct communication with parents (face-to-face, telephone) is a goal			

Chapter 5
Organizational/Systems Change

The move toward population-focused mental health work in schools requires a very difficult paradigmatic change involving systems (Weist, 2003b). Systems change demands challenging shifts in thinking and changes in how things are done in schools (Schrag, 1996). The key components of systems change require a shared vision, strong leadership, structure in the form of a team, and commitment of stakeholders. It requires support for integrating changes into the general fabric of the school or district and funding that is steady. It is critical to appreciate that systems change takes time. A consensus is that systems change takes *3–5 years* (Schrag, 1996, p. 494). Change is messy. "Change is about adaptation and resiliency" (Glor, 2007, p. 2). The capacity of a system (a school) to change, and also to maintain itself, is one indicator that the system is "fit." Fit systems are complex and the various components interact with one another. As components interact, change can emerge.

Organizational change is necessary in a healthy system and involves people working together to make change work (Knoff, 1996). An organizational team can work to facilitate the process of change. In order for schools to integrate evidence-based practices into schools, for example, there must be considerable change at the organizational level as well as at the individual level (Austin & Claassen, 2008). In order for schools to move from reactive to proactive, or to embrace a preventive mental health practices model, change is needed.

School culture is constructed as adults in the school interact with others, including personnel within the school and those in the community (Hinde, 2004). Culture has to do with meanings (assumptions, values, beliefs, stories, and symbols) that are shared throughout the organization (Austin & Claassen, 2008). School administrators and school teams must make both ideological and cultural changes. Homogenous cultures may have better success when changes are attempted, or on the other hand, a homogenous culture may interfere and block attempted change more easily than a disparate school culture. Organizational factors have to do with how much change is needed and the structures that may facilitate or block attempts to change.

The ways in which schools are governed affect the school culture. Schools are managed within a hierarchy (Hinde, 2004). The most potent barrier to change has to

G.L. Macklem, *Preventive Mental Health at School: Evidence-Based Services for Students*, DOI 10.1007/978-1-4614-8609-1_5, © Springer Science+Business Media New York 2014

do with power relationships in a school. The culture of the school can be positive, problematic, or even toxic. In order for school change to be successful, it must take the culture of the particular school into consideration. A number of assumptions underlie school culture including the expectations staff members have for children's behavior, the process of decision-making in the school, the roles and responsibilities of various staff members, the structure of the school, the typical practices of individuals within the school, and professionals' attitudes toward change. Assumptions need to be understood and analyzed to determine whether or not change will be embraced or resisted.

Factors that affect organizational culture include how consistent the points of view of the staff may be, the views of subcultures within the school, and whether or not the practices of the organization are consistent. In order to make cultural changes, school systems must appreciate that practitioners need time to conduct the research needed to determine what changes they may want and need guidance in regard to making decisions based on large volumes of information. A good deal of what we know about organization change comes from the business world. Whether or not a change can be sustained depends upon:

- Whether or not the change is better than what was done previously
- How consistent the change may be with what was done before
- Whether the change is simple or complex
- Whether or not the change can be implemented in concrete and clear steps
- Whether or not the change has an immediate effect versus effects over time (Austin & Claassen, 2008, p. 331)

It is the individuals within organizations who manage systems change. These change leaders may be different in terms of their self-competence and may react differently to change. If change is to be successful, members of the school staff must be ready for change. It is important to consider to what degree those who will be affected by a change understand the change, and whether or not the new procedures may be easy to put in place. Opinion leaders in an organization are very important. Others respect these individuals in the organization. Some are considered experts and others simply relate well to others and are trusted. If they embrace change, they are critical resources.

O'Connor and Freeman (2012) described several stages of change. These include building consensus among stakeholders, developing structures to support the change, and sustainability. In the case of response to intervention (RtI), a three-tiered model growing in popularity in schools, a significant amount of supports are necessary for success. Professional development is needed. District support is also needed particularly around resources, measurement procedures, and how to use the data. These variables each affect culture and beliefs, which may need to change. Strong leadership is a critical variable.

Top-Down Versus Bottom-Up Change

School reform efforts require changes that are extremely hard to achieve. Top-down federal and state mandates have increased the accountability of schools. However, top-down change tends to be cosmetic (Knoff & Curtis, 1996). Changes in education are often fleeting. This occurs when the focus is on the next new idea rather than on the system itself. Educational fads are both familiar and frustrating to school staff. In order for change to last, there must be ongoing support, skills development, and attitude changes.

Top-down change conflicts with local control and is considered a less desirable approach for organizational change (Grimes & Tilly, 1996). In bottom-up change, staff members are more likely to be actively engaged and may be able to generate support at all levels of the school. When change comes from within schools, staff members who implement the new practices "own" the change (Fullan, 1996). When new practices are tried out and deemed valuable, policy changes can follow. When policy changes are made first, they do not typically engender support. If a model for change is part of the change process, staff members must understand how activities and services fit together.

Also to be considered is the fact that local control of students' education and health service priorities are strongly influenced by changes in leadership. Leadership changes can decrease the likelihood of a good preventive program being sustained as new ideas come into favor affecting programs previously in place (Weist, 2003a). Change is experienced as difficult both by individuals in schools and also by the system itself. Change creates discomfort. Change challenges beliefs and past practice. Change can create discord among staff and systems within and around a school. Change can raise opposition and barriers. When change is top-down, those affected may raise strong concerns around government control versus local control and local rights. Top-down mandates can be interpreted as too complex to implement or as too vague to be understood and implemented. Staff members in a school may feel that mandates sacrifice excellence (Ysseldyke & Geenen, 1996). Change is never a straight road; it is nonlinear. When change is mandated, the risk is that it will be superficial. Change needs to take place at the ground level, at the individual school, or at the school system level (Fullan, 1996). Staff members working together can create a vision and can take action to make changes.

Change Agents

When comprehensive mental health programming is the goal, a strong and active leader is needed to jump-start system organizational change (Grimes & Tilly, 1996, p. 469). The ability to be a *change agent* takes place in relation to others in a system (Fullan, 1996). Change in schools requires enormous energy to get started but once a critical point is reached, the process is easier. Change agents must be involved in implementation and measure change in comparison to where the school was before the work was implemented, using that state of affairs as the baseline. Communication of both successes and problems is critical. Change agents must not criticize past practices or get rid of them too quickly.

A change agent must have effective skills in communication that are not judgmental and do not change the power structure among members of the school community. Major stakeholders must work together in an atmosphere of mutual respect and trust (Curtis & Stollar, 1996). Both problem solving and planning with attention to "people" and relationships are necessary.

Champions or change agents can be extremely effective in motivating others, in adopting new roles, in offering good ideas, and in recommending practices. All of these variables take place during the first phases of implementation of a prevention program (Hendy & Barlow, 2012). At the early stages of implementation of a preventive program, change is centered within a small group. Once the process involves the whole system, change will be more successful if the change process is lead by a team. Practically, it is critical for a school team to conduct in-depth interviews with those who will be the recipients of preventive interventions (Montano & Kasprzyk, 2008). Only in this way can practitioners determine the outcomes, barriers, and facilitators that are relevant to stakeholders. Underlying beliefs must be understood in order to predict attitudes, uncover perceived norms, determine participants' self-efficacy, and predict whether or not the change will take place.

One of the change agent's roles is to keep the process from stopping by recognizing difficulties and preventing them from interfering with the change process (Van de Ven & Sun, 2011). To increase trust between change agents and those affected by change, change agents need to share and discuss issues. Resistance to change is a result of interactions between change agents and those affected. Some change agents manage resistance better than others depending on how they interpret behaviors. Resistance is a *socially constructed reality* that depends on perceptions and points of view (Ijaz & Vitalis, 2011). Change agents who see themselves as coaches or "champions" have more success in helping perspective participants in the change process move toward acceptance (Bouckenooghe, 2010).

Readiness for Change

Research into organizational change has involved examining the effects of change and the process of change over time (Bouckenooghe, 2010). Readiness to change has to do with motivation to change (Cohen, Beliner, & Mannarino, 2010). Readiness or openness to change involves the degree to which those who will be affected by change believe in the need for change and believe that the proposed changes will be positive for them and for the whole system. Attitudes toward change are fostered by the work environment, the process of change itself, and the proposed type of change. Attitudes toward change develop as people try to make sense of the change. This is a form of "collective sense-making" (Cohen et al., 2010, p. 519).

Individuals in a system who are open to change will support the change and believe it will work (Bouckenooghe, 2010). A goal for change agents is to build a strong collective readiness to make the changes desired. Readiness for change involves not only beliefs about the need to change but also the belief that the school system can make the changes successfully. Unfortunately, assessment is often skipped when organizational change is attempted (Austin & Claassen, 2008). When school change is planned, it is very important to *measure* readiness for change because readiness precedes changes in behavior.

The scientific basis of the idea of organizational readiness for change as compared to individual change is limited (Weiner, 2009). Readiness for change has to do with commitment to implement a preventive program and belief that the program will make a difference or "change efficacy." Implementation is often a "team sport" according to Weiner. Organizational readiness is promoted when the change is valued. The task demands must be reasonable and resources available. Time is needed to put the change in place and there must be support for the change. Additional considerations affecting readiness involve how flexibly the change can be managed, whether or not the change conflicts with the organizational culture, and whether or not past practice with changes were positive. It may be helpful to communicate and promote a positive view around resources, task demands, and situational factors. It may be helpful to create a feeling of urgency in some situations and involve stakeholders both in the design of the change and also in implementation planning. Visits to other sites may be helpful to help staff members see that change can make a difference. These activities can move a school toward acceptance of the process.

In school change efforts, the critical factors include organizational readiness, support for staff training, a plan for monitoring change, supervision, and staff support. When these are in place, the new program can become an excepted component of the general/overall school program (Hoagwood & Johnson, 2003).

Importance of Theory in Implementing Preventive Programs in Schools

Darnton (2008) prepared a guide listing social–psychological models along with theories of behavior change. Models assume that behavior is based on "intention" and the outcomes that the individual expects. Attitudes are influenced by beliefs and values. Social norms have to do with the perception of what others think one should do or not do. "Agency," or the sense that one can successfully change, makes a difference. Models show what can influence behavior, but models do not explain how to change behavior.

Theories of change explain the process of change. Theories explain why someone acts (Darnton, 2008). Theories of change include why change occurs at all, stages of change, learning-based models, organizational learning models, systems thinking models, and diffusion models showing how behavior spreads in a network. Peirson, Boydell, Ferguson, and Ferris (2011) describe systems change as a process of transformation (p. 308). This transformation affects a system's structure, function, and culture. Change can be thought of as a series of evolving strategies instead of steps in a straight line. Shared beliefs must become shared action and shared responsibility. "Systems thinking" can be very useful when applied to complex behavior.

A theory of change is a tool. Theory guides program designers, researchers, and practitioners when developing preventive interventions to prevent, diminish, or resolve social problems of students or schools (Harris, 2005). Theory can be thought of as a way to think about values, points of view, and the underlying assumptions about why change would occur or why change would be the result of the preventive effort (Vogel, 2012). Theory provides the framework for the change process. A theory of change can strengthen the focus of a preventive program and provide the framework for decision-making. It makes all of these more explicit. A theory of change supports critical thinking (Vogel, 2012, p. 4). Darnton (2008) described 60 social–psychological models and theories of behavior change. However, not all models fit health behaviors of students or are relevant for schools.

Before examining the several relevant models for school change, it is helpful to understand why theory is important in the first place. Theory helps identify the *active ingredients* of a program by comparing findings from a set of studies. When theory is not used, it is very hard to generalize results from one study to different groups, settings, and times (Glanz & Rimer, 2008, p. 150). Interventions using theories are more successful. In fact, five of seven meta-analyses comparing studies found that theory-based interventions were from somewhat to clearly better than interventions not based on theory.

Glanz and Rimer (2008) cite a meta-analysis of hundreds of studies focused on a particular behavior. They wanted to determine common theoretical constructs positively affected by interventions. Several of the constructs that were common included perceived barriers, perceive risk, self-efficacy, and readiness to change. In actual practice, it is not unusual for prevention program developers to combine theories. Theories help school teams determine "how" the intervention works. There is not a great deal of evidence to suggest that one theory is better than another. Because there is no definitive data to say that one theory is best, practitioners need to choose theories based on how well a particular theory fits the behavior the school wants to change.

If prevention programs are going to be sustained, the programs must be effective when implemented. They must work consistently. The theory of change of the program must be convincing (Burns, 2011). Theory is also important because it gives meaning to the outcomes. The structure of a theory helps a school team know what to do when there are problems. Change theory also helps practitioners adapt programs to fit settings without losing effectiveness.

Rimer and Glanz (2005) described a number of influential theories of health-related behaviors. The theories they described are used widely. Using theory for program planning, development, and intervention helps practitioners bring evidence-based interventions to school populations. Theory helps explain why people engage in risky or healthy behaviors; it explains how to design strategies to change behaviors that cause problems. Theory explains how to measure change. Theory tells us why problem behaviors occur.

Change theory can tell us what to work on, where to spend time and energy, and how to measure change that occurs (Darnton, 2008). The process of making change in a school involves a number of steps. The school team first identifies the population and the behavior to change. Next, the team makes a short list of factors influencing the behavior. Then the team identifies the *relevant change models* (which can be accomplished easily by contacting the developers of the programs).

Objectives are written. Intervention techniques that have worked in the past are located. The team analyzes the participants' perceptions and engages them perhaps using focus groups. The program is piloted. The pilot is evaluated. The preventive intervention or program is implemented. Feedback and data is collected along the way and after the program has been implemented.

To help select a change theory, Darnton (2008) provides tables to help match behaviors that a school may want to change to various models. For example, if the goal is giving up drug use such as smoking, this behavior fits with Prochaska and DiClemente's Transtheoretical Model (1983) to be discussed, whereas eating vegetables, use of condoms, and increasing exercise fit better with the Theory of Planned Behavior (Ajzen, 1991).

Choosing a theory begins with a detailed analysis of the problem including the cultural background and life experiences of the students who will be affected by the change (Rimer & Glanz, 2005). There are differences in rates of mental health problems to consider as well as differences in prevalence of risk behaviors and determinants of behaviors for students and families of different races and ethnic backgrounds. Theory helps practitioners ask the right questions and zero in on what is causing a problem.

French et al. (2012) suggest four steps to develop a theory-informed preventive intervention:

- Step 1 identifies the behavior and the players. This step helps identify the behavior change needed.
- Step 2 requires a literature search to *choose the theory* or theoretical framework likely to help the team move ahead. Barriers and enablers need to be identified and measured.
- Step 3 requires determining which program will allow a team to manage the barriers and also what might facilitate change. This involves which components will be delivered and how each activity or technique must be delivered. The team must determine what is feasible for the particular school.
- The final Step 4 has to do with measurement. The school team must ask what outcome measures will be measured.

Successful prevention efforts require behavior change, but changing behavior is complicated and involves many variables interacting with one another (Michie & Johnston, 2012). Currently, effective change strategies are underused and practitioners don't always know how they work. To increase the effectiveness of behavior change, it is important that behavior change strategies (also known as active ingredients) be clearly communicated and *linked to theory*. Behavior itself must be precisely defined because a specific theory may be more successful in predicting some behaviors more than others. Behavioral change techniques are the components that match the active ingredients of the prevention program or the proposed mechanism of change. Theories delineate the constructs, relationships, and the scientific explanations of *how change occurs*. Theories describe the how, the when, and the why change occurs. They are "fundamental." Active ingredients must be linked to the theory explaining why behavior changes.

In reviews of hundreds of implementation studies, it was not typical to find that theories of behavior change were actually used (Cane, O'Connor, & Michie, 2012).

Yet, there is fairly strong evidence that preventive interventions built on behavior change theory will be successful (Beckman, Hawley, & Bishop, 2006). In prevention work around obesity, strategies that affect nutrition and physical activity work better than information-based programs. In a pilot program with 11- and 12-year-old children and their families, researchers identified behavior change techniques such as goal-setting, increasing self-efficacy, and readiness for change. They demonstrated that theory-based health behavior change techniques could be applied to obesity prevention.

It is important to understand that one theory is seldom sufficient to explain most health behavior concerns (Brewer & Rimer, 2008). Theories of change have a lot in common but they differ in scope. Some theories come from disease prevention, and some are easier to use than others. Theories of change are not perfect. Fullan (2006) pointed out that most change theories do not emphasize capacity building. Capacity building has to do with strategies that increase the effectiveness of all members of an organization to get involved. Without an investment in capacity building, a preventive effort may fall short and not get the hoped-for results.

The benefit to using theory appears to be understated, as those researchers who suggest they do not use theories may actually have used theories without being aware of having done so (Brewer & Rimer, 2008). There are several theories that are used frequently for planned changes in schools, and it may be helpful to examine the theories of change that are most frequently used in health promotion. Of the many theories of change, those written about most frequently include The Health Belief Model (HBM; Rosenstock, 1966), The Theory of Reasoned Action (TRA; Fishbein & Ajzen, 1975), The Theory of Planned Behavior (TPB; Ajzen, 1991), Social Cognitive Theory (SCT; Bandura, 1988; Miller & Dollard, 1941), and the Transtheoretical Model (TTM; Prochaska & DiClemente, 1983).

The Health Belief Model

The HBM has a long history. It was developed by social psychologists working in public health to explain why people did not participate in a screening program designed to identify tuberculosis. Today it is used to identify which beliefs need to be changed to help an individual develop positive behaviors (Carpenter, 2010). There are four components of the model (Redding, Rossi, Rossi, Velicer, & Prochaska, 2000). Perceived susceptibility explains that a person will avoid negative behavior if he or she feels susceptible to a disorder or problem. Perceived severity asks how serious is the person's perception of consequences of his/her behavior. Perceived effectiveness or benefit has to do with motivation. This will depend on whether or not the person believes that there is a link between the behavior and consequences and if taking action will reduce risk. Perceived cost or perceived barriers have to do with how much work will be involved. Self-efficacy, or a person's confidence in his/her ability to take action and succeed, is a complicating factor recognized by those who support this theory.

One problem with the theory is that it doesn't explain how these beliefs affect one another alone or in combination. There have been a number of studies that have gathered empirical support for predicting behaviors such as exercise and safe sex behaviors (Baban & Craciun, 2007; Brewer & Rimer, 2008). These studies suggest that beliefs can motivate behavior. Yet, the HBM does not address social, interpersonal, and contextual concerns. Carpenter (2010) conducted a meta-analysis of 18 studies involving 2,702 people to determine how effective this theory might be. Benefits and barriers were the best predictors of behavior, but other variables were not very strong. Carpenter questioned continued use of the model.

Theory of Reasoned Action

The Theory of Reasoned Action takes a social–behavioral approach (Redding et al., 2000). The goal of this theory is to predict behavior. It suggests that a person's *intention* to perform a behavior is related to whether or not the person will actually engage in the behavior. Intention depends on norms, attitudes, and self-efficacy. This theory suggests that people behave because they choose to do so based on rational decision-making. The more a person wants to do something, the more likely that the person will do it (Baban & Craciun, 2007). Significant others can influence behavior when the social norm is to conform to the opinions of others who are important to the individual.

Theory of Planned Behavior

The Theory of Planned Behavior is an expansion of previous theories. It addresses a person's perceived control of behavior and suggests that risky behavior could be changed if one changed one's beliefs (Baban & Craciun, 2007). Perceived behavioral control is the perception about the degree to which action in regard to a risky behavior is easy or difficult. A person is more likely to do what he or she has some degree of control over, and this in turn has to do with one's skills, abilities, emotions, and also the opportunities one has to change behavior. Attitudes, intentions, and behaviors are linked, and this makes preventive interventions easier. Changing attitudes, perceived control, or norms could in turn change a person's intentions. There are two types of beliefs: normative, which affect subjective norms; and behavioral, which influence attitudes (Redding et al., 2000). Unfortunately, the correlation between behavior and intention is not very strong.

The Theory of Planned Behavior includes aspects of intention, i.e., behavioral willingness and implementation intention (Brewer & Rimer, 2008). Implementation intention specifies exactly when and under what conditions people will act. This has a strong influence on behavior. The intention–behavior relationship is not thought to be as strong as it has been considered in the past, particularly in regard to risky behaviors in social interactions, behaviors that are deeply habitual, and when intentions are not closely tied to action. Attitudes can affect behavior, but many beliefs and attitudes can be changed when targeted by preventive interventions. This theory is supported by laboratory and field studies as well as interventions to change health behaviors.

Social Cognitive Theory

Social learning theory morphed into the SCT when it became associated with health behavior (Elder, Ayala, & Harris, 1999). SCT stresses the interaction between cognition and behavior through the expectancy that something good will happen as a result of engaging in a particular behavior. Redding et al. (2000) indicate that this theory is a comprehensive clinical approach to behavior change. In SCT, a key concept is an interactive relationship between behavior, the individual, and the environment. Environmental situations, or context, can help or interfere with behavior. Past experience can also influence behavior. Modeling is an important strategy associated with this theory as are developing coping skills.

Self-efficacy and outcome expectancies are central in this theory (Baban & Craciun, 2007; Redding et al., 2000). Self-efficacy influences feelings, thoughts, and behaviors and is very important in the behavior change process. Strong self-efficacy is tied to good health. Poor self-efficacy is associated with internalizing symptoms. Action–outcome expectancies relate to the idea that actions lead to results. Two of the strategies associated with this theory are mastering skills and engaging in behavioral rehearsal. There is some data to indicate that SCT explains a small to medium amount of variance in a person's behavior. Self-efficacy is a better predictor of behavior change than other factors in weight control, resistance to drug use, and preventing unprotected sexual activity. Self-efficacy is also stronger than past performance in influencing behavior.

The Transtheoretical Model

The TTM is a multistage model as compared to the models already described, which are considered continuum theories. Stage models move people along a continuum toward health or toward learning a new behavior (Baban & Craciun, 2007). Because health behavior is complicated, one stage or level may not be adequate to explain behavior. In a stage theory, not only are there different influences at each stage, but the barriers may be different at each stage. The idea of a stage theory is that interventions can be designed to match the stage in which the person is functioning, by addressing the barriers appearing at that stage. The TTM comprises five stages:

- Precontemplation (no intention to change)
- Contemplation (beginning to consider change, but no action yet)
- Preparation (ready to change behavior and preparing or planning to act in the immediate future)
- Action (initial steps to engage in the new behavior, risk of relapse is high)
- Maintenance (behavior change has been reached but there may be relapses although the risk is lower) (Baban & Craciun, 2007, p. 54; Elder, Ayala, & Harris, 1999; Redding et al., 2000)

Elder, Ayala, and Harris break down the precontemplation stage into three phases. "Unaware" is the first phase in which the individual has no idea that his or her behavior is problematic or risky. "Uninvolved" is next, in which the person knows the behavior needs changing but at the moment it isn't high priority. "Undecided" is the third phase. Here the person starts to consider the benefits and cost of behavior change (Elder, Ayala, & Harris, 1999, p. 281). A practitioner could determine the particular stage in which a student is functioning by determining how the student responds to suggestions for change.

The TTM appreciates the idea that a student can revert to an earlier stage or get stuck at a particular stage, as well as move continually forward through the five stages (Baban & Craciun, 2007). The model can be described as spiral (Redding et al., 2000). In practice, a student can be included in a preventive intervention based on the stage in which he or she is functioning at the time. Determining the stage the person is in at a particular time can reduce dropping out of a preventive intervention.

The model recommends different interventions for each stage. In the earlier stages, decisional balance, or the weight of reasons for changing or not changing, determines the decision to move out of the precontemplation stage (Redding et al., 2000). Motivational interviewing can be used as a strategy in the early stages (Elder et al., 1999). Motivational interviewing helps to move students to act on their behavior. Empathetic reflection is used as reinforcement and helps the student see the issues around his or her risky behavior. Cognitive approaches are helpful to begin the change process. In later stages behavioral-skills training would be a better fit.

Brewer and Rimer (2008) report that TTM does not seem effective for changing some behaviors and argue that the support for the model has been overstated. Norcross, Krebs, and Prochaska (2011) conducted a meta-analysis of 39 clinical studies to assess the ability of the model and to predict psychotherapy outcomes. They found a significant relationship between stage of change and outcomes. The TTM model has been used successfully to stop smoking and drug use, for stress management, increasing exercise, and changing eating habits. Most of the studies have been cross-sectional (Baban & Cracuim, 2007; Redding et al., 2000). Measures of the stages of change are similar to measures of intention (Brewer & Rimer, 2008). The need for students to move through all of the stages has not been proven. More or fewer stages may fit some students better. The model has generated considerable discussion. At the same time, the model has several advantages. Behavior change is described as a process. Tools are available for intervention development. TTM emphasizes measurement.

The Transtheoretical Model in Practice

TTM has been used with at least 48 different behaviors and has been used with individuals from many countries (Prochaska, Redding, & Evers, 2008). The most disappointing work has been in universal programs with adolescents dealing with substance abuse. Social influence models do not appear to be effective with this population for this problem. On the other hand, studies to prevent bullying at all school levels have produced strong positive results using TTM. Smoking prevention studies with adolescents have successfully used TTM.

Van Marter, Dyment, Evers, Johnson, and Prochaska (2007) evaluated the effectiveness of a bullying prevention program at the elementary level. The program was designed to increase respect and decrease involvement in bullying behaviors. The program was delivered using the Internet in 12 schools. Changes in stages of the TTM determined that the program was effective. Evers, Prochaska, Van Marter, Johnson, and Prochaska (2007) also designed an Internet intervention to address bullying in middle and high schools. The intervention was based on determining changes in stages of TTM. Researchers reported significant treatment effects.

TTM has been used in regard to prevention of obesity, which requires multiple behavior changes (Driskell, Dyment, Mauriello, Castle, & Sherman, 2008). Risks for obesity include low physical activity, avoidance of eating fruits and vegetables, and excessive television viewing time. When students completed questionnaires, high school students had the most behavioral risks for obesity. For students at all grade levels, risk for one behavior such as low physical activity increased the odds of risk for another behavior.

Mauriello, Sherman, Driskell, and Prochaska (2007) implemented a web-based, multimedia obesity prevention program for adolescents. They piloted it using TTM as a framework. The program offered individualized feedback based on a student's readiness to engage in behavior contrary to weight gain and unhealthy eating (Mauriello et al., 2006). Effectiveness trials were published in 2010. Students in eight high schools in four states were randomly assigned to no treatment or to a multimedia intervention. Data was collected on student movement to action and maintenance stages and the degree to which these changes were stable. Effects were strongest for changes in eating behaviors. Students who changed one behavior were more likely to make similar gains in a second behavior. The program therefore initiated behavior change *across* behaviors.

Evers et al. (2012) used an Internet intervention based on TTM to address drug use in middle school students. Using random assignment by schools, researchers found students reduced their use of drugs. Students were asked to indicate their intention to stop using each of a variety of substances and were assigned an overall stage of change based on the data collected. Students in the intervention group were more likely to reach the maintenance stage than control students by 3-month follow-up. Finally, Xu et al. (2011) used TTM to evaluate a program to reduce sedentary behavior in elementary and middle school children. Measuring stages of change, they determined that the intervention program decreased sedentary behavior of children on weekends.

The Most Commonly Used Theoretical Models in the Health Field

Glanz, Rimer, and Viswanath (2008) found that the theories used most often in the health field were the TTM, SCT, and the HBM models. Norcross et al. (2011) suggested the Social Ecological model was used often as well. The constructs that many theories for understanding behavior change have in common include the idea that behavior change is a *process*. Motivation is more important than intention, intention is stressed over action, and the emphasis is on changing behavior in many theories rather than maintaining change.

Different theories fit some behaviors better than others. Ramos and Perkins (2006) point out it is necessary to find out whether or not the *components* of a prevention program match the program developers' theory of change and therefore produce results. In a study of the Pennsylvania State University's Alcohol Intervention Program Level 2 (AIP2), Ramos and Perkins identified five different behavior change theories that were connected to the major components of the AIP2 program. They connected the program elements including the information taught, the skills, and the activities to the five theories of change. They recommended strategies and activities to strengthen connections between the program activities and the theories. For example, they suggested matching feedback from a readiness-to-change tool to the participants' stage of change to strengthen the connections between the activity and TTM stages of change theory.

Theories of Organizational Change

Change in organizations takes place at the individual level, team level, and organizational level (Butterfoss, Kegler, & Franciso, 2008). When change is needed system-wide, major restructuring may be needed requiring a change in organizational culture. The Stage Theory of Organizational Change suggests that organizations must pass through a series of steps as they change. Each stage requires its own accompanying strategies to negotiate the change process. Educators seldom, if ever, adopt new programs until the organization has accepted it. Similar to individual change, organizational change strategies are connected to the stage in which the organization finds itself at a given time. Organizational capacity, organizational culture, and school climate are important variables that can be stable and resistant to change.

Organizational development theory involves several steps:

- Identification of the problem(s) and the underlying causes
- Planning to develop strategic interventions to address the problem(s) based on organizational readiness to implement strategies

- Identification of barriers, problem solving, and implementation of the new program
- Progress monitoring and evaluation to determine if the new program or structure has been fully implemented and change is taking place (Butterfoss et al., 2008, p. 345)

Organizational theories can help school teams understand how to facilitate the acceptance and sustainability of an evidence-based preventive intervention in a school system. A school or school district can use organizational theory. Integrated approaches to prevention utilize resources more efficiently, increase chances that a change will be sustained over time, and eliminate duplication (Butterfoss et al., 2008).

Sternberg's Theory of Organizational Modifiability suggests that how easily an organization will change depends on the degree of desire for actual change, the desire for the appearance of change, and the perceived quality of the organizational culture. Sternberg (2002) contrasts surface-structural change in comparison to deep-structural change. Surface-level change builds on structures already in place. These changes do not affect the organizational culture. Deep-level changes require more time and energy in order to get success. They require more scaffolding for changes to work.

Diffusion of Innovations Theory

Currently there is more and more interest on the part of researchers on implementation and diffusion of programs that work. The change theories that are utilized today originated with Kurt Lewin's stage model (Lewin, 1951) which consisted of unfreezing of the ways of doing things, taking action as a result of being exposed to new ideas, and refreezing the new behavior (Butterfoss et al., 2008). Current theories are derived and built upon both Lewin's writings and Roger's Diffusion of Innovations Theory. Unfortunately, preventive programs diffuse throughout the school slowly as the rewards are not immediate (Rogers, 2002).

The Diffusion of Innovations Theory helps practitioners understand the process that is needed to implement preventive programs because even when schools have an evidence-based and effective prevention program, implementing it properly in the manner in which it was designed can remain elusive. Diffusion can be thought of as the process through which a preventive intervention is communicated among members of the school (Oldenburg & Glanz, 2008). The Diffusion of Innovations Theory was proposed by Rogers in 1976, so the theory is not new. The work of interest here has to do with health promotion and the individual and organizational changes that result in prevention. The key to whether or not a preventive intervention will be accepted in a school system or single school building is the presence of a champion and some influential early adopters. In addition the program needs to be considered important to those who will be involved or affected by the program.

The Diffusion of Innovations Theory has to do with the process through which programs become part of the general school program (Dusenbury & Hansen, 2004). The theory assumes that interventions are accepted by different staff members and spread at different rates in subgroups among school staff (Oldenburg & Glanz, 2008). The characteristics of a program that make a difference in whether or not the preventive innovation spreads throughout the whole school staff include:

- Relative advantage of the program over what exists
- How compatible or how well the innovation fits the values, norms, and needs of the school
- How easy or complex the program may be, with easier to implement programs more acceptable
- Whether or not a pilot program can be conducted
- How observable are the results (Berwick, 2003)

Ryan and Gross (1943) first described categories of individuals in a system in regard to how readily they adopt new inventions. Today, five categories of subgroups are identified in regard to how a change is adopted in an organization (Rogers, 2003). These categories are descriptive. They are not useful for making predictions or explaining the success or failure of new programs. These so called "adopter" categories can refer to a single person's network or can apply to an entire social system (Valente, 1996). They are helpful in appreciating the importance of people in a system. They are also helpful in appreciating the time it takes to work toward acceptance of a preventive program in a school. The five categories label groups as innovators, early adopters, early majority adopters, later majority adopters, and laggards.

Because individuals adopt new programs over time, they can be classified into categories based on their innovativeness (Rogers, 2003). The innovators are the first group, which theoretically would make up 2.5 % of the population of teachers implementing a new program. Innovators are interested in new ideas they can understand and apply complex knowledge and can cope with uncertainty. Innovators may not be respected in an organization, however. The early adopters would make up 13.5 % of the total population. This group is respected by others in an organization and has high "opinion" leadership. Change agents look for the early adopters because this group can trigger a critical mass when they buy-in to innovative programming.

The members of the early majority make up 34 % of the membership of an organization (Rogers, 2003). Although it may take more time for them to buy-in, they are important. This group provides the interconnectedness between the various subgroups in a school. They tend to have more formal education than late adopters. They are more empathetic, more scientific, more rational, and are better connected. They have higher aspirations. The late majority group comprises 34 % of teachers. They buy-in because of peer pressure. They are more skeptical and wait until the culture of the organization seems to accept the new program before they feel "okay" about it. They wait until any uncertainty left is gone before buying-in.

The laggards would comprise 16 % of the school community and are suspicious of change (Rogers, 2003). They need to be sure that the preventive effort will not dissolve when the change agent leaves, or fail completely. Understanding this model helps innovators and the early adopters from getting discouraged when attempting change.

The Diffusion of Innovations Theory has been recommended for use in prevention of abuse of alcohol, tobacco, and drugs. *Smart Choices,* a school-based tobacco prevention program (Brink et al., 1995; Parcel, 1995), is based on Social Cognitive Theory and Diffusion of Innovations Theory. Sharma and Kanekar (2008) feel that overall the Diffusion of Innovations Theory is a robust theory. It certainly helps those who want to change schools appreciate how long it may take to effect change and why they may meet resistance.

Resistance to Change

Ford and Ford (2010) claim that more than half of the efforts to change systems do not succeed. In fact, 70 % of all efforts to change organizations fail (Van de Ven & Sun, 2011). The common explanation for failure is staff resistance. Resistance is described as not buying-in, as stonewalling efforts, or as pushback when change is attempted. When school administrators label school staffs' behavior as resistant because they don't want to fail, resistance to change may appear to them an acceptable explanation of difficulties implementing change.

Schools prefer stability to change because stability allows them to be efficient. However, forces external to schools such as laws and regulations, technology, and the economy demand change. Coercion and manipulation to make teachers change is likely to backfire. Administrative processes, poor performance such as an increased school dropout rate, or a sudden increase in drug use among students can trigger change. School change can trigger a number of reactions. There may be initial denial that a problem exists, there may be resistance, or there may be gradual exploration and hopefully buy-in (Bovey & Hede, 2001). Resistance is a normal reaction to proposed change. The ability to handle resistance is the most critical skill required for school leaders attempting change. Whether or not resistance will rear its head depends on the amount of impact the change has on *individual* adults in the school system. School change can generate strong negative feelings when those affected experience loss attributed to change in the ways in which they have been doing their job.

Change does not mean the same thing to everyone involved. Some teachers and mental health staff members may look at school change as dictatorial while others see it as innovative (Margolis & Nagel, 2006). Unfortunately teachers are often blamed when there is resistance to change rather than determining why they appear resistant or investigating what might make it easier for them to accept and implement changes. Teachers may feel ignored when change is top-down. Teachers may feel that those demanding change do not understand the constraints with which teachers must cope on a daily basis. It is important for change agents to observe and attend to problems as teachers see them. Teachers need prevention efforts that are powerful and of high quality. Preventive interventions must match their students and be easy to implement. Teachers need training and professional development that demonstrates new ways of teaching in concrete steps. They need all materials provided so they don't need to create them. They need experiences that model techniques and demonstrate the program's value. Teachers need opportunities to use and practice skills. It is important for change agents and coaches to listen to teachers respectfully and give credit for effort. Offering choices helps teachers accept change, so it is important that new programs are flexible. School change that ignores the value of teachers as controllers of opinion in a school will run into trouble (Forman, Olin, Hoagwood, Crowe, & Saka, 2009). When a critical mass of school staff feel disheartened, a negative morale can emerge (Margolis & Nagel, 2006, p. 155). Teachers need to hear that change agents appreciate how difficult their work is on a daily basis. Teachers are central in universal prevention efforts (Schaeffer et al., 2005).

An increasing number of schools are implementing school-wide positive behavior support (SWPBIS; Sugai & Horner, 2006). In order to understand some of the problems involved in implementing SWPBIS and in particular to determine why there may be resistance to the changes imposed by this model, researchers interviewed 14 technical assistance providers from 10 states. All of those interviewed faced resistance in their attempts to support universal implementation of SWPBIS. The barriers this group encountered included lack of administrative leadership, skepticism regarding need, hopelessness around the change, philosophical differences, and feeling disenfranchised (Lohrmann, Forman, Martin, & Palmieri, 2008, p. 262). Among the strategies the technical assistants used to counter resistance included building a case for change, use of a buy-in vote, helping school staff see that change was possible, looking for common ground, and helping members of the school staff become part of the process. For SWPBIS in particular, teachers needed to believe that they were actually responsible for changing student behavior. They needed to understand that it was part of their job and was their responsibility. Teachers also needed to feel safe and not too stressed.

Emotional resistance is contagious and may threaten leaders in a school attempting change. Emotional conflict may relate to previous change attempts rather than the current effort and this must be resolved for change to progress. Resistance is a product of the relationship between change agents and those affected by change.

Interestingly, studies suggest that when asked about behavior that appeared resistant, individuals did not interpret their behavior as undermining (Ford, Ford, & D'Amelio, 2008). If barriers can be identified, it is more likely that the change process can proceed more smoothly (Landaeta, Mun, & Rabadi, 2008). Researchers recommend that change agents investigate the *reasons for resistance* so that they can try to implement strategies that fit the problem (Lohrmann et al., 2008) (Table 5.1).

The Positive Side to Resistance

Huang and Huang (2009) suggest that the idea of resistance to change itself should be challenged. Resistance to change can play a positive or a negative role (Van de Ven & Sun, 2011). On the positive side, resistance can increase awareness and can focus school professionals on the school's stated purpose or mission. Resistance can

Table 5.1 Possible causes of resistance to systems change in schools

Lack of a clear vision	Embedded routines in conflict with changes
Refusal to accept practices that are not wanted or are not expected	Lack of teamwork
Perpetuation of old practices	Discomfort with the change process
Assumptions not reorganized or ignored	Overutilization of some members of the staff and/or resources needed for other priorities
Communication barriers (information distortion, blocked flow of information)	Pessimism around whether or not the change effort will succeed
Costs that are too high	Lack of knowledge, skills, abilities, resources, norms, tools, or processes necessary to implement the change
Too much loss	Requirement for tedious work
Lack of motivation for change because of different interests or beliefs and values	Change seen as incompatible with the instructional content
Too many changes so staff members feel overwhelmed	Lack of time to make the change
Reactive mind-sets	Lack of belief that change will make a difference
Lack of administrative support	Loss of status
Power structure changes	Concerns about loss of pay
Disagreements around the problem or the solutions	Loss of cultural comfort
Lack of belief that the organization is capable of making effective changes	Expected results not forthcoming
Expectations not met	Return on investments is not acceptable
Role incompatibility	Past experiences of change were negative
Staff believe there is no need for change	The need for change is not clear
Lack of belief that goals can be achieved	Goals are not agreed upon
Lack of confidence in change leaders	Perception of role incompatibility
School changes occur so frequently that acceptance of change is undermined	Too many competing priorities
Lack of belief that change will positively effect student learning	Staff turnover
Staff lack skills to effect change	Lack of flexibility of change leaders
Loss of perceived fairness	Lack of belief that change will help diverse students
Loss of trust	Loss of a psychosocial factor
	Loss of a comfortable organizational structure
	No incentive for change

Sources: Forman et al. (2009), Glover and Dent (2005), Jansen (2000), Landaeta et al. (2008, pp. 77–854), Lohrmann et al. (2008), Margolis and Nagel (2006), Van de Ven and Sun (2011), and Yue (2008)

build participation, help the organization learn from past errors, generate improvements in the change plan, and result in change. Resistance can actually help the change process by bringing some energy into the discussion.

Avey, Wernsing, and Luthans (2008) surveyed 132 employees from a number of different organizations with different jobs. They found the positive resources of workers could combat negative reactions. Instead of talking about resistance, it may be helpful to consider behavior in response to change such as an attempt to make sense of the change. One way to deal with behavior that appears resistant is to ask about it directly. Studies suggest that when asked about behavior that appeared resistant, individuals did not interpret their behavior as undermining the effort (Ford et al., 2008).

Resistance can be thought of as a necessary and positive energy. Instead of blaming resistance, resistance can be thought of as a type of feedback that can provide information to those attempting change. Another way to think about resistance is that it could simply be a "stage in the process" of change (Ford & Ford, 2010). There is a social aspect to change as participants talk with each other and determine how they will understand and think about the change as a group (Jansen, 2000). Resistance needs to be appreciated as part of the process. Complaints, questions, criticisms, and objections can make people more aware of, and more knowledgeable about, the change. These behaviors can encourage discussion, keeping everyone talking and engaged. They can keep the ideas alive. They can facilitate discussion about why change is needed.

Resistance is better than apathy (Van de Ven & Sun, 2011). Those trying to make changes in schools need to consider resistance as something to be used. Resistance points out problems that need to be addressed. The first step to changing schools is to identify the weakest constraint or barrier, and change it, so it is more effective. Then, move to the next weakest barrier as the process of change spreads throughout the organization or system. The factors that overcome resistance to change include educating staff and communicating with school staff *around data*. It may also be possible to develop psychological capital through training interventions (Avey et al., 2008). Providing more support for change, inviting staff into the decision-making process, increasing communication, and negotiating directly with those who appear to be resistant will help decrease perceived resistance.

Gatekeepers of change must be identified, such as the principal or the most influential teachers. These individuals must be committed to the proposed changes. In addition, if all stakeholders are not involved, meaningful change will not occur (Curtis & Stollar, 1996). Teachers, parents, support staff, and students need to be involved. When changes are made, adult learners need practice, coaching, and ongoing mentoring feedback if they are going to actually use the skills on which they are trained through professional development activities (Fullan, 1996). When members of the organization can participate in the change, their points of view are accepted, and they feel that can influence the change. They are more likely to react positively to change (Kykyri, Puutio, & Wahlstrom, 2010). Involvement and feelings of ownership make a huge positive difference when change is attempted.

Planned Change

Planned change involves setting goals, implementing the change, evaluating the changes made, and making modifications as needed (Van de Ven & Sun, 2011). Breakdowns can occur when there are multiple changes going on in a system at the same time. Careful planning allows the school to respond to issues or concerns. When

Table 5.2 Questions for discussion with school professionals

1. Which students or families are we targeting and why?
2. Who are the groups that influence a change in students' behavior?
3. What are the most important long-term changes we want?
4. What is our vision for change as a school/district?
5. Who and what needs to change in order to reach our goals, including communities, families, school schedules, and school policy?
6. What specific changes need to take place in these groups?
7. What are our core beliefs about how we can make these changes happen? What are our assumptions?
8. What are the risks that might prevent change? What are the barriers we need to address? Does any group need protection?
9. How will we know if change has occurred? How will we measure the effects of the program? How will we communicate what we have learned?

Adapted from Vogel (2012, pp. 26, 27)

change is contemplated, the stakeholders addressing it need to thoroughly analyze the unique needs and characteristics of the particular school. This includes the school's strengths and resources as well as the negative problems the staff members want to address (Curtis & Stollar, 1996). Strategies that help school staff become more accepting of the changes include conducting workshops, bringing in or providing technical assistance, and staff training (Oldenburg & Glanz, 2008). In planning for change it is helpful for a group of colleagues to have something with which to save time. Time is important in school settings. Communication exchange rather than persuasion or edict works better. When everyone is engaged in a group discussion, differing views can be communicated and differences resolved (Table 5.2).

Prevention in Action Challenge: Four Challenges

1. Think of change that has occurred in a school you know well. Was this a top-down change or a bottom-up change? How well did it go? What difficulties were encountered? How were they resolved?
2. Examine the various *readiness-for-change* tools that are available and determine which tool may be most useful for a school system that may be contemplating change. (For example see: http://sisep.fpg.unc.edu/, http://www.wmbridges.com/, http://www.watsonwyatt.com/, http://teamstepps.ahrq.gov/, and many others online.)
3. Review the various theories of change and determine which theories might fit the following behaviors:

    (a) Giving up smoking or drug use
    (b) Increasing activity to combat depression
    (c) Teaching children to make better food choices

(continued)

(continued)

    (d) Reducing school dropout
    (e) Reducing delinquency
    (f) Preventing suicide attempts
    (g) Stopping student harassment in school areas of low supervision
    (h) Deterring students from joining gangs
    (i) Reducing anxiety associated with high stakes testing

4. Identify a student behavior about which you have some concern and select a theory of change that might help you address the problem. Make one statement to sum up the theory of change. Make sure that the theory of change makes sense in light of the problem and the changes needed.

Chapter 6
High-Risk Behaviors and Mental Health

Adolescence is a critically important time for prevention work to decrease substance use, inactivity leading to obesity, unprotected sexual activity, and exposure to violence (Swahn, 2012). There is a range of high-risk activities that adolescents engage in across countries. Using the 2003 National Survey of Children's Health, researchers looked at eight risk factors for students and found that decreasing health was associated with increasing numbers of risk factors (Larson, Russ, Crall, & Halfon, 2008). Risk behaviors among adolescents lead to many negative outcomes in adulthood (Hesseler & Katz, 2010). Multiple risks have a cumulative effect on children's mental health.

The Youth Risk Behavior Surveillance System (YRBSS) includes a national school-based survey, which is used in part to evaluate school and community preventive interventions (http://www.cdc.gov/healthyyouth/yrbs/brief.htm). The various categories of risk behavior in this survey include tobacco use, alcohol and drug use, dietary behaviors and low physical activity, sexual behaviors, and activities that foster violence. The statistics for adolescent risky behaviors change from year to year and can be accessed through the most recent YRBSS data. Of interest is the increase in risky behaviors at adolescence and the fact that most preventive efforts take place in schools (Steinberg, 2008). Early adolescence is a time of important changes in the tendency of young people to engage in risky behaviors. The increased tendency to seek sensation may be due to brain changes in the reward system so that young adolescents are more willing to take risks, although it is clear that all adolescents do not respond to this maturationally driven phenomenon to engage in risky behaviors.

There are times during student development that stand out as time periods that may be an important focus of preventive work. Adolescence is a period of life when experimenting with risk behaviors is not uncommon. When risk behaviors are seen in adolescence but not before, intervention outcomes appear to be better than for students who exhibit persistent conduct difficulties from a young age (Monshouwer et al., 2012). During adolescence, studies indicate that students involved in one type of risky behavior are often involved in other types of risk behaviors. Tilleczek and Ferguson (2007) reviewed 100 international reports, academic papers, and policy

G.L. Macklem, *Preventive Mental Health at School: Evidence-Based Services for Students*, 109
DOI 10.1007/978-1-4614-8609-1_6, © Springer Science+Business Media New York 2014

reports to examine the many "nested" transitions from childhood to adolescence, or from elementary to secondary school. This critical developmental transition is complex as risk factors cross individual schools, families, and cultures. Students facing multiple risks experience effects that are compounding. Some of the risk factors at this juncture include daily hassles, class and poverty issues, gender differences, visible minority status, a need to belong, lack of attention on the part of the school to social issues, exposure to new groups, dating, risk of social isolation, changing family relations, decreased teacher–student relationships, academic stress, identity issues, adjustment patterns, and overlooked mental health concerns. Transition programming may relieve some of these stresses.

Individual differences may make some adolescents more likely to engage in risky behaviors. Students who do not have strategies for working through negative emotional experiences may turn to substance use (Hesseler & Katz, 2010). Emotion-avoidant strategies are related to an increased likelihood of substance use. Emotion regulation is a critical variable in vulnerability to risky behaviors. If students have not developed strategies to deal with their emotions in middle childhood they may turn to negative, risky, and impulsive behaviors to reduce the intensity of those negative feelings in adolescence. Prevention of risky behaviors needs to involve developing emotional competence. Students who have weaknesses in emotion regulation and especially in regulating anger, along with poor awareness of anger, are at increased risk for use of hard drugs. Difficulties regulating loneliness is hypothesized to lead to efforts to connect to others through sexual activities. There is an important correlation between depression and risky behavior leading to delinquency in teens. Urban high school students have been surveyed yearly to determine why this was the case (Hooshman, Willoughby, & Good, 2012). These researchers found that self-medication explained the connection between higher levels of depressive symptoms in grade nine and faster trajectories for drug use across the high school period.

Some adolescents are at higher risk than others. For example, 12- to 18-year-old girls who report same-sex attraction, behavior, or orientation are at high risk for substance abuse (Marshal et al., 2012). In fact they are 400 % more likely to say that they are involved with substance use. Girls in this group have clearly higher rates of substance use as compared to their peers. As an aside, school-based mental health workers need to emphasize privacy and confidentiality policies when they encounter students like these when they experience difficulties in school.

There are gender differences in risky behavior. Researchers suggest that there may be actually more unmet mental health needs among girls than boys. Girls are less satisfied with their lives and experience more psychosomatic illnesses in adolescence than boys (Swahn, 2012). There are also environmental differences that contribute to risky behaviors. Researchers have identified a relationship between neighborhood disorder and the likelihood that teens will engage in risky behaviors (Furr-Holden, Milam, Reynolds, MacPherso, & Lejuez, 2012). Neighborhoods with property damage, graffiti, and individuals using drugs constitute a high-risk environment for young people. This type of disordered living situation provides too many opportunities for engaging in risky behaviors.

The Idaho State Department of Education published information listing the risk and protective factors for unhealthy adolescent behaviors. This publication divides risk factors into four domains. Rebelliousness, friends involved in problem behaviors, a positive attitude toward problem behavior, and early involvement in risky behaviors were listed as one domain. A family domain included family history of risk behaviors, poor parental management, family conflict, parent excuses for risk behavior, or adults who engaged in risky behaviors. These increased risks for students. Risks associated with school included persistent aggressive behaviors, academic failure, and weak commitment to schooling. Community risks included availability of drugs and firearms, local norms in favor of risk behaviors, high mobility, community disorganization, and both economic and social deprivation (http://www.sde.idaho.gov).

Key Risky Behaviors to Address in School-Based Prevention

Risk behaviors leading to violence is a serious concern across the U.S. Negative and inappropriate behaviors affect the educational process in schools for all students and staff. As misbehavior increases in schools, attachment to school decreases. Students become less committed and less involved in school (Peguero, Popp, Latimore, Shekarkhar, & Koo, 2011).

Peer contagion has been described as a process involving mutual influence. This process includes behaviors and emotions that could cause harm to others (Dishion & Van Ryzin, 2011). The behaviors that may be affected by peer contagion include deviancy training, aggressive behaviors, violent behavior, carrying weapons, disordered eating, use of drugs, and depression. An understanding of peer contagion can present opportunities for prevention. Some peer groups can become involved in risky behaviors through peer contagion. Peer contagion can undermine secondary prevention efforts when similar students with problem behaviors are placed in small groups. Fragmented communities of marginalized groups can foster gangs where behavior can escalate into violence. Prevention efforts that strengthen connections to positive peers and adults may be helpful.

Data suggests that ethnic minorities are both victimized and more likely to be aggressors than White youth. Of particular concern is the fact that girls age 12 and older are considered to be most at risk (Rodney, Johnson, & Srivastava, 2005). There are additional variables such as differences in schools that must be considered when considering prevention activities. For example, school-based strategies that have been effective in preventing delinquency include culturally relevant activities, extracurricular activities, strengthening academic performance, and strengthening commitment to school.

Self-injury is a risky behavior of serious concern. Suicide prevention has been addressed in preventive efforts. Cusimano and Sameem (2010) identified 36 suicide prevention programs for middle school and high school students designed using randomized controlled trials and time series analyses with comparison groups, and follow-up questionnaires. Unfortunately, none of the studies showed a reduction in suicide rates although there were significant changes in knowledge, attitudes, and willingness to seek help. Miller, Eckert, and Mazza (2009) located 13 studies, most of which were universal programs in schools. Consistent methodological weaknesses were found in the universal and selected programs. At the same time, some evidence was found to support strategies such as providing information, teaching problem-solving skills, and reinforcing protective factors in suicide prevention efforts. Teaching coping strategies and problem-solving strategies are important in the few more promising programs. The authors conclude that there is a "significant need for school psychologists to identify and disseminate effective prevention programs generally" (p. 182).

Sexual activity can lead to teen pregnancy and illness due to infections. Some of the factors involved in sexual activity that begins early on, and also for pregnancy during teenage years, include poverty, family stress, having been exposed to violence, poor parental supervision, weak educational or career opportunities, high mortality rates in neighborhoods, minority status, and father absence (Ellis et al., 2003). Father presence in a family is a protective factor. Early father absence is a risk factor. Teen pregnancy was 7–8 times more likely among girls whose dads were not involved early on, as compared to girls whose fathers were not available later in their development.

Eating disorders are typically first seen in adolescence with a ratio of 10–15 to 1, girls to boys. Eating disorders are seen in students of all social classes and races. Negative self-judgment is the most common risk factor. Minority students who are heavier, and who identify with White, middle-class values and beliefs, are at greater risk than those students who are less influenced by these values. A randomized, controlled trial of the *Planet Health* intervention for reducing obesity (http://www.planet-health.org) was implemented in four metropolitan area communities at the middle school level in Massachusetts. The intervention was successful for girls, but not for boys (Gortmaker et al., 2011). Regular classroom and gym teachers ran the program, which focused on reducing television viewing, increasing physical activity, and eating fewer high-fat foods, while increasing fruits and vegetables in the diet.

Tobacco use is a concern for prevention efforts. Interviews with sixth to tenth grade students in the Chicago schools determined that positive initial sensitivity to smoking tobacco predicted continued smoking, leading to dependence (Hu, Grielser, Schaffran, & Kandel, 2011). Differences in sensitivity and subjective learned experiences are involved in nicotine dependence. Once students are smoking regularly, conduct problems become risk factors, more so for boys than girls. Peer smoking is an important risk factor for depressive symptoms. Smoking correlates with depressive symptoms in that as smoking increases in 12- to 19-year-olds, depressive symptoms increase as well. Smoking predicts depression among younger adolescents in particular (Galambos, Leadbeater, & Barker, 2004). Researchers hypothesize that students who are at risk for depression due to family history, or emotional experiences, are more likely to *initiate* smoking. Prevention work addressing tobacco use needs to also include strategies to cope with sad and irritable feelings.

Kelder et al. (2001) examined the connections between depression and substance use in predominantly Hispanic 12- to 14-year-old middle school students. The association was strong. This argues for early identification of depressive symptoms and for addressing motivational issues in prevention programs. A common problem in students who experience depression is lack of motivation.

Drug and Alcohol Use and Abuse

The risky behaviors that constitute the greatest concerns for teens include sexual risk-taking, substance use and misuse, risky driving, and violence (Anglin, Halper-Felsher, Kaplan, & Newcomer, 2011). Work in schools on drug and alcohol prevention has been extensive. A history of conduct problems is related to substance abuse (Monshouwer et al., 2012). Data from the Tracking Adolescents' Individual Lives Survey (TRAILS) indicate that involvement in externalizing behaviors from 11 years of age results in consistently high levels of problem behaviors. The externalizing behavior by itself can trigger early use of substances. Because the pattern begins at about age 11 years rather than earlier, a student's vulnerability interacts with other risk factors associated with adolescence. Additional factors include low effortful control, seeking high intensity activities, and family issues. The development of substance use and abuse is associated with externalizing behaviors.

Swendsen et al. (2012) found that both alcohol and use of drugs is not unusual in the US adolescents. Diagnostic interviews of teens determined that there is a large increase in drug and alcohol use between 13 and 18 years of age. Greater rates of drug abuse than alcohol abuse were found, as well as high rates of regular use. Tolerant attitudes around use of marijuana have increased among students. The median age of beginning to abuse alcohol and drugs is 14 years of age in the United States. Researchers feel their data indicates a higher incidence risk than has previously been estimated. Risk of reaching "abuse levels" is greatest in 13- to 14-year-olds, likely compromising brain-based developmental processes during this period. Rates of use were lower for other racial/ethnic groups compared to White or Hispanic adolescents although African American adolescents were more likely to transition to abuse from dependence than their white peers. Gender differences were not significant until after 15 years of age. Both risk and protective factors influence substance use and mental health issues. Contextual factors are important in poor adjustment and in treatment for adjustment difficulties. A study of students aged 12–18 in British Columbia determined that adolescents who engaged in substance use at lower levels reported fewer symptoms of emotional difficulties and considered their parents and peers more protective (Barnes, Mitic, Leadbeater, & Dhami, 2009).

Timing is an important consideration in planning preventive interventions for risky behaviors in school-aged students. There is a higher prevalence of drug use for eighth and ninth graders, as compared to sixth and seventh graders, which suggests that the middle school period is a critical period for prevention efforts (Nichols, Mahadeo, Bryant, & Botvin, 2008). Some prevention programs include emotion regulation strategies (approximately 25 %) and others do not. Those programs, which do include emotion regulation skills, focus on anxiety reduction and this appears to be helpful. Studies suggest that girls in particular respond to emotional problems and family issues by smoking and/or using substances. A study of middle school students in sixth grade, with a follow-up survey in seventh grade, determined that anger levels predicted initiation of drug use in multiethnic city students. Drug use constituted a coping strategy for these students. Anger management needs to be included in prevention programs.

It is important for mental health workers in schools to try to identify students at risk for becoming involved in peer relationships that facilitate risky behaviors. The period between age 10 and 15 years is considered to be *early* adolescence and is a time of critical transitions (Nichols et al., 2008). Many developmental tasks are encountered during this period. There are changes in brain structure and function affecting biological, emotional, and behavioral functioning. Abilities to plan, to hold information in one's mind in order to solve complex tasks, self-regulation, and inhibitory control begin to increase during this period. Psychopathological conditions increase during this period as well. These cognitive changes along with peer relationships affect relationships with parents, although parents remain highly influential. Peers more easily influence adolescents who have problematic relationship with their parents. Young adolescents are influenced by cultural messages and values through various media and peer groups. Alcohol-specific risks include a positive family history of alcoholism, having friends who use alcohol, use of alcohol within the family or by older siblings, positive alcohol expectancies, and starting to use alcohol early. Cross-sectional data from the Health Behaviors in School-Aged Children U.S. Survey indicated that bullying and victimization was connected to use of alcohol, tobacco, and marijuana use in tenth grade students, both male and female (Luk, Wang, & Simons-Morton, 2010). Depression was connected to bullying victimization for both boys and girls. Depression was also associated with substance use—more so for girls. This suggests that victimization for girls may lead to symptoms of depression.

Alcoholism runs in families because addiction has a genetic component. When the father in the family is dealing with alcoholism, sons are at high risk. There is some data to suggest that depression is also associated with alcoholism, and this relationship is stronger for women. There are differences in rates of alcoholism associated with different cultures. Norms vary among cultures. Drinking patterns are modeled in families. Skills for drinking responsibility are taught, or not taught, in various cultures (Falo-Stewart & Klostermann, 2008). Children of alcoholics are at risk for negative mental health outcomes (Ellis, Zucker, & Fitzgerald, 1997). Particularly concerning is the risk for children of parents with comorbid illnesses along with alcohol dependence. Poor problem solving within families is a particularly negative factor for children of alcoholics. Many beliefs about the effects of alcohol, along with rates of use and abuse, are strongly influenced by ethnicity.

It is important to look at schools themselves as risk factors, because individual and neighborhood factors do not fully explain differences in use of substances by themselves (Tobler, Komro, Dabroski, Aveyard, & Markham, 2011). Schools are considered risky environments for some adolescents (Mason & Korpela, 2009). Schools are located in neighborhoods. Neighborhoods that are disordered, with poor social controls, influence the schools that exist nearby. When schools are disordered along with the neighborhoods in which they are located, this relationship convinces students that social institutions cannot enforce standards. Urban students already using substances were interviewed in a relevant study. These students felt that the risky environments for drug use included school as well as friends' homes and movies. In a study of *Project Northland Chicago*, a 6-year prevention program to reduce alcohol misuse in racial and ethnic minority students, researchers determined that in schools with academic achievement that was stronger than expected (given the profile of students), there was a concomitant lower incidence of alcohol, tobacco, and marijuana use (Perry et al., 1996; Tobler et al., 2011). In addition, there was a decrease in behavioral problems. Researchers identified a 25 % reduction in use of drugs and in delinquent behavior. Schools have a clear role in decreasing risk behaviors in youth.

Racial/Ethnic Considerations in Drug and Alcohol Use and Abuse

The demographics of the United States are changing quickly, especially in schools. School professionals need to attend to the fact that there are differences in prevalence rates for drug and alcohol abuse among youth with various cultural backgrounds. There are differences in background and current risk factors across racial/ethnic groups. Predictors of drug and alcohol abuse differ according to student backgrounds. For these reasons, prevention programs must carefully consider cultural sensitivity in program development and program choice for prevention work in schools (Resnicow, Soler, Braithwaite, Ahluwalia, & Butler, 2000). The strength of the relationship between perceptions of peers drinking and use of alcohol is present in all cultures (Demetrovics, 2012). The strength of this relationship also depends on differing cultural norms. There has been useful data collected for African American, Hispanic, and Asian students.

Important variables for drug use among African American students include peer risky behavior, which is the only factor consistently mediating all drug use for this group of students. However, there are other important factors to include parental monitoring, important in use of alcohol and also in drug refusal (Clark, Belgrave, & Abell, 2012). Parents play an extremely influential role in the drug use of their children especially in neighborhoods where peers are involved in risky behaviors. Boys appear to be more likely to use marijuana when their friends use this drug. The relationship of African American girls aged 11–14 years with their fathers predicted confidence to refuse drug use (Boyd, Ashcraft, & Belgrave, 2006).

A study of 12- to 14-year-old urban middle school students who were predominantly Hispanic determined that there was an association between depression and five types of substance use (Kelder et al., 2001). This data makes it clear that prevention efforts need to begin in middle school or earlier, and that depression needs to be addressed in addition to refusal skills. Asian and Pacific Islander students have less risk for drug use, although the rates in more recent studies are not as low as has been assumed (Harachi, Catalano, Kim, & Choim, 2001).

Prevention Efforts to Reduce Risky Behaviors

Universal prevention programs that teach students emotional regulation skills support appropriate behavior and strategies to deal with negative peer influences (The Multisite Violence Prevention Project, 2009). When programs are schoolwide, they involve teachers to reinforce the goals of various interventions and model skills. For children with few risks, prevention programs need to stress strengthening assets or resources. For children in the high-risk group, due to the number of risk factor to which they are exposed, programs need to focus on reducing risks while resources are strengthened. When a number of risk factors occur at the same time, mental health problems increase dramatically.

Jepson, Harris, Platt, and Tannahill (2010) conducted a meta-analysis of intervention studies involving six health-related behaviors. These included eating behaviors, exercise, smoking, alcohol misuse, sexual behaviors, and drug use. Researchers were interested in studies preventing the risk behaviors and in those studies aimed at helping individuals change negative behaviors. In the case of smoking, the data indicated that providing information by itself was not effective. Smoking restrictions in schools and restricting tobacco sales to minors together appeared to be more effective with girls than boys. Moderate evidence was found for school programs designed to increase physical activity over the whole day. School-based interventions for teens involving the family and interventions that had many components were found to result in an increase in physical activity in teens. School-based programs designed to teach children not to ride with drivers who had been drinking showed some positive results, but there was insufficient evidence to say that efforts of peer organizations, or social norming campaigns, could decrease alcohol consumption in students. On the other hand, there was evidence that motivational interviewing could change eating behaviors. None of the school-based programs met the criteria in the Jepson et al. study for effectiveness in deterring drug abuse. Interventions to promote condom use, reducing the number of partners, and frequency of sex were found to be effective, particularly if they promoted use of contraception versus abstinence. Long-term effectiveness of interventions in general is lacking, but Jepson and colleagues concluded that school-based efforts are effective overall.

Prevention Systems Involving Schools and Communities Working Together

Fagan and Eisenberg (2012) determined that considerable progress has been made in preventive efforts to reduce antisocial behaviors and in implementation of preventive practices at low cost, thanks to federal initiatives. *Project Northland* is a multicomponent community prevention system to prevent early alcohol involvement of students in grades 6–8 in urban areas (Komor et al., 2004). It includes a social–behavioral curriculum, peer leadership, extracurricular activities, and a task force involving the community. The first efficacy data showed significant effects on the likelihood of students beginning to use alcohol, or using alcohol, by eighth grade in the intervention communities.

Researchers have continued to follow the original efficacy study of *Project Northland* with yearly surveys, records of alcohol purchase attempts by students, and parent telephone surveys. Long-term results show that *Project Northland* was most successful when students were young. At this developmental period, social skills and peer influence were emphasized. The project was re-implemented when students were in grades 11 and 12. However, during the period when students were in grades 9 and 10, alcohol use significantly increased. When the program was re-implemented, and access to alcohol and changing community norms were targeted, the program was again effective in reducing the growth rate in alcohol use and in binge drinking, although the program was not as effective as the initial effort when students were younger. Researchers conclude that efforts must be *continual and age-appropriate* to maintain interest and involvement. They recommended a continued press to change the community culture.

Communities That Care (CTC) is a prevention system providing training and materials to communities in which collaboration between community groups and schools takes place (Hawkins et al., 2009). CTC does not require that a specific program is chosen, but rather allows the local stakeholders to choose a program from an established group of programs that have empirical support. The focus is on reducing risk factors that predict risk behavior such as initiation of alcohol use and delinquency. The Center for Substance Abuse Prevention (SAMHSA) provides the materials, all of which are available on the Internet. The theory of change connected to CTC predicts that it takes 2–5 years to see changes in risk factors, and 5–10 years to see community-level changes in teen alcohol use, smoking, and delinquency. The Hawkins et al. study looked at effects of CTC among students followed from fifth through eighth grade. Forty-one communities in seven states (12 pairs of matched communities) participated in the study. Researchers were able to demonstrate that the incidence and prevalence of alcohol use and binge drinking could be reduced through the efforts of community stakeholders trained in this system. In addition, both the incidence of tobacco use and also delinquent behaviors were reduced among students by age 14.

In consideration of the recent discussions among researchers around the effectiveness of prevention programs for different subgroups, the Community Youth Development Study (CYDS) looked at differential effects of subgroups of students involved in CTC (Oesterle, Hawkins, Fagan, Abbott, & Catalano, 2010). Researchers found that the effect was stronger for boys than girls, and students who were not delinquent benefitted more than eighth grade students who were delinquent at baseline. It was hypothesized that boys may be more receptive to reductions in risk factors and therefore benefitted more than girls. CTC had a stronger effect on reducing the use of smokeless tobacco than on smokers. Smokeless tobacco use is elevated in small communities as compared to urban communities. Overall, the differential effectiveness of CTC on reducing substance use and reducing delinquency was fairly equal across subgroups.

Most prevention programs implemented in schools are time-limited and address one behavior at a time. The *Aban Aya Youth Project* (AAYP) is a curriculum for urban African American students (Flay et al., 2004). This program targets students in grades 5–8, has a community program, and addresses violence prevention and delinquency associated with school, substance misuse, provocative behavior, and sexual behavior. This culturally sensitive program has been demonstrated to be successful for boys in a randomized controlled study, especially when the program included strengthening family and community ties. There were no significant effects for inner-city African American girls.

Difficulties with emotional coping and emotional expression are associated with relational aggression, in predominantly low-income African American fifth and eighth grade students (Sullivan, Helms, Kliewer, & Goodman, 2010). Difficulty regulating anger was significantly connected to physical aggression for boys in the Sullivan et al. study. Poor ability to cope with the intensity of anger can lead to emotional disinhibition and result in increased levels of aggressive behaviors. This study found similar rates of relational aggression among boys and girls. When exploring the functions of relational aggression, researchers suggested that feelings of sadness might be driving this type of aggression. Dealing effectively with sadness may be important when developing prevention curricula in addition to teaching students about anger regulation.

Hecht et al. (2003) examined a culturally grounded intervention for substance use for 6,035 middle school students in 35 schools. This intervention taught anti-drug norms and resistance skills along with other social skills. A media campaign and booster sessions were included. Three versions of the program were implemented. One version targeted Mexican American students, another combined African American and European American students, and the third was considered to be multicultural. The interventions were determined to work in that gateway drug use was decreased and student skills and attitudes improved. Although cultural matching did not appear to be helpful, the Mexican American and multicultural versions resulted in the most outcomes. Use of substances among eighth grade Latinos/as students is higher than their white or black peers and is related indirectly to perceived discrimination through acculturation stress (Kam, Cleveland, & Hecht, 2010). Prevention programs for this group of students may be more successful if efforts include coping strategies to deal with discrimination and acculturation stress.

School-Based Efforts to Prevent Substance Use

Alcohol is the "drug of choice" for teenagers and is normative among students of this age group. Given starting drinking alcohol occurs around age 10 years, most school-based interventions have been targeted for middle schools with the goal of preventing onset of alcohol use, reducing risk factors at the individual level, and/or addressing environmental risk factors. There are high rates of alcohol use by young adolescents and preteens with significant consequences. Rates of use are high in

Table 6.1 Promising school-based interventions

Elementary level	Middle school level
Seattle Social Development Project (Hawkins et al., 1992; Hawkins, Von Cleve, & Catalano, 1991)	*Project Northland* (Perry et al., 1996, 2002)
Linking the Interests of Families and Teachers (Eddy, Reid, & Fetrow, 2000; Eddy, Reid, Stoolmiller, & Fetrow, 2003)	*Project STAR*, or *Midwestern Prevention Project* (Chou et al., 1998; Pentz et al., 1989, 1990)
Raising Healthy Children (Brown, Catalano, Fleming, Haggerty, & Abbott, 2005; Catalano et al., 2003)	*Keepin' it REAL* (Hecht et al., 2003)
Preventive Treatment Program (Tremblay, Mâsse, Pagani, & Vitaro, 1996)	

rural settings and among Hispanic students, and more programming is needed for these populations (Stigler, Neusel, & Perry, 2011).

Given the work that has been conducted on prevention programs, there are now available a number of "reviews of reviews." Nation et al. (2003), for example, conducted a review-of-reviews to look at prevention programs involving substance abuse, risky sexual behavior, school failure, and delinquency. Researchers examined different types of drug prevention programs and determined that "interactive" programs were clinically and statistically superior to non-interactive programs (Tobler & Stratton, 1997).

Spoth, Greenberg, and Turrisi (2008) identified 400 interventions designed to reduce underage drinking. Of these, only 12 met the criteria for "most promising" for school-aged youth, yet there has been good progress in developing effective programming. Underage drinking is serious as it is associated with depression, suicidality, behavioral programs, academic difficulties, health problems, risky behaviors, and even deaths. Spothe and colleagues evaluated prevention programs for different age groups, different settings, and different subgroups. They used strict criteria for research designs, specification of the samples used, manualization, effects, and outcome assessments. In the case of school-based interventions, many were short-term (6 months), and data was very limited for late elementary age students or for high school students.

Stigler et al. (2011) summarized the Spothe et al. research in regard to the school-based interventions that were most promising on the basis of their literature search, and also in regard to determination of the rigor of the research. Elementary and middle school interventions have been identified (Table 6.1).

Unfortunately, only one intervention was considered "most promising," the *Project Toward No Drug Abuse* (Sussman, Dent, & Stacy, 2002). Although *Project Northland* has been implemented and shown to be successful with high school students (Perry et al., 2002), the data for other prevention programs such as *Promoting Alternative Thinking Strategies* (Kam, Greenberg, & Kusché, 2004; Riggs, Greenberg, Kusché, & Pentz, 2006) and *LifeSkills Training* (Botvin, Baker, Dusenbury, Botvin, & Diaz, 1995; Spoth, Randall, Shin, & Redmond, 2005) did not meet the full criteria. Hopefully, they may at some point as research continues. There are specific characteristics, which make some programs more effective than others (see Table 6.2).

Table 6.2   Characteristics of effective programs for alcohol prevention

- Comprehensive programming with multiple interventions in multiple settings
- Social norms are addressed
- There is adequate staff training and support
- Parents, peer leaders, and community connections are made
- Personal and social skills including resistance are trained
- Varied teaching methods are used. Teaching approaches are active, skills-based, and hands-on. They include small group activities, role-plays, and practice instead of information or group discussions
- There is sufficient dosage or program intensity. There is sufficient quantity and quality of contact hours. There are multiple sessions over multiple years. Follow-up or booster sessions are included
- Preventive interventions are culturally and developmentally appropriate for the local population
- The programming is theory-driven with a focus on social influences versus past practice or logic
- Positive relationships are emphasized

Sources: Cuijpers (2002), Komro and Toomey (2002), Roona, Streke, and Marshall (2003), Stigler et al. (2011), Tobler et al. (2000), and Tobler and Stratton (1997)

In addition, programs that were appropriately developmentally timed, socio-culturally relevant, had well-trained staff, and conducted outcome evaluations were important.

Motivation to change is an important consideration when working with individual students. Motivational interviewing is a technique for helping students help themselves as it affects desire to change (Falo-Stewart & Klostermann, 2008). In this process students are helped to resolve their ambivalence, which is critical because one of the most effective factors in the success of interventions is the motivation to change one's behavior.

A Case Addressing a Risk Behavior

Some of the tasks involved in selecting and implementing a preventive program in schools includes:

- Investigating the risk and protective factors involved for the risk behavior.
- Determining the strengths and limitations of the local school system.
- Locating a short list of evidence-based programs, from which to select a program that fits the particular local community.
- Determining the readiness of the school to implement the program.
- Collaborating with all stakeholders.
- Implementing the program with fidelity.
- Evaluating outcomes.

Although there are additional steps involved, these steps provide a demonstration of the approach needed to address risk behavior in students. Tobacco use is used as an example for this discussion. Envision a high school in which cigarette smoking has become a serious problem among students and a few faculty members. In addition, the student population in this example is predominantly Hispanic.

It is important to first understand the risk behavior. In an effort to help update the U.S. Preventive Services Task Force (USPSTF) recommendations around prevention of tobacco use in children and adolescents, Patnode et al. (2013) conducted three systematic reviews of the tobacco prevention literature through September of 2012. Researchers located 19 controlled trials that were designed to prevent tobacco use initiation or promote cessation (or both) in youth 11–17 years of age. Most trials examined cigarette smoking alone, and many studies were not recent. However, pooled analyses from a random-effects meta-analysis found a 19 % relative reduction in smoking initiation among students who received behavior-based prevention interventions to prevent smoking initiation over 12 months. Behavior-based interventions did not improve cessation rates. However, results from the 2010 National Survey on Drug Use and Health (SAMHA, 2012) indicated that more than 3,800 children and adolescents under age 18 smoke their first cigarette. Every day, approximately 1,000 students start to smoke on a daily basis. The rate of past month tobacco use has recently declined in White and African American students aged 12–17, but not for Hispanic students, Asian students, or American Indian and Alaska Native youths. Most new cigarette smokers as of 2010 started smoking before they were 18 years old.

According to data from 2007, the CDC Youth Risk Behavior Surveillance found that 49.7 % of high school students who were already smoking had tried to stop. The National Institute on Drug Abuse indicates that nicotine is addictive and that for some smokers there is a genetic predisposition to tobacco addiction (Volkow, 2009). Individuals with behavioral and mental health disorders have a 2–4 times higher incidence of tobacco use than their peers. Even intermittent smoking in adolescence can result in addiction. Adolescents may be more sensitive to the reinforcing properties of nicotine than students in other age groups. Tobacco use can be the result of peer influences. Johnson et al. (2007) reported that programs teaching skills such as refusal, communication, and decision-making might be helpful to those adolescents who lack these skills.

The environment or school culture makes a difference. Aveyard et al. (2004) found that authoritative schools in the UK had stronger effects on student behaviors as they provide the support and control that might keep students from smoking. Another group of researchers in Scotland determined that a focus on caring and inclusiveness was protective (Henderson, Ecob, Wight, & Abraham, 2008). Still another group determined that when schools were intolerant of smoking, students were less likely to start smoking (Pabayo, O'Loughlin, Barnett, Cohen, & Gauvin, 2012). A question for a school prevention team involves determining whether or not school staff members would support a norm of anti-smoking.

Another important question for schools is whether or not the effort to affect use of tobacco is worthwhile? Cuijpers (2003) determined that school-based programs using interactive teaching approaches have a small effect on reducing use of substances. All prevention programs increase knowledge. However, many smoking prevention programs do not work over time, and many programs are promoted when they don't have solid data. Flay (2009) points out that even effective programs may not work when the local student body does not match the efficacy study group, the implementers, the school setting, or the culture of the students and the community.

The next step is to determine the prevalence of the problem in the local school. Clearly a needs assessment should be considered. School staff might consult with various state and federal agencies to find an appropriate tool. It is important to determine the support available in the community to address the issue. Next, school capacity to implement a program needs to be determined. Realistic goals must be set. The school team needs to determine at what point or points (K-12) the preventive work should take place. Since most programs to reduce student initiation and to reduce smoking take place at middle school, this would be a reasonable level to target. Data collection points and procedures need to be planned as well.

What Types of Programs Are Effective?

Another important question for schools is what types of programs are effective? Drug prevention programs have different goals such as increasing information and knowledge, reducing use of drugs, preventing students from starting to use drugs, reducing drug abuse, and/or diminishing the effects of use (Cuijpers, 2003). Cuijpers (2002) concluded that programs must focus on norms and commitment not to use substances. Even intensions to use must be influenced which may direct a school team to an appropriate theory of change. Additionally, interactive approaches, community components, peer leaders participation, and training refusal skills are necessary. Flay's (2009) inclusive analysis of prevention programs determined that school-based smoking prevention programs can be effective. More effective programs were interactive, taught skills, involved 15 or more sessions (data is available up to the ninth grade), and resulted in *substantial* short-term effects. Information by itself is not effective in tobacco prevention. Unfortunately there is little evidence of long-term effectiveness of prevention efforts.

Individual differences matter in tobacco use prevention. Nilsson and Emmelin (2010) found that early adolescents said that they started to smoke as a way to get control of their feelings and to get control over stressful situations. For this reason, researchers felt that consistent talk about tobacco use from both parents and schools would be helpful. The risk of starting to smoke cigarettes was determined to be significantly higher for youth with high hostility, symptoms of depression, and for students who were both bullied and were also victims of bullying. Strategies to manage negative feelings must be included in prevention of smoking programs (Weiss, Cen, Mouttapa, Johnson, & Unger, 2011). Clearly program effects depend on the program content, the school climate, school culture, fidelity of implementing the prevention program, and individual student characteristics (age and personality) (Flay, 2009). All of these variables need to be considered when searching for a program that matches a local school or district.

Examining Local School Culture and Demographics Issues

A particularly critical variable and challenge for a school-based team is to match programs with the local school culture. Student and community culture makes a difference. Caution is needed when attempting to select or implement programs with different ethnic or cultural populations (Flay, 2009). In a school in which students are predominantly, but not completely, Hispanic, a program would be needed which would be helpful for a Hispanic or a multicultural population. The leading causes of mortality among Hispanics living in the United States are smoking-related (Webb, Rodriguez-Esquivel, & Baker, 2010). Hispanic middle school level young people are more likely to smoke than their peers. Individual factors, as opposed to family and school factors, have been found to make a difference as some Hispanic students have reported that their confidence to say "no" is low. Additionally this group of students lack information about the negative effects of smoking (Shih, Miles, Tucker, Zhou, & D'Amico, 2010). One study found that Hispanic students have higher exposure to the perception that smoking is common (Davis, Nonnemaker, Asfaw, & Vallone, 2010). Another individual factor is intention to smoke. Jimba and Sharma (2012) examined this phenomenon. They found that Hispanic adolescents had significantly stronger intentions to smoke over the past 12 months when asked, than their White peers.

For a school in which Hispanic students are the majority, school professionals would need to find studies in which Hispanic students made up a majority of the population of students in efficacy studies for specific programs. It would be important to locate programs, which include skills training, since this has been demonstrated to be effective. Hispanic students 12–15 years of age need to learn how to avoid engaging in tobacco use. Elder et al. (1994) demonstrated that Hispanic students were particularly interested in refusal skills training and responded well to this approach. Students needed to understand possible outcomes when they engage in smoking. They needed decision-making skills and positive relationships with trusted adults. Students need to understand peer pressure to smoke and develop skills to resist environmental pressure.

Johnson et al. (2007) studied the effects of a school-based smoking prevention program in middle schools in which students were either heterogeneous or where Hispanic/Latino students were in the majority. In schools in which most students were Hispanic/Latino, both individualistic (stop smoking for my own health) and collectivist (stop smoking for my family) programs worked well for depressed and hostile adolescents. In schools in which there was a cultural mix of students, the individualistic program worked better. However when smoking initiation was considered, only the program that was culturally sensitive (collectivist) was successful for students in large schools in which the Hispanic students were the majority. Culturally adapted prevention programs have an effect on smoking initiation for Hispanic students (Kong, Singh, & Krishnan-Sarin, 2012).

Project FLAVOR, a culturally sensitive program, was effective for Hispanic students in schools in which they were in the majority (Johnson et al., 2007). *Project FLAVOR* (Fun Learning About Vitality, Origins, and Respect) is a multicultural interactive program with activities such as making a "Wheel of Life" collage and acting out a soap opera (Unger et al., 2004). The program was effective for delaying smoking in Hispanic boys but not in boys from other groups (Johnson et al., 2005). The program was effective when the school population was predominately Hispanic. In schools with predominantly multicultural or Asian students, the program was not effective for Hispanic students. The authors concluded that smoking prevention in culturally diverse students is a very complex affair. Culturally sensitive programs may work better although the risk is that they may work differentially for students of the several cultures involved (Flay, 2009).

Selecting a Program That Will "Fit" the Local School and Community

It is important to determine whether the goals of a potential program include smoking cessation or delay of initiation as different programs have different outcomes. Consultation with administrators and stakeholders will help establish goals. Once a school team has an idea about what is needed and what might work or not work, a short list of programs needs to be developed that have the particular characteristics desired. The programs must be evidence-based. The program must include interactive components. The programs must address a diverse, but primarily Hispanic, population. Training in specific skills must be included to include decision-making skills. The programs must show at least short-term effects.

A list of evidence-based tobacco prevention programs can be located at Intervention MICA (http://health.mo.gov). This website is run by the Missouri Department of Health and Senior Services. The list can be broken down to identify programs implemented in school-based settings. A further breakdown to address children, teens, Hispanic, and "All" races will result in a shorter list. The Wisconsin Department of Public Instruction also publishes a list of evidence-based programs (2007). NREPP and the California Healthy Kids Resource Center provide lists of programs as well. One approach is to see which programs are listed by more than one agency (Tables 6.3 and 6.4).

The programs listed by more than one agency during one search included *Not On Tobacco* (N-O-T) *Program* (Dino et al., 2001), *Project Towards No Tobacco Use* (TNT) (Dent et al., 1995; Sussman, Dent, Stacy, Hodgson, et al., 1993; Sussman, Dent, Stacy, Sun, et al., 1993), the *LifeSkills Training Program* (Botvin, 2000), and *Project ALERT* (Ellickson, Bell, Thomas, Robyn, & Zellman, 1988). Of note is the fact that *Project ALERT* was removed from the list of promising programs by the Center for the Study and Prevention of Violence Institute of Behavior Science in 2009. It is important to keep in mind that programs get re-evaluated periodically and the listings change. Practitioners need to keep their data up-to-date. The next task is

Table 6.3 Determining multiple agencies listing several tobacco prevention programs

Program	Agency/institution recognition
Not on Tobacco Program (N-O-T)	CDC National Registry of Effective Programs (PDF)
	Substance Abuse and Mental Health Services Administration's (SAMHSA's) Evidence-based "model" program
Project Towards No Tobacco Use (TNT)	Substance Abuse and Mental Health Services Administration (SAMHSA) "model" program
	Helping America's Youth (HAY) Programs: Level I
	Office of Juvenile Justice and Delinquency Prevention (OJJDP) Exemplary "model" program
	Blueprints "model" program
	Health Canada: "Exemplary" program
The Life Skills Training Smoking Prevention Program	Blueprints "model" program
	Center for Substance Abuse Prevention (CSAP) "model" program
	Department of Education—Safe Schools "exemplary" program
	Communities That Care—Developmental Research and Programs "effective" program
	National Institute of Drug Abuse (NIDA) "effective" program
	Sherman et al. (1997) "effective" program
	Surgeon General's Report (2001) model 2
	Title V (OJJDP) "exemplary" program
Project Alert	Blueprints "promising" program
	Center for Substance Abuse Prevention (CSAP) "model" program
	Department of Education—Safe Schools "exemplary" program
	Communities That Care—Developmental Research and Programs "effective" program
	Mihalic and Aultman-Bettridge (2004) "favorable" program
	Sherman et al. (1997) "effective" program
	Title V (OJJDP) "exemplary" program

Source: National Center for Mental Health Promotion and Youth Violence Prevention, http://www.promoteprevent.org

to locate the efficacy studies for each of these programs along with the most current studies for each program. Once located, the rigor of the studies needs to be evaluated in order to determine the strength of the program, by evaluating the study designs. The school team also needs to look carefully at the study subjects to determine if they included diverse, and especially Hispanic, students. Supplemental materials available may make a difference to a particular school. Once these questions are addressed the local team can prepare an argument to support their program choice and share it with all stakeholders.

There are several additional issues to consider, such as strategies to monitor smoking in the building and in the area immediately around the build. A school policy about smoking and increased supervision might be areas to explore. Planning how the program might fit into the general school program can be a considerable challenge. Health courses are a logical place to implement programs in middle and secondary schools. Gaining schoolwide and parental support for the program needs to be addressed and an implementation process needs to be developed.

Table 6.4 Expanded data collection from a literature search

Intervention	Population		Setting	Outcomes	Research designs	Quality of research ratings	Agency listings
	Age	Race/ethnicity					
Not on Tobacco (N-O-T) program	13–17 years	All	School	Smoking reduction (more effective for boys) Smoking cessation (more effective for girls) Equally effective regardless of stage of readiness	Quasi-experimental	NREPP (2/08) 3.5/4.0 for reduction, 3.6/4.0 for cessation Centers for Disease Control and Prevention-Model Program National Cancer Institute 4.5/5.0	NREPP, Children's Aide Society, Centers for Disease Control and Prevention, National Cancer Institute, American Lung Association
Project Towards No Tobacco Use (TNT)	10–14 years	27 % Latino	School	Reduced initiation by 26 % and weekly use by 60 %	Randomized block design	Office of Justice Programs-promising	California Healthy Kids, Children's Aide Society
The Life Skills Training Smoking Prevention Program	13–17 years	All (Spanish version)	School	Reduced initiation of cigarettes after 3 and 6 years over control group. Six-year reduction of 44 % over controls	Experimental	NREPP (9/08) 3.9/4.0 Social Programs That Work-Top Tier Office of Juvenile Justice and Delinquency Prevention-effective	NREPP, Promising Practices Network, Children's Aide Society, National Institute on Drug Abuse, Office of Juvenile Justice and Delinquency

Project alert	13–17 years	All (Spanish version)	School	Current and occasional cigarette use was 20–25 % lower, regular and heavy use was one-third to 55 % lower	Experimental	NREPP (12/06) 4.0/4.0 Office of Juvenile Justice and Delinquency Prevention, 6/11	California Healthy Kids, NREPP, Promising Practices Network, National Institute on Drug Abuse, National Center for Mental Health Promotion and Youth Violence Prevention

Sources: http://www.nrepp.samhsa.gov, http://www.californiahealthykids.org/rvalidated, http://www.drugabuse.gov, http://www.promisingpractices.net, http://evidencebasedprograms.org, http://www.ojjdp.gov, http://www.promoteprevent.org

Implementation

Implementation fidelity is critical. The California Healthy Kids Resource Center has fidelity guidelines and a checklist to use with *Project TNT* (http://www.california-healthykids.org). The checklist includes questions about delivery, dosage, setting, materials, target population, and provider qualifications and training. *Project TNT* also has an implementation manual, pretest and posttest student surveys, and suggestions for their use. The developer of the *N-O-T* program indicates that sessions must be delivered completely by a trained individual. Process forms are included in the curriculum. The *LifeSkills Training Program* (LST) has manuals, student guides, and pre- and posttests as well as online training workshops. Finally, process and outcomes assessment are critically important and need to be planned before any program is implemented. Again, an Internet search may provide materials in addition to that which the program developers and disseminators provide. This effort is time-consuming but tasks can be divided among team members to reduce stress. The process itself increases the likelihood of success and, when the process is documented and shared, the likelihood that the program once implemented will be sustained is increased.

Prevention in Action Challenge: Choose One of the Two Cases to Analyze

Case Study A

A high school is located in a blue-collar community where the primary occupation of the men is fishing. Fishing is an extremely dangerous occupation and deaths are not unusual. There are many mothers who are "head of the household" due to either the men in the family being away fishing for long periods of time or fishing-related deaths. An additional stress is that, in recent years, fishing jobs have been going overseas and unemployment has become a problem. The superintendent of schools describes families as pressured and defeated.

Community stress has affected the high school. This year there are 17 high school girls who are expecting babies. The school administrators are frustrated because they feel they have provided both prevention and support to reduce teen pregnancies. Sex education is provided for freshman. There is a clinic connected to the school. There is a day-care center connected to the school for young mothers. So far this year, the high school clinic has administered 150 pregnancy tests. Clinic workers have petitioned the school committee to allow them to provide contraceptives to high school students.

The school committee is torn about whether or not to allow the clinic to provide contraceptives in light of the fact that the community is *strongly opposed* on religious grounds. Some students feel that the girls have no better

(continued)

(continued)

options than to become mothers giving them some status. The principal has asked the school psychologist and other mental health professionals to evaluate the school's current efforts, determine if current prevention efforts are adequate, and if not, to recommend what should be done. She is particularly interested in universal, evidence-based preventive programming but is worried about the political ramifications depending on which program might be selected and implemented.

Case Study B

This high school has a student population that comprises 49.9 % Hispanic students, 25.5 % African American students, and 18.3 % white, non-Hispanic students. Last Friday evening, there was a serious disruption during which two students were stabbed. School officials reported that the incident was gang-related. City officials consequently pledged "zero tolerance" for gang violence. School officials have formed a collaboration with local police to discuss what can be done to address gang violence. The school superintendent has established an in-house team to address positive approaches that can be taken within the school district itself.

Taking a comprehensive preventive mental health services approach, locate evidence-base preventive programming for Tiers 1, 2, and 3 at each school level (elementary, middle, and secondary). Additionally, recommend ways to involve parents and the community in this effort.

Chapter 7
Evidence-Based Prevention of Externalizing Disorders

There is substantial agreement among both researchers and practitioners to classify behaviors into internalizing and externalizing categories (Cosgrove et al., 2011; Guttmannova, Szanyi, & Cali, 2007). Externalizing behaviors are identified as "undercontrolled" behaviors. Children whose behavior is undercontrolled have difficulty with peers, break rules, tend to be irritable, and are typically belligerent. Physical fighting, bullying, using weapons, making verbal threats, and impulsive aggression are externalizing behaviors (Rappaport & Thomas, 2004). Antisocial behavior predicts failure at school, rejection by normative classmates, making increasing connections with deviant peers, and getting involved in negative acts (Berkout, Young, & Gross, 2011). This may be the easiest way for some students to get rewards from their environments.

Loeber and Burke (2011) describe externalizing behaviors as persistent disobedience, stealing, aggression, vandalism, gang fighting, and homicide. The disruptive disorders described by APA range widely in intensity, and include attention deficit-hyperactivity disorder (ADHD), oppositional defiant disorder (ODD), and conduct disorder (CD). All three disorders are characterized by poor behavioral self-control, but beyond this, the three disorders differ.

Children and adolescents with ADHD have particular difficulty with impulse control, behavioral control, and also with attentional skills (Loeber & Burke, 2011). Students with ADHD who exhibit social problems are at risk for depressive symptoms (Drabick, Gadow, & Sprafkin, 2006). In fact, mood disorders along with symptoms of depressive thinking and behavior have been associated with ADHD in adolescence. This is particularly true for those students who regulate their emotions poorly (Seymour, 2010). ODD involves negative, hostile, and oppositional behaviors directed toward authorities. ODD has been shown to predict behavioral difficulties that persist. CD involves rule breaking, violating norms, lying, truancy, and cruelty. It has most often been seen more in boys than girls. Children with CD symptoms also experience depressive symptoms when their family life is characterized by high conflict and poor cohesion.

G.L. Macklem, *Preventive Mental Health at School: Evidence-Based Services for Students*, 131
DOI 10.1007/978-1-4614-8609-1_7, © Springer Science+Business Media New York 2014

Witkiewitz and the Conduct Problems Prevention Research Group have indicated that there is an underlying *continuum* of externalizing behaviors in the research on adult externalizing disorders. Tackett (2010) argued for better integration of childhood and adult disorders and more appreciation for developmental concerns in the *spectrum* of externalizing disorders.

Externalizing problems are seen quite early. Berkout et al. (2011) conducted an impressive search of the several literatures on conduct disorder. They report that externalizing behaviors are seen as early as 17 months of age, with more boys displaying a medium level of physical aggression. They note that early onset of antisocial behaviors is more typical for boys in general, although some studies indicate that that the onset for girls is as early as 7 years of age. When girls exhibit antisocial behavior at an early age, CD tends to be seen later on.

The Risks for Externalizing Behaviors

The etiology of externalizing behaviors is complex, with both biological and environmental variables operating. Externalizing behaviors appear to be moderately heritable (Cosgrove et al., 2011). One example of genetic influence is the finding that early onset of puberty has been connected to disruptive behavior disorders (Berkout et al., 2011). Early onset of puberty is associated with adolescent onset of CD. Attentional difficulties are also characteristic of both boys and girls with CD. There has been recent interest in traits of children and adolescents with externalizing disorders. Children who evidence high levels of callous and unemotional traits, including low guilt and empathy and a narrow range of emotions, tend to exhibit more intense forms of CD behaviors (Canino, Polanczyk, Bauermeister, Rohde, & Frick, 2010). A biological risk factor specifically for girls is prenatal nicotine exposure (Rappaport & Thomas, 2004; Snethen & Van Puymbroeck, 2008).

Social cognitive variables are involved in risk for externalizing disorders. Children who are aggressive tend to misread cues and interpret ambiguous situations as involving individuals with hostile intent (Rappaport & Thomas, 2004). In externalizing disorders, as in internalizing disorders, there is a relationship between anger, frustration, and irritability (Eisenberg et al., 2009). Externalizing children are more rejected by peers and have difficulty in school. When they are aggressive, they become angrier than their peers and increasingly hostile over time. Children, whose externalizing behaviors increase over time, exhibit low effortful control and higher impulsivity than peers. The relationship between effortful control and externalizing behaviors is seen when children are very young and becomes stronger as children age. When effortful control remains problematic between the ages of 3 and 10, children exhibit higher rates of externalizing behavior (Chang, 2009).

Emotional competence involves emotion appraisal, emotion expression, and emotion understanding (Bohnert, Crnic, & Lim, 2003). Children who exhibit aggressive behaviors are not as competent in their ability to express negative feelings, they tend not to exhibit empathy, or they exhibit a narrow range of emotions.

They have more difficulty understanding their emotions and regulating them. In 7- to 10-year-olds more intense and frequent anger added to difficulty expressing how they feel with words is connected with more externalizing behaviors. Aggressive children have difficulty recognizing feelings in themselves, have difficulty describing causes of emotions, and have difficulty preventing themselves from verbally expressing negative emotions in negatively stimulating situations. Negative emotionality is risk factor that is seen for both internalizing and externalizing disorders (Guttmannova et al., 2007). Daredevil behavior is associated with externalizing problems but not with internalizing behaviors.

Environmental variables are significant risks as well. Modeling by family, peers, admired people, neighborhoods, and media plays a role in the development of externalizing behaviors. Peer influences are particularly important in low socio-economic (SES) neighborhoods (Snethen & Van Puymbroeck, 2008). Children and adolescents tend to select friends who are equally aggressive. Direct, vicarious, and self-reinforcement increases the likelihood for future aggression. Intermittent reinforcement for participating in inappropriate behaviors provided by parents is a factor (Berkout et al., 2011). Poor neighborhoods do not always provide positive reinforcement and in fact may offer reinforcement for inappropriate behaviors.

Low nurturance and use of both harsh and inconsistent management of child misbehavior is connected to increasing externalizing at the time. This parenting style predicts future externalizing behaviors (Berkout et al., 2011; Deutsch, Crockett, Wolff, & Russell, 2012; Mrug & Windle, 2008). It may be that parent discipline practices are more influential when youngsters also associate with deviant peers, or that parenting practices influence susceptibility to being drawn to negative friends. In any case, harsh punishment and low warmth is associated with an increase in CD. Negative discipline and antisocial behavior of parents presents a risk factor for both boys and girls for development of CD. When parenting is less negative it can serve as a protective factor. There may be an exception for African American families, in that strict control and authoritarian parenting practice do not appear to be detrimental (Deutsch et al., 2012). Authoritarian parenting may be protective for African American children in dangerous environments. In fact, there appears to be increased benefit in the case of strict parental practices for African American youngsters. When adolescents have a good deal of freedom, the result can be the development of deviant friendships and a higher level of negative behavior the following year. Parental support, including kin networks, is critical to reduce delinquent behavior for African American students because negative peer associations have greater impact for this group of children. Even for European American families, parental controls are protective in high-risk neighborhoods so this parenting style may actually be less associated with racial factors than it is with neighborhood risk.

By following children from age 6 to 9, Lansford et al. (2011) found when parents used physical discipline, antisocial behavior increased the next year. This relationship was stronger than the phenomenon of negative child behavior influencing parent practices. Interestingly, both mild discipline and harsh discipline have been connected to more externalizing behaviors. When parents model negative social interactions, and do not provide consequences for antisocial behavior, children are at risk for antisocial behavior (Berkout et al., 2011). Parents may be totally unaware of their influence on their child's behavior (Rappaport & Thomas, 2004). This presents an opportunity to talk about parental management when students are acting out in schools.

There is some indication that stronger connections to school, and commitment to learning, are protective factors. Students more connected to school, and to their teachers, tend to exhibit less deviant behavior. Well connected students are less violent and less involved with alcohol and other substances (Mrug & Windle, 2008). However, this variable may not be as strong when preadolescents also experience harsh parenting, experience negative peer influences, and have been acting out since they were preschoolers. There are additional school factors. For example, when children experience conflicts with their teacher at the time of school transitions, externalizing behaviors increase in elementary school (Silver, Measelle, Armstrong, & Essex, 2005). Teacher–child closeness can be a protective factor for children who begin their school career *already* exhibiting externalizing behaviors as they enter school for the first time.

Risk factors include exposure to violence and easy access to guns (Rappaport & Thomas, 2004). Boys carrying guns exhibit the most aggressive behaviors and tend to believe that their behavior is justified. They believe their friends accept violent behaviors as normative. Use of illegal drugs, including alcohol, is associated somewhat with violent behaviors; each behavior predicts the other. The association between drug use and violent behavior is complex as it is connected to family history of alcohol use, drug abuse, gang connections, impulsivity, and symptoms of depression. Deviancy training and peer pressure are risk factors. These behaviors establish norms that both drive and support antisocial behaviors (Deutsch et al., 2012). Yet another risk factor is social ostracism, which can lead to aggressive behavior. This is the case for some students who are bullied or who bully others (Rappaport & Thomas, 2004). Warm parenting can decrease the influence of negative peers.

Risk factors interact to produce effects on behavior (Rappaport & Thomas, 2004). In addition, they are cumulative. Their effects also depend on the specific stage of development in which they are present. When students are exposed to risk factors that are ongoing, aggressive behaviors are reinforced and influenced, and this results in aggressive behavior remaining stable.

Gender Differences

Research examining gender and ethnicity in relation to externalizing behaviors is fairly recent. Unfortunately, much of the research has been centered on Caucasian boys with neglect of girls (Mrug & Windle, 2008). Prior studies have indicated that rates of externalizing behaviors are higher in boys than girls. Boys appear to be more affected by deviant and substance-using adolescents than girls.

Gender differences in externalizing behaviors have generated considerable interest among researchers of late. Reports that girls primarily use relational aggression with the goal of damaging relationships have been commonly reported. Relational aggression is driven by intent to hurt others and "meanness." Additionally, if aggressive behaviors include both physical and relational aggression, there is little gender difference in externalizing behavior. Use of physically aggressive behaviors has increased for girls in recent years, as well as participation in gangs.

The gender difference has been called the "gender paradox" (Berkout et al., 2011). Although the research on girls is new and there is a great deal more to learn, there is some information available of interest. CD is one of the most severe externalizing problems for adolescent girls (Rappaport & Thomas, 2004). For girls, childhood onset of CD is seen more often than previously reported. Girls with CD around ages 7–9 years are more likely to have family members with emotional disorders than boys. When girls have characteristics of unhelpfulness and high sensitivity to reinforcers they are at risk of developing CD. "Unhelpfulness" is not related to CD for boys. Interpersonal problems associated with ODD are a predictor of CD for boys but not for girls. When CD is more severe, girls tend to experience "comorbid" internalizing difficulties; i.e., externalizing and internalizing behaviors occurring together. Anxiety is an important complication for girls whereas under-arousal and behavioral disinhibition are more commonly seen in boys. Girls with CD bully others more than boys, and are more callous toward others. Environmental disadvantage is related to CD in girls. Girls show a greater sensitivity to punishment, which is related to the development of CD. Some girls develop CD in spite of a tendency to be behaviorally inhibited. Finally, girls with CD demonstrate more severity of symptoms and more pathology when they have CD as compared to boys with the disorder. Additionally, CD is associated with depressive symptoms and sometimes precedes depression in girls in adolescence (Hipwell et al., 2011). Girls' depression and family conflict have been connected to later antisocial behaviors (Rappaport & Thomas, 2004).

Girls exhibiting antisocial behaviors are at considerable risk for experiencing a range of psychiatric consequences as compared to boys (Rappaport & Thomas, 2004). A study of diverse groups of teens exhibiting severe behavior disorders determined that the girls in the group, as compared to the boys, exhibited posttraumatic stress disorder. Girl "gangs" tend to behave in a more violent manner than boy gangs. Girls in gangs are hypothesized to consider gangs a refuge from other overwhelming stresses in their lives.

Ethnic Differences in Externalizing Behaviors

Ethnic differences in externalizing behaviors are challenging to study. It is difficult to isolate various risk factors such as cultural differences, effects of poverty, neighborhood characteristics, differing parenting practices, and the methodological differences of the studies published on this topic (Canino et al., 2010). Ethnic minority students are more likely to live in disadvantaged neighborhoods or neighborhoods with high crime rates than other groups. They experience more stress associated with poverty. They may experience more physical abuse related to poverty and stressed families. All of these are risk factors for ODD and CD. There are also cultural differences in expectations for behavior among parents of different ethnic groups, as well as cultural differences in ways of expressing psychopathology. When researchers study ethnic differences the definitions used for externalizing behavior may not be the same. In fact, the definitions of disorders such as CD have changed over time; i.e., the degree of "clinically significant impairment" required for diagnosis. Research comparing different subgroups is sparse. Interestingly, higher rates of ADHD in a population are identified using the Diagnostic Statistical Manual, fourth edition (DSM-IV) than the International Statistical Classification of Diseases and Related Health Problems, 10th edition (ICD-10) resulting in inconsistent data across research studies that have been completed to date (Canino & Alegria, 2008). This situation may improve as classification systems are updated. Although ethnicity and neighborhood factors are confounded, delinquency is found in all ethnic groups but studies show that the details differ (Deutsch et al., 2012).

Students living in poverty attend schools with fewer qualified teachers and have decreased access to textbook and computers. Their schools tend to be underfunded with higher student–teacher ratios, and with differences in school policy and practices. These students' parents tend not be able to be involved in their child's education for a variety of understandable reasons. They are more likely to drop out of school. Racial–ethnic minority students are also exposed to more severe punishments when they exhibit misbehavior in schools. Unfortunately they are judged more harshly for the same infractions that others commit, and are referred to administrators for less serious behaviors than other students. They are twice as likely to be retained at grade level and more likely to be suspended than Caucasian students. Losen and Martinez (2013) disaggregated suspension rates in 26,000 American schools by race, gender, English language learner, and disability. They found that one in every nine students was suspended during the 2009–2010 school year. Suspension rates for African American and Latino students doubled between 1973 and 2010. Thirty-six percent of all Black male students with disabilities at middle and secondary school levels were suspended at least once. Research shows being suspended even once in ninth grade is associated with a 32 % risk for dropping out of school. Racial discipline *disproportionality* is a very significant problem in American schools (Gregory, Skiba, & Noguera, 2010; Williams & Greenleaf, 2012).

Racial disproportionality cannot be attributed to demographic factors, SES, single-parent households, family income, *or* to the hypothesized differential behavior of some racial and ethnic groups (Skiba, Poloni-Staudinger, Simmons, Feggins-Aziz, & Chung, 2005; Tobin & Vincent, 2011). Research on classroom processes has determined that the problem of disproportionality begins with the teacher in the classroom, where the teacher's expectations and beliefs clash with the culture of some ethnic minority students. These students may have a different way of communicating which can lead to conflict with their teachers. Current studies suggest that African American students are sent to the office and then given consequences by administrators that are different from children in other groups. This is differential selection and differential processing to the detriment of one group of students.

Discrimination is an important factor in determining ethnic differences in externalizing behaviors. For example, both gender and racial discrimination affect African American adolescents. In one study, African American boys reported more gender discrimination than girls but both boys and girls were found to be well aware of the fact that both gender and racial discrimination were operating in their environments (Cogburn, Chavous, & Griffin, 2011). These experiences affected boys' emotional adjustment and academic performance. Racial discrimination affected girls' self-esteem and depressive feelings more than their school performance. In the case of African American adolescents, not having strong connections with school is somewhat associated with externalizing behaviors (Mrug & Windle, 2008). All of this is interesting, when major differences in school behaviors between African American and White students have not been found. For example, the literature suggests that African American students are less likely to experiment with substances in middle school than their white peers (Thompson et al., 2011).

A study of Puerto Rican adolescents examining rates of disruptive behavior disorders determined that rates of disorders increased with age for girls but not boys in New York City (Bird et al., 2006). Disruptive behavior disorders in this group were often seen associated with ADHD. The precursors of disruptive behaviors among these adolescents were low parental warmth, low parental approval, conflicts in peer relationships, and parental reports of aggressive behavior when the students were toddlers.

The Different Developmental Pathways of Externalizing Behaviors

Behavior problems during childhood predict continuing difficulties including substance abuse, underachievement, risk of dropping out of schools, and antisocial acting out. Studies suggest that there are significant numbers of children exhibiting externalizing behaviors and to a high degree in early childhood, although there is notable variability in regard to persistence of externalizing behaviors for subgroups of children (Guttmannova et al., 2007). In general, however, when externalizing behaviors are seen early on, children tend to be at risk for continued difficulties (Hill, Degnan, Calkins, & Keane, 2006). When young children exhibit externalizing behaviors these behaviors tend to include aggression, opposition, and destructive behaviors.

Although most young children improve in coping skills, and in ability to deal with situations that might otherwise trigger misbehavior as they get older, some children do not improve. In fact, researchers have proposed a number of behavioral trajectories in children (Hill et al., 2006). One group of children is described as showing high initial externalizing behaviors and maintaining this level of misbehavior. Another group with high levels of externalizing behavior improved. A third group exhibited moderate levels of externalizing behavior and improved. A fourth group continued to show both initial and also continuing low levels of externalizing behavior. Studies of trajectories may not adequately reflect girls or minorities, and may differ according to age group (Rappaport & Thomas, 2004). Hill and colleagues found that lower SES placed boys, but not girls, at risk for exhibiting high levels of externalizing behaviors and maintaining those behaviors. Girls, but not boys, between ages 2 and 5 years, who improved in emotion regulation, decreased their externalizing behaviors. Inattention was a risk factor for higher levels of externalizing behavior for both boys and girls in early childhood, but especially for girls.

Multicultural studies suggest a distinction between proactive and reactive aggression (Rappaport & Thomas, 2004). When students act proactively, they are looking for rewards and dominance. When they are aggressive in reaction to perceived threat, they are exhibiting reactive aggression. Additionally, reactive aggression is triggered by impulsive and explosive anger. Students may feel irritable and hyperaroused. In proactive aggression, information processing may be involved. This distinction may be helpful in that children exhibiting reactive aggression may be helped with cognitive behavioral therapy, whereas those exhibiting proactive aggression need increased monitoring and consistent consequences.

Berkout et al. (2011) describe several trajectories of negative behaviors. One trajectory involved bullying, progressing to physical aggression, and finally violent offending. This described boys only. A second trajectory progressed from lying and shop-lifting, to vandalism and offenses against property rights. For this trajectory, boys also were involved with deviant peers. Girls needed the additional variable of poor monitoring by parents. A third trajectory for boys progressed from stubbornness to illegal behaviors.

Thompson et al. (2011) identified five trajectories of externalizing behaviors. These were low, low-medium, moderate, increasing to high, and high. The increasing-high group exhibited a moderately low level of behavior problems when they were 4 years old, but increased in externalizing behaviors quickly. By age 10 years this group was exhibiting more negative behaviors than the high externalizing group. Externalizing behaviors were found to be relatively stable during childhood, except for one subgroup, with most children exhibiting only low levels of behaviors. 83.3 % of children in the study did not change their behaviors significantly. Students in the moderate, or increasing-high externalizing group, were at risk for delinquent behaviors. Participants of the high group were at risk for substance abuse. Those with a consistently high or increasingly high degree of externalizing behaviors were most likely to engage in risk-taking behaviors later on.

Bullying

Concerns about externalizing behaviors in schools have focused primarily on violence prevention for many years but since 2000, the focus of research and the literature has shifted to a subtype of aggression in which there is an imbalance of power. In this case a more powerful student aggresses toward a less powerful student

(Guerra, Williams, & Sadek, 2011). This behavior, well known as bullying, is often repeated against a victim and is considered a pervasive behavior. The previous focus on general aggression has shifted to bullying prevention with federal and state mandates to implement prevention programs to deal with bullying.

Nansel's seminal study (2001) of 15,686 children in grades 6–10, surveyed throughout the United States, determined that 29.95 % of students reported that they were involved in bullying in one way or another. A smaller sample of 1,985 Latino and African American students in sixth grade, from 11 low SES urban schools, described a high rate of bullying. As many as 22 % of students were identified as bullies (Juvonen, Graham, & Schuster, 2003). These "bullies" had high social standing among peers. Students both bullied and also victimized (bully victims) had the highest rate of behavior problems as well as school and peer relationship difficulties. The Monitoring the Future (MTF) project involves a nationally representative study of adolescents. Each year, eighth, tenth, and twelfth grade students take a survey addressing a variety of issues. The report addressed here included more than 50,000 12th graders interviewed from 1989 to 2009 (Johnston, Bachman, O'Malley, & Schulenberg, 2010). Although the proportion of 12th graders exposed to bullying decreased over the long term, there was an upsurge in bullying exposure between 2002 and 2009. Students from single-parent and no-parent families, students with poor school performance, students with less-educated fathers, and students with African American backgrounds were especially targeted. Intense victimization was higher for girls in this study.

Bullying behaviors begin very early, probably as early as when children first form groups. It increases from elementary to middle school (Guerra & Williams, 2010). A high level of bullying continues into secondary school for verbal bullying and cyberbullying. Physical bullying decreases once students are in high school. The average incidence of bullying and bystander behavior that is *not helpful* for stopping bullying occurs at about the same level in rural districts as in city schools. It is about the same in schools with a dominant ethnic or racial group of students as it is in diverse schools. And, it is about the same in schools in which many students are eligible for free or reduced lunch as it is in schools with lower numbers of eligible students.

Being a victim of bullying in the first few years of school can result in early adjustment difficulties (Arseneault et al., 2006). Students who were victimized at 5 years of age had more internalizing issues by the time they were 7 years of age, although girls who were victimized also exhibited externalizing behaviors. Children who were both victims and bullies had more internalizing and externalizing problems by the time these students were 7 years of age. Many researchers have looked at the consequences of having been bullied. The consequences of bullying can be profound. Consequences range from psychosomatic problems (Gini & Pozzoli, 2009) to suicidal thoughts (Winsper, Lereya, Zanarini, & Wolke, 2012). Children bullied between 4 and 10 years of age are at risk for suicidal ideation by age 10 or 12 years. This is the case for both victims and bully/victims. Chronic victims and bully/victims are at elevated risk for self-injurious behaviors. In a study of 6,042 children in England, the group of children bullied over long periods of time had the highest prevalence of suicidal ideology and self-harm. Bully/victims have been found to exhibit three times the risk of suicidal ideation. There is correlational data to support long-term effects of having been bullied (Staubli & Killias, 2011). One retrospective study found that children bullied before age 12 were still negatively affected when in young adulthood.

Bullies do not do well either. Bullies have been found to lack moral compassion (Gini, Pozzoli, & Hauser, 2011). A longitudinal study of 557 German children involved in bullying determined effects 5 years later. There were small but highly significant correlations between bullying and later antisocial behaviors. Bullies are often involved in other problem behaviors such as drinking alcohol and smoking. They experience school adjustment issues (Nansel et al., 2001). Bully/victims have the greatest adjustment difficulties and the worst outcomes including social isolation and academic difficulties. This group is at high risk.

Bullying is often a strategy to establish status in the peer culture. Bullying prevention programs need to teach students how to negotiate peer networks without resorting to bullying (Guerra & Williams, 2010). An interesting study was conducted with 2,678 school-aged students in grades 5, 8, and 11 as part of a 3-year bullying prevention initiative in Colorado (Guerra et al., 2011). Students in 21 elementary schools, 30 middle schools, and 8 high schools were surveyed. Additional students who were not surveyed participated in focus groups to explore prevalence and variability of bullying. Through this research effort, it was clear that many children bully others occasionally, while a smaller group of students are more regularly engaged in bullying. Contrary to many studies with cross-sectional designs, this study attempted to determine how bullying changes over a year's time in a school. The survey data indicated that as students perceived their school climate in an increasingly negative manner student self-esteem declined. A general decrease in self-esteem predicted an increase in victimization over a school year. Increases in normative beliefs supporting bullying predicted an increase in bullying as the year progressed. Students in schools or grade levels that considered bullying acceptable were more likely to bully others. When students perceived their school climate positively, bullying and victimization decreased. This is important for school-based mental health practitioners planning interventions. The school climate needs to be addressed in prevention efforts.

Older students shared that bullying was "entertaining." Students related bullying to sexuality (Guerra et al., 2011). All middle school and high school students shared that bullying was associated with popularity and sexuality through the semi-structured focus groups. Male bullies were described as increasing their status by overpowering other boys and by lowering the status of girls by negatively labeling them. Adolescent girls considered bullying as a way to eliminate competition for attractive boys through gossip, rumors, cell phones, the Internet, and exclusion. Researchers reviewed their findings with teachers and students as a way to determine the validity of their conclusions. Given the fact that bullying is so common, the researchers recommended use of universal programming as a first step in reducing bullying. Additionally they recommended diversity training, addressing the sexualized nature of bullying in adolescence, and working with both boys and girls together when providing preventive programming.

Considering bullying from a social network perspective is intriguing. Faris and Felmlee (2011) suggest that peer status can be viewed as "social network central-ity." When the goal of an adolescent is to reach the center of her/his social network or once the adolescent is there, aggressive behaviors increase to maintain one's central position. Data was collected from 3,772 adolescents in grades 8, 9, and 10 across 19 schools in North Carolina. Researchers found that the more popular the student, the greater likelihood that the student would be involved in aggressive behaviors. Changes in popularity, described as a *shift in centrality*, increased aggres-sion in general. This was particularly the case for students who were already popu-lar and were vying for top positions in their group. The student(s) at the top no longer needed to be aggressive, but those *near* the top were 38 % more aggressive than those at the bottom of the network. As peer status increased, aggression and competition increased. Even in schools in which boys and girls were separated, some students who moved toward the center of their social network became particu-larly aggressive toward students of the same sex.

A current and increasing interest in bullying behaviors has to do with the Internet or cyberbullying. School-aged students are more and more involved in using the Internet for bullying. In Colorado, a large survey of students in grades 5, 8, and 11 completed questionnaires that included items to address Internet bullying (Williams & Guerra, 2007). Researchers determined that Internet bullying was at its highest point among middle school students, with no differences between boys and girls. Internet bullying was related to approval of bullying, a negative school climate, and negative peer support, in the same way as other types of bullying. The Growing Up with Media Survey is a national cross-sectional survey of 1,588 students, 10–15 years of age, measuring Internet harassment among other behaviors. Sixty-four per-cent of children experiencing Internet harassment reported that they were not bul-lied in school. Data from the Health Behavior in School-Aged Children (HBSC) 2005 Survey involving a nationally representative sample of students in grades 6–10 determined that school bullying was more prevalent than cyberbullying (Wang, Iannotti, & Nansel, 2009).

A survey of 20,406 high school students in Massachusetts identified that 59.7 % of students who experienced cyberbullying were also bullied in school. Only 36.3 % of students bullied in school were victimized by cyberbullying (Schneider, O'Donnell, Stueve, & Coulter, 2012). Students experiencing both types of bullying reported the most distress. Being victimized by either form of bullying produced elevated distress. More students reported school bullying than cyberbullying (25.9 % reported school bulling over the past 12 months as compared to 15.8 % reporting cyberbullying). Olweus, seminal researcher of bullying behavior, has crit-icized the research reporting prevalence of cyberbullying (Olweus, 2012). He reports data from several large studies in the United States and in Norway, to the effect that students involved in cyberbullying are involved in school bullying for the most part and cyberbullying has not resulted in "new" victims or bullies. When a student experienced both types of bullying, the added effect from cyberbullying is not significant according to Olweus. Cyberbullying depends on student access to computers and to lack of supervision of children and adolescents, as well as to how data is collected. For these reasons, prevalence data can be confusing. International studies are seen with increasing frequency on the prevalence of cyberbullying, and on issues related to bullying and cyberbullying.

Using data from the 2009 Youth Risk Behavior Survey, researchers found when girls or boys, who are bullied in school, are also depressed, they are at risk for suicide attempts (Bauman, Toomey, & Walker, 2013). The mediating role of depression (but not suicide attempts) did not hold for boys in cyberbullying, although it held for girls. Certainly there needs to be more preventive work conducted with high school students along with detection of depression in students experiencing bullying. Students targeted online have been found to be eight times more likely to report bringing a weapon to school in the previous month (Ybarra, Diener-West, & Leaf, 2007).

Prevention of Bullying Behaviors

Efforts to prevent bullying, specifically, have resulted in a large number of programs and curricula. Many programs are based on the work of Olweus (1993), who developed a well-researched whole-school program in Norway (Felix & Furlong, 2008).

The *Olweus Bullying Prevention Program* (OBPPP) was first evaluated in a longitudinal study involving 2,500 students in 1985. The goals included reducing bullying, preventing new bullying problems, and improving peer relations by restructuring the school environment. The program addressed the behaviors of adults by improving school discipline and modeling positive behaviors. The first evaluation of the program resulted in a reduction of victimization by 62 %, and bullying by 33 % (Olweus, 1994). After 2 years of implementation, bullying decreased by 50 %. Teachers fully implementing classroom rules, classroom meetings, and using role-play had more success in reducing bullying than when the program was not fully implemented. School climate improved as well. As the program has been used more widely and overtime, implementation has varied widely (Olweus & Limber, 2010). In order for the program to work in the United States, cultural adaptations have been needed to include establishment of a coordinating committee, and teacher training. Eight components are considered critical. A coordinating committee, staff training, a questionnaire, staff discussion groups, adoption of specific rules about bullying, a supervisory system, a kick-off event, parent involvement, posted rules in classrooms, classroom meetings, serious talks with students involved and their parents, and involvement of the community are core program components. Studies using extended cohorts designs have shown positive results. US studies have evaluated the effectiveness of the OBPP in both elementary and middle school populations.

A collaborative of agencies and researchers selected OBPP to implement in Philadelphia, PA. When implemented with fidelity, the OBPP showed modest evidence of success. The program required effort to implement. Particularly important was posting school rules, targeting problem areas of the schools, staff training, classroom meetings, and positive incentives. In addition a coordinating committee and needs assessment were determined to be necessary.

There are many additional programs that have some research support. The Alberti Center for Bullying Abuse Prevention prepared a guide focusing specifically on school-based bullying prevention programs. The guide selected programs that focused on universal school-based bullying prevention alone or combined with social–emotional skills, programs based on solid research and theory, programs that were researched and evaluated in the United States, programs published by at least one peer-reviewed publication, or programs that were part of a comprehensive evaluation report (Serwacki & Nickerson, 2012). Eight programs met the criteria. The eight listed were:

- *Al's Pals*: *Kids Making Healthy Choices*, for prekindergarten and first grade
- *Bully Busters*, for kindergarten through eighth grade students
- *Bully prevention in Positive Behavioral Interventions and Supports*, for elementary and middle school
- *Bully-Proofing Your School* for prekindergarten through twelfth grade
- *Creating a Safe School* for sixth through twelfth grades
- *Get Real About Violence* for kindergarten through twelfth grade
- *OBPPP* for kindergarten through eighth grade
- *Second Step: A Violence Prevention Curriculum*, for prekindergarten through eighth grade students

Some states also list programs that they feel are evidence-based.

School-based practitioners need to carefully research, evaluate, and match a program to their local school needs and resources. In addition, it is important to stay on top of the research as new programs, new studies, and new findings may alter original decisions that are made when selecting a program. Although a program may be successful in highly controlled research studies, it may not work in the "real" world where there is competition for limited resources or the needs of the local population may be different. Controlling all variables may be extremely challenging such as guaranteeing an adult will respond if a child complains of bullying (Black, Washington, Trent, Harner, & Pollock, 2010).

Four meta-analyses exploring the effectiveness of bullying prevention programs in schools have been published with mixed results. Vreeman and Carroll (2007) reviewed school-based bullying prevention interventions that had been carefully evaluated looking for direct and indirect outcome measures around bullying issues. They determined that many interventions did decrease bullying. Better results were identified in interventions that involved multiple disciplines. Curriculum interventions alone were less successful, and indirect efforts did not produce consistent effects. The same year Ferguson, Miguel, Kilburn, and Sanchez (2007) also published a meta-analysis. This meta-analysis of school-based bullying prevention programs showed a significant prevention effect, although the effect was not strong enough to meet criteria for *practical* significance. When programs targeted at-risk students, the effects were slightly better. The authors concluded that, in general, bullying prevention programs have an effect that is hard to discern.

Merrell, Gueldner, Ross, and Isava (2008) conducted a meta-analytic study of bullying prevention interventions. They found that the studies they reviewed had positive effects for only one-third of the variables included in the studies. Most studies evidenced no meaningful change in outcomes. From this analysis, Merrell et al. concluded that bullying prevention efforts produced "modest positive outcomes." Specifically, the changes that occurred tended to be in regard to knowledge about bullying and attitudes toward bullying, rather than influencing bullying behaviors.

Farrington and Ttofi (2009) conducted a fourth meta-analysis of the effectiveness of bullying prevention programs. These researchers conducted a more extensive literature search than in the previous efforts, including only the programs that were directly focused on bullying outcomes rather than on aggression *and* bullying. They looked at research designs that included randomized studies, experimental–control studies with before and after measures, other experimental–control comparison studies, and quasi-experimental age-cohort study designs comparing students of the same age after the prevention program with students of the same age before the intervention in the same school. This meta-analysis indicated that school-based anti-bullying programs *were effective* in reducing a student's chance of "being bullied." Generally bullying was reduced by 20–23 %. Victimization was reduced on average by 17–20 %. Interestingly, effects were greatest in studies using the age-cohort designs and were lowest in the studies using randomized designs. In some of the research using randomized designs only three to seven schools were randomly assigned. Farrington and Ttofi concluded that the results of their meta-analysis were "encouraging."

Researchers were particularly interested in which elements of bullying prevention programs resulted in various outcomes (Farrington & Ttofi, 2009). Decreases in both bullying and victimization were found in programs that included parent training or parent meetings, discipline of incidents, for longer program duration (number of days) and stronger program intensity (number of hours). Programs need to be implemented over time and be intensive to reduce bullying in schools. Older programs and those in which measures were taken as frequently as twice per month worked better. When school staff members supervise the playground, results of programs improve. It appears that whole-school programs reduce bullying but not being bullied. Researchers point out that the way bullying is measured affects outcomes and more frequent assessment is needed. In addition, bullying needs to be carefully defined, and research designs need to be improved to avoid contamination of control students by experimental students.

Positive Behavior Interventions and Supports

Given the common concerns about school behaviors and the fact that estimates of lost instructional time are as high as 80 %, a school-wide effort to reduce problem behaviors is considered to be critical (Sullivan, Long, & Kucera, 2011). Many of the problems associated with school discipline can be ameliorated when schools use school-wide preventive strategies involving a multicomponent and multi-layered approach. The overarching goal of school-wide prevention efforts to deal with inappropriate and dangerous behavior is to make the learning climate more positive so that all students can be successful socially and academically, and teachers have adequate teaching time (Flannery, Sugai, & Anderson, 2009).

Positive behavior interventions and supports (PBIS) or school-wide positive behavior support (SW-PBIS) is a *systems* approach to improve school culture. This makes it more likely that all students will be academically and socially successful (Horner et al., 2009). The foundation for this approach is the use of applied behavior analysis school-wide to improve school success for all children (Utley, Kozleski, Smith, & Draper, 2002). Additional theoretical influences include social learning theory and organizational theory (Sullivan et al., 2011). The use of SW-PBIS in schools is a positive alternative to popular but ineffective approaches such as zero tolerance, and other restrictive and punitive approaches. Punitive practices such as zero tolerance and expulsion have little impact on student behavior. SW-PBIS proponents recommend schools chose outcomes, data practices, and systems that fit their particular school (Simonsen, Sugai, & Negron, 2008). Meaningful outcomes for all students are identified and data is collected. Practices include rules, teaching skills, and a school-wide reinforcement system. Additional behavior supports for students having difficulty are put in place along with data collection procedures including office referrals, a point system, and other measures. The third (tertiary) prevention level of the system includes data collection and individualized behavioral plans. The key is support for all students across all settings. A systems coach is identified and staff members are trained well.

SW-PBIS is implemented at all three levels or tiers (Horner et al., 2009). Tier 1, the primary prevention level, includes work by classroom teachers teaching, monitoring, and rewarding the behavioral rules and consequences that have been set in place and published school-wide. Data about student behaviors is collected in an ongoing manner and the data is used to make important decisions. Students are also expected to help support appropriate behaviors of peers. All members of the school must be invested in preventing problematic behaviors. Responses to negative behavior of a particular student, or of groups of students, are addressed according to previously agreed upon actions, which may involve structural changes or individual re-teaching of appropriate behaviors. In addition to primary prevention, secondary prevention practices are established involving interventions for students at risk, and tertiary individualized strategies for problem students based on functional behavioral assessment. Implementation of SW-PBIS typically takes ±3 years of staff training, and school-wide efforts to change the school culture. SW-PBIS has been implemented with success in elementary schools, middle schools, and high schools, although less often at the high school level (Flannery et al., 2009). Importantly there is data to indicate that SW-PBIS can be sustained in schools in which it has been successfully implemented. In some schools SW-PBIS has been sustained for almost a decade (Horner et al., 2009). Outcome studies indicate that SW-PBIS has resulted in significant behavioral and social gains, and, of importance, gains in academic areas.

Horner et al. (2009) were interested in the effectiveness of SW-PBIS when implemented by school staff at the elementary level. They involved 30 schools in a treatment group and 23 schools in a delay group in two states (Hawaii and Illinois).

State personnel provide training and technical assistance. SW-PBOS was implemented with fidelity over a 3-year period. Not only were the experimental schools seen as safer, but third-grade reading improved as well. This demonstrated the effect of improved school organization, school climate, and discipline practices on academics.

A 5-year longitudinal randomized controlled effectiveness trial of SW-PBIS conducted in 37 elementary schools indicated that staff training resulted in implementation with high fidelity (Bradshaw, Mitchell, & Leaf, 2009). Importantly this study resulted in significant reductions in both exclusion of students through suspensions, and office referrals for inappropriate and dangerous behavior. The impact of SW-PBIS on school organizational health was also examined in this study (Bradshaw, Koth, Bevans, Ialongo, & Leaf, 2008). School staff members were asked to report on the school's overall organizational health over a 3-year period. The 2,507 school staff members felt that SW-PBIS had had a significant effect not only on the health of the organization but also on staff affiliation. SW-PBIS implementation was measured using the School-wide Evaluation Tool to collect data over 3 years for 21 schools randomly assigned to receive training, and 16 schools that did not receive training. Trained schools implemented PBIS at significantly better levels (Bradshaw, Reinke, Brown, Bevans, & Leaf, 2008).

State departments of education and local school systems are increasingly interested in implementing SW-PBIS. Iowa is implementing SW-PBIS statewide with promising results (Mass-Galloway, Panyan, Smith, & Wessendorf, 2008). New Hampshire has started a statewide systems change involving SW-PBIS. Early efforts resulted in a reduction of 6,010 office referrals for discipline and 1,032 for suspensions. Middle and high schools benefitted most. School-wide gains in math have been found in the majority of schools who carefully implemented SW-PBIS (Muscott, Mann, & LeBrun, 2008). The state of Maryland has developed a model and collected both summative and formative evaluation data from 467 schools that were trained to implement the model. Researchers determined that the structure that was developed for implementation promoted high-fidelity implementation (Barrett, Bradshaw, & Lewis-Palmer, 2008). Illinois is implementing SW-PBIS and early results indicate that strong implementation fidelity had the effect not only of improved social outcomes but also of additionally improved outcomes in math (Simonsen et al., 2012).

An interesting study looked at the impact of SW-PBIS on bullying (Waasdorp, Bradshaw, & Leaf, 2012). Data was collected involving 12,344 students in 37 Maryland elementary schools in a 4-year trial. 45.1 % of students were African American. Teacher reports indicated that students in the schools implementing SW-PBIS reported decreased bullying and peer rejections. The effects were stronger for younger students participating in SW-PBIS. The expected and typical increase in bullying and peer rejection at middle school was reduced. The study was unable to identify which elements of SW-PBIS accounted for the reduced risk for bullying behaviors. However, given that SW-PBIS does not typically target bullying, if specific lessons relating to bullying were added to SW-PBIS, the effect might be stronger.

Management of the school playground is a specific problem that has attracted researchers. Too many students, too few adults, adults who have not been trained, and a space that is too large to effectively monitor children contribute to inappropriate behaviors at recess. A study examined the results of a plan developed by a behavior support team to reduce behavioral incidents on the playground (Todd, Horner, Anderson, & Spriggs, 2002). Systems level school improvement goals, team management, and data-based decision making were involved to support the changes implemented at recess. Not only were changes successful in reducing inappropriate behaviors but school climate improved, and staff satisfaction increased. Lewis, Powers, Kely, and Newcomer (2002) looked at the effects of directly teaching playground behaviors, along with group contingencies, in a school using SW-PBIS. The frequency of problem behaviors decreased across three recess periods. Office disciplinary referrals in an elementary school in Oregon showed that 46 % of all behavior problems were taking place on the playground (Leedy, Bates, & Safran, 2004). Again, using a systems-based approach, practicing and reviewing appropriate recess behavior resulted in a 78 % decrease from baseline data.

Researchers have additionally examined how to apply a cost analysis to the use of SW-PBIS (Blonigen et al., 2008). Barriers to implementing SW-PBIS (Lohrmann, Forman, Martin, & Palmieri, 2008) have been investigated. Use of office discipline referrals (ODRs) to collect data (Spaulding et al., 2010) has been examined. SW-PBIS at the preschool level has been explored (Frey, Park, Browne-Ferrigno, & Korfhage, 2010).

ODRs are easy to collect and can be used to measure progress in use of SW-PBIS as school discipline improves. When ODRs are examined they tend to show that they involve child–child problems at the elementary school level and adult–child problems in middle school. At the high school level they are more likely generated when students skip school or are chronically late. SW-PBIS proponents and researchers have generated tools for school districts to use when implementing SW-PBIS, making it easier to implement (George & Kincaid, 2008).

SW-PBIS researchers have also looked carefully at disproportionality in discipline. One of the strongest strategies for identifying whether or not a school district may need to rethink their policy and procedures is to disaggregate discipline data. The Relative Rate Index (RRI) is a measure of disproportionality recommended by the office of Juvenile Justice and Delinquency Prevention (OJJDP: http://www.ojjdp.gov). School teams can total the number of each group of students by race/ethnicity in the school district. For each group, divide the number excluded by suspension or expulsion by the number enrolled. Then, divide the rate for each minority group by the rate for White students. Tobin and Vincent (2010) examined the data collected by schools that were able to reduce their discipline gap, and reported the top ten strategies of the top ten schools. The three most common strategies involved regular chances for improving staff skills in active supervision, quarterly evaluation of data, and booster training for students depending on the data collected. The remaining strategies were used equally often by four of the ten schools. These included involving family and/or community when it made sense to do so, training on positive parenting strategies for parents, and teaching expected behaviors in areas other than the classroom. Additional strategies mentioned by some of the schools included use of consistent consequences, continuing instruction when negative behavior occurred, developing procedures for emergencies, and a budget for the school-wide support team.

Secondary Prevention Strategies

A secondary prevention effort often connected to SW-PBIS is *Check & Connect* (Christenson, Stout, & Pohl, 2012), a manualized prevention program. The program has two components. The "check" component is designed to assess the engagement of a student in an ongoing basis by closely monitoring the student's attendance, behavior, grades, and credits. The "connect" component involves giving the student attention, partnering with teachers and the family, and partnering with community services, if the student is involved with a community agency. A monitor implements the program with a caseload of students. The monitor meets with students once a week at the elementary level, and twice a month at the secondary level. The monitor and student discuss progress made to date. They problem-solve when there are challenges. Sinclair, Christenson, Evelo, and Hurley (1998) explored the efficacy of the program using a randomized controlled trial with students participating from Minneapolis secondary schools. Students who received *Check & Connect* in seventh and eighth grades, and continued to receive the program in ninth grade, were significantly less likely to drop out of school by the end of the first follow-up year. Students also earned significantly more credits toward graduation than control students. Currently, a number of studies are underway to further explore the efficacy of the program through the American Institutes for Research at the University of Minnesota.

The *Check, Connect, and Expect* (CCE) program (Cheney et al., 2010) combines the *Check & Connect* program just described, and the Behavior Education Program (Crone, Horner, & Hawken, 2004), also known as *Check-in, Check-out*. Both programs utilize supervision of targeted children daily, with monitoring and coaching. Both include frequent feedback about functioning in the school environment. Both include reinforcement, connection with an adult role model, and skills training and/or problem solving when needed. Both are promising programs. About 70 % of students improve behavior and do not develop further problems using CCE. Preliminary studies indicate that CCE prevents further difficulties and less than 20 % of students require tertiary prevention services.

Parent Training

Parent training is considered an effective prevention tool for reducing externalizing behaviors in children. Parent training involves direct instruction for parents so that they actively acquire skills (CDC, 2009). Skills are taught to parents using modeling, practicing skills through rehearsal or role-play, practicing skills with one's child, and homework. Training may include active role-playing, discussion, and watching videotapes demonstrating skills (Lochman, 2000). Outcomes include decreased rates of aggressive behaviors, lower rates of placements in special classes, and a decreased degree of severity of problem behaviors in children. Positive parenting improved as well.

Working with preschoolers to prevent the development of externalizing behaviors is both important and likely to be successful (Chang, 2009). Early identification of oppositional behavior, and also of negative conduct, is particularly important (Mrug & Windle, 2008). Because about 50 % of children exhibiting significant problems in behavior when they start school will demonstrate increasing behavior and academic difficulties as they progress through elementary school, helping parents of these children is critical (Brotman et al., 2011). Parenting practices can protect children, or can exacerbate misconduct, adding emphasis to the importance of including parents when planning preventive efforts. This is critical when planning secondary prevention for at-risk children who live in neighborhoods with deviant youngsters. An effort to increase "positive" parenting is important because this could prevent externalizing behaviors in children (Berkout et al., 2011).

Kaminski, Valle, Filene, and Boyle (2008) completed a meta-analysis of training programs for parents of young children. Their goal was to identify specific skills that work, along with how parents of young children might teach them effectively. The parenting skills that they identified that had better results included emotional communication and positive interaction skills. The discipline skills that were most effective in various programs to reducing externalizing behaviors included correct use of time out, responding consistently, and interacting positively with children. Whether teaching general parenting skills, or teaching specific skills for management, explicit instruction and practice with their child were more effective than simulating practice. When programs addressed other skills, externalizing behaviors did not decrease and in fact distracted parents from more effective practices.

In another meta-analytic study, Dretzke et al. (2009) conducted a review of randomized controlled studies involving students already in school. This analysis determined that parent-training programs were effective in changing inappropriate behaviors, although most of the studies were of short duration and the number of participants was not very large in any of the studies. Efforts to determine what might interfere with the success of parent training included critical or harsh parenting techniques, mothers' depression, substance abuse on the part of fathers, poor adjustment of the adult partners, and/or internalizing disorders in the children.

The efficacy of parent training is considered "established" (Bert, Farris, & Borkowski, 2008, p. 243).

The *Incredible Years* (IY) is a series of parent-training programs that have been demonstrated to work by various review groups (Broderick & Carroll, 2008; Letarte, Normandeau, & Allard, 2010; Webster-Stratton & Herman, 2010). The *BASIC* parent-training program, targeting four different age groups, teaches parents interactive play techniques and how to manage children's behavior "peacefully" (Webster-Stratton, 2000). The training program for parents of students 6–12 years is a multicultural program, which includes video vignettes utilizing age-appropriate diverse families, and children with several different temperaments. It features logical consequences, monitoring, and problem solving. The *ADVANCE* training deals with family risk factors and ways parents can support academics. The several programs each have a manual to facilitate implementation with fidelity. Studies indicate that IY has a positive impact on parenting skills and on parents' understanding of child behavior. Randomized controlled trials have shown that parents of White, Latino, African American, and also Asian families had positive outcomes. The programs run 18–20 weeks.

The IY parent-training program for the 2- to 8-year-old groups diagnosed with ODD or conduct disorder has been shown to be effective in seven randomized control group studies (Webster-Stratton & Herman, 2010). Program developers completed this group of studies. In addition, five independent research groups have published studies with existing staff. The IY parent-training program has been implemented utilizing a randomized controlled trial in an urban area to assist disadvantaged parents (McGilloway et al., 2012). Program results were seen up to 6 months later. The IY program has been successful for children with conduct disorders with comorbid ADHD (Jones, Daley, Hitchings, Bywater, & Eames, 2007) and also for families whose children were involved with a child protection service agency. Trained leaders in the UK implemented the Incredible Years BASIC parent program for 12 weeks and effects were maintained up to 18 months (Bywater et al., 2009). In addition, IY includes a child-training curriculum for children aged 3–7 years with conduct disorders and a teacher-training program. This universal school-based preventive curriculum has been demonstrated to be efficacious. Aggression was reduced at recess, children exhibited improved self-regulation and social competence, behaviors improved, and teachers used more positive teaching strategies (Webster-Stratton, Reid, & Stoolmiller, 2008; Webster-Stratton, Reinke, Herman, & Newcomer, 2011). As in all prevention interventions, children at greatest risk showed the most improvement. The intervention has worked equally well for preschool as with elementary school-aged students. IY can be integrated with positive behavior supports to facilitate the development of consistent environments between home and school (Webster-Stratton & Herman, 2010).

Prevention in Action Challenge: Locate Agencies Listing Evidence-Based Programs for Prevention of Risky Behaviors

Select a behavior in which you are interested and build a table to determine the agencies listing the programs that relate to the behavior. Consider programs to prevent:

Delinquency	Prevention of PTSD
Violence prevention	Prevention of harassment
Depression prevention	Dropout prevention
Preventing dating violence	Drug and alcohol abuse
Suicide prevention	Anxiety prevention
Obesity/eating disorders prevention	Prevention of cyberbullying

---

(continued)

(continued)

Locate several evidence-based programs (EBPs) to address one of these behaviors. List the several most promising programs and check to determine how many agencies list each of the programs.

Behavior:

List of EBPs	CASEL	BVP	DFSs	OJJDP	PPN	NREPP	Other

(CASEL) The Collaborative for Academic, Social, and Emotional Learning, http://www.casel.org/programs/selecting.php

(BVP) Center for the Study and Prevention of Violence, Blueprints for Violence Prevention, http://www.colorado.edu/cspv/blueprints/index.html

(DFSs) Exemplary and Promising Safe, Disciplined and Drug-Free Schools Programs, http://www.ed.gov/admins/lead/safety/exemplary01/index.html

(OJJDP) Office of Juvenile Justice and Delinquency Prevention Model Programs Guide, http://www.dsgonline.com/mpg2.5/mpg_index.htm

(PPN) Promising Practices Network on Children, Families and Communities, http://www.promisingpractices.net/programs.asp

(NREPP) Substance Abuse and Mental Health Services Administration's (SAMHSA's) National Registry of Evidence-Based Programs and Practices, http://nrepp.samhsa.gov/

Chapter 8
Social–Emotional Learning

As important as academic competence may be, children and adolescents also need to be able to interact with others in respectful ways, master good work habits and values, contribute to society, and be good citizens. Many educators and parents are in favor of a broader educational mission for our schools that includes social–emotional competence, character development, mental health, and involvement in one's community (Greenberg et al., 2003). Schools must do more than ever before, while at the same time dealing with a multitude of challenges as a result of a changing school population and limited resources. Many preventive efforts have been initiated in schools, but in the past they have not been linked to the school's mission and have been fragmented in their approach. Frustrated at the lack of success of preventive health *promotion* efforts, the Fetzer Institute, a nonprofit foundation focused on relationships between people, held an important meeting to address this concern. The term *social and emotional learning* (SEL) was first presented at the 1994 Fetzer Institute, which was designed to focus on disjointed efforts to improve children's well-being and positive interrelationships (Elbertson, Brackett, & Weissberg, 2010). One outcome of the Fetzer Institute was the formation of the Collaborative for Academic, Social, and Emotional Learning (CASEL). The goal of CASEL has been to establish evidence-based SEL programming preschool through high school. CASEL has become the guide to school-based SEL-preventive efforts. And, since 1990, SEL has become a major emphasis in American education (Hoffman, 2009).

In 1997, the original members of CASEL identified the skills which they felt would be the key skills that students would need (Elias & Weissberg, 2000). These skills included effective communication with others, willingness and skills to cooperate with others, empathy, self-awareness and optimism, goal setting and planning, problem solving, and a reflective approach to life. These and other skills have to do with relationships because school-based learning is relational. The importance of active learning was recognized early in the thinking of CASEL members. Active practices, such as role-playing, were considered critical. Practice with school staff and parents using cues, self-monitoring using checklists, and shared language throughout the entire school, and full integration into the general curriculum was considered essential

G.L. Macklem, *Preventive Mental Health at School: Evidence-Based Services for Students*,
DOI 10.1007/978-1-4614-8609-1_8, © Springer Science+Business Media New York 2014

for generalizing SEL skills. More than an isolated curriculum, SEL concepts, and skills must be part of all academic learning. Finally a caring school community was considered the best protection against social, emotional, and physical problems.

Students' academic achievement improves in schools in which there are caring relationships with peers and school staff members, and when they develop a strong sense of belonging (Elbertson et al., 2010). Elias and Weissberg believe that SEL could be an organizing and integrative framework for broader school prevention goals. SEL has been described as fitting nicely with other prevention work in schools to include SW-PBIS which fosters consistent expectations in the whole school, cooperative learning, differentiated instruction, and service learning (Elbertson et al., 2010). As long as there is a school-wide commitment, this type of integration would affect multiple outcomes.

The social–emotional domain is broader than simply behavior. The domain includes concepts such as affect, emotional resilience, social competence, and pro-social behavior (Merrell, 2002). This broader view addresses bigger problems through prevention programs, consultation, and interventions that affect the entire classroom. Class-wide and school-wide programs are now the preferred approach to addressing problems that affect students. When service delivery occurs on a class-wide or school-wide basis, children can remain in class. Service delivery to mixed groups, rather than pulling out students that are similar in poor skills, has advantages. Students have opportunities to model a wider range of appropriate behaviors and skills. The teacher remains as part of the intervention. The advantage here is that the teacher has the opportunity to help students generalize skills.

Kress and Elias (2006) point out that SEL is part of the popular discussion among researchers and practitioners. SEL has a strong base of interest. It has gained momentum because of an emphasis on emotion and spirituality, progress in brain research, and because SEL addresses what researchers consider mediators of academics. The push for evidence-based preventive interventions has moved SEL forward in educational circles.

Social–Emotional Competencies

SEL addresses five areas of social–emotional competence. These are self-awareness, self-management, social awareness, relationship skills, and responsible decision-making (Elias, O'Brien, & Weissberg, 2006). These are considered "core" SEL competencies (Weissberg & O'Brien, 2004). SEL competencies additionally include 17 skills and attitudes (Payton et al., 2000). These are organized into four groups: awareness of self and others, positive attitudes and values, responsible decision-making, and social interaction skills. Beyond this there are 11 program features which SEL researchers consider extremely important if implementation is to be successful. These include the design of the curriculum presented in classrooms, coordinating SEL into the larger system, teacher training and support, and program evaluation. An anachronism was developed to help educators understand what makes a program successful, S.A.F.E. The "S" stands for sequenced set of activities.

The "A" stands for active learning. The "F" stands for focus on developing personal and social skills. The "E" stands for explicit targeting of skills.

SEL instructional programs target social–emotional competence, but additionally SEL targets prevention of risky behavior such as substance abuse and violence (Greenberg et al., 2003). Some programs deal with volunteer service. Some combine academics and community service. Still others are multi-year and multicomponent, adding parent training and making connections with the local community. Those programs lasting 9 months, or more, have been more successful than shorter programs.

Theory Supporting SEL

The theory on which SEL programming is based suggests that learning takes place in the context of relationships. SEL skills and competencies impact academic functioning and success because students who participate cooperatively and actively in school learning activities, and have positive relationships with adults and peers, are more successful (Elbertson et al., 2010). Many prevention programs implemented in schools could be coordinated with school-wide SEL programming but in the past they have been implemented without an overarching plan. SEL offers an overall framework into which many school efforts can be coordinated. The SEL framework addresses school and class climate, SEL programming from K-12, and system-level planning and commitment. The model involves obtaining commitment from administrators and all stakeholders, a shared vision, assessment of school needs and resources, an action plan, staff training, curriculum implementation, family involvement, and program evaluations.

Lazarus and Sulkowski (2011) point out that SEL actually has a two-pronged approach. The first has to do with teaching and modeling SEL skills and practicing SEL skills in multi-environments. The second has to do with establishing a positive and caring school environment to support attachment and learning SEL skills. There is a reciprocal relationship between SEL skills and school climate (Elias et al., 2006, p. 11). Elias (2012) connects social–emotional learning and character development (SECD). He describes SECD as a set of skills and attitudes that become essential life habits. The same skills and habits mediate multiple outcomes. Elias recommends that every child receives at least one half hour of instruction in skills per week, as part of a comprehensive sequenced curriculum. Instruction would be provided by a trained educator, either a teacher or a counselor. It takes 2 years of cuing and prompting to internalize skills so all members of the school community must work together to guarantee that students will learn.

Need for SEL and Legislative Support

A serious effort is being made to improve the learning environment in schools, but unfortunately these efforts are being made without planning or a coordinated design involving the whole school or system (Elbertson et al., 2010). The strong demand for academic outcomes has focused efforts on performance of basic skills. The problem is that ignoring SEL is making it less likely that students' achievement will increase. SEL facilitates attendance, appropriate behavior, and engagement in learning. The focus on academic achievement alone interferes with acceptance of SEL programming. Educators and decision-makers need to understand the benefits of the SEL model. They need to understand the factors within a school that facilitate the integration of SEL efforts with other programming.

One factor that brings SEL into schools is legislation. In 2003, Illinois State Learning Standards integrated SEL into their curricula through the Children's Mental Health Act (Public Act 93-0495) (Elbertson et al., 2010). Illinois was the first state to design and adopt a comprehensive package of SEL principles, which have become part of the official state learning standards (Gordon, Ji, Mulhall, Shaw, & Weissberg, 2011). Schools must endorse sequential and developmentally appropriate skills training, along with coordinated implementation and ongoing professional development throughout a school system, if SEL programs are going to be effective. Skills must be reinforced throughout the environment and at home to generalize. Families and schools must work together in order for students to become competent and successful.

The Children's Mental Health Task Force made up of 100 organizations started the movement to promote a new approach to addressing the emotional well-being of children (Gordon et al., 2011). They produced a report consisting of a number of important recommendations that included creating a mandate for addressing SEL. This effort led to the passage of the Illinois Children's Mental Health Act. A committee worked with CASEL and other organizations to develop the SEL Learning Standards. Illinois stands as a model. Other states have begun a similar process such as Idaho and Pennsylvania. States in the USA came together to develop national standards for math and English language arts known as The Common Core Standards for Language Arts. Most states have adopted the national standards, which include SEL content. Individual school districts within states have some flexibility as long as they comply with the overall goals of the state standards (Dusenbury, Zadrazil, Mart, & Weissberg, 2011). CASEL recommends that every state has at least one standard for "personal" development and one standard for "social development." Illinois remained the only state with standards from K-12 as of 2011, but a number of states are moving toward development of SEL standards.

Complications and Impediments to Implementing SEL in Schools

Large-scale efforts to implement SEL programming in schools require considerable effort and time. This type of systemic change is challenging. It has not been easy for schools. Very few teachers or administrators have received preservice exposure to SEL programming or the skills necessary to implement this service (Elbertson et al., 2010). Various schools use different approaches for adopting, combining, and adapting SEL programming, some with unsatisfactory results. Schools may string a variety of programs together from elementary to middle and then to high school without thinking things through. The program content and teaching strategies may be poorly matched. When schools have limited resources and little time, they may implement a prevention curriculum on a short-term basis without sufficient staff training or monitoring (Weissberg & O'Brien, 2004). Schools that are implementing SEL program are not doing so with uniform quality (DeAngelis, 2010).

Overcoming time constraints, dealing with funding issues, and providing teacher training may be necessary in order to implement a number of SEL programs with fidelity (Elias, Bruene-Butler, Blum, & Schuyler, 1997). SEL programming can be integrated with existing efforts if curricula or programs are compatible and if the existing efforts are evidence-based and are working. Schools can start with a small pilot project to gather data to obtain funding. Teacher training can take place through staff development efforts with the support of staff already on board such as school psychologists.

Critics of SEL

In spite of the rapid growth of advocacy for SEL programming in schools, SEL is not without its critics. There is some objection to SEL on the basis of family privacy (Craig, 2007; DeAngelis, 2010). Some claim that SEL programs are too broad-based. Still others argue that the burden SEL programming places on teachers is too much.

Arguments with the evidence itself include the difficulty of determining the effectiveness of programs with enormous differences in design, goals, and methodology. Watson and Emory (2010) have expressed concerns about what they feel is a lack of consensus about exactly which of the SEL capabilities are essential, and how to measure them. Although overall findings from various meta-analytic studies demarcate the benefits of SEL programming, Duncan et al. (2007) presented an alternative point of view. This group of researchers conducted a meta-analysis of studies that related school-entry skills to later academic achievement. They concluded that attention skills, rather than either social skills or problem behavior, predicted achievement after ruling out knowledge and cognitive ability. However, these researchers conceded the idea that improvements in behavior and social skills might predict engagement, motivation, self-concept, or school adjustment. These are important school outcomes. An additional criticism of SEL is the fact that often, many programs are implemented simultaneously, so it is difficult to establish efficacy results (Hoffman, 2009). The average number of activities being implemented in schools simultaneously was 14 (Elbertson et al., 2010).

More than 200 types of classroom-based SEL programming have been implemented in schools across the USA (Hoffman, 2009). The rise of SEL programming has been in response to a behavioral crisis in our schools. However, Hoffman argued there had not enough large-scale independent evaluations of many of the SEL programs. Reviews of SEL programming included studies with questionable research designs.

Studies of sustainability were needed. The effects of SEL programs on promoting competencies was not yet clear. Further, programs taught skills rather than focusing on emotions, when "emotion" was considered by SEL advocates as the means to academic and social competency.

Hoffman (2009) argued that the SEL approach focuses on behavioral control strategies. This would lead implementers to attend to remediating deficits when SEL goals have to do with the relational aspects of classes and schools. Hoffman feels that the original ideals of SEL are not connected to the actual practices of SEL implementers. An example given was that a major focus of SEL programming is the regulation of negative and disruptive emotions. But, when teachers remove a child who is disruptive from class, this is not an emotionally responsive approach that would increase a child's sense of belonging. Hoffman additionally notes that in her mind SEL had not dealt with cultural diversity and the politics of power.

Problematic behaviors of children and adolescents are interrelated and complex (Weissberg & O'Brien, 2004). They develop over time. Problems such as drug use, bullying, sexual promiscuity, and school alienation can be addressed if preventive efforts are interrelated, coordinated, connected, and placed under one prevention umbrella. There is ample data to indicate that such efforts can be successful in schools. Given that there has been some criticism of the SEL movement, and that the drive to include SEL in general education is taking place in the USA, Great Britain, and Wales, it is vital to look at the research that has been published on the impact of SEL-preventive programming.

Impact of SEL Violence Prevention and Drug Prevention Programs

Meta-analyses are helpful in determining generic intervention approaches as well as distinct models (Wilson & Lipsey, 2007). Additionally a meta-analysis is helpful in determining the kinds of students who benefit most. A meta-analysis can identify the most effective programs. Nine meta-analyses have looked at the effects of SEL programming on behavior. These programs are discussed in order of publication because the studies available for meta-analysis depend on the time periods during which studies were reviewed and analyzed.

Tobler and Stratton (1997) completed a meta-analysis of 120 school-based prevention programs involving tobacco, marijuana, and alcohol use. Universal interactive programs for adolescents (including minority students) had significant effects when the intervention population was smaller in size. Implementation of larger programs is complex. Higher intensity, system-wide comprehensive programs that included not only restructuring of the school itself but also taught refusal skills, goal setting, assertiveness skills, coping skills, and communication skills were more successful than programs teaching different skills (reported in Greenberg et al., 2003). This analysis found that mental health practitioners had better results than when instruction was delivered by teachers.

Durlak and Wells (1997) reviewed 177 programs and reported that the average student participating in a program to prevent behavioral and social problems does better than 59–82 % of students in control groups. Greenberg, Domitrovich, and Bumbarger (2001) examined 34 universal and targeted studies that used quasi-experimental or randomized designs. They found that the best programs were multi-year designs, focused on multiple domains, addressed school climate, changed teachers' and parents' behaviors, developed strong home–school relationships, and reached into the community for support.

A meta-analytic study of 165 school-based experimental and quasi-experimental studies examined the connection between bonding to schools, social competency, academic performance, and problem behavior (Najaka, Gottfredson, & Wilson, 2001). When measures of competence were based on others' observations, rather than self-report, a strong relationship was found. Improvements in social competency skills and improvements in problem behavior worked together. When students' attachment to school improved, problems decreased. Interventions with social competency instruction significantly decreased delinquency, decreased alcohol and drug use, and decreased conduct problems. When students were more attached to school and more committed to learning, they behaved better so researchers recommended implementing prevention programs that would increase bonding to school.

Hahn et al. (2007) described 53 violence prevention programs implemented in schools. Some programs provided information about the causes of violence through discussion while other programs helped students to become more sociable. Still other programs were based on social learning theory (Bandura, 1977). Some involved the whole school in the program to change school climate. At the elementary level, programs tended to focus on disruptive behavior. In the upper grades programs tended to cover general violence or specific types of violence using additional skills training. Some programs included student peers or involved university teams. Of the 53 studies only seven had the strongest designs and were implemented with fidelity. For all grade levels, the median effect was a 15 % reduction in violent behavior for program participants (p. 6). All school-based antiviolence program approaches whether informational, cognitive/affective, or training social skills, were effective in reducing violent behavior. Programs were effective in lower SES or high crime areas. Programs were not equally effective in schools in which the student population was predominately minority, i.e., in schools in which the student population was more than 50 % African American, the effects were lower.

Wilson and Lipsey (2007) conducted a meta-analysis of 249 experimental and quasi-experimental studies of school-based SEL programs. They were also interested in programs designed to reduce aggressive behavior. Overall both universal and targeted school-based programs were effective. Most universal programs used cognitive approaches. Programs that also included a behavioral approach tended to be somewhat more effective. The decreases found in aggressive and disruptive behaviors were statistically significant. A 25–30 % reduction in inappropriate behaviors was estimated. Effects were greatest for at-risk students as is the case in most prevention programs. Effects were more significant for students from economically disadvantaged backgrounds. More comprehensive programs involving the entire schools were long-term and were not determined to be more effective in this study. Researchers speculated that this result might relate to the fact that over time programs become diluted. Selecting a program that school staff members feel would be easy to implement is critical.

Although most school-based drug prevention studies were completed in cities, Brown, Guo, Singer, Downes, and Brinales (2007) were interested in programs conducted in rural schools. Their meta-analysis determined a modest but consistent positive impact of drug prevention programs on later use. In addition, programs impacted level of use. Program approaches that worked well were interactive. Effects were stronger for students who had never used drugs. Results were stronger for marijuana compared to alcohol, tobacco, or inhalant use. Effects were most pronounced 6 months post-intervention and then declined. When school-based programs were evaluated to determine their effect on illicit drug use, another meta-analysis determined that successful programs were highly interactive, time intensive, and were delivered to all middle school students (Soole, Mazerolle, & Rombouts, 2008). Contrary to previous reports, booster sessions and multifaceted programs had little impact.

Yet another meta-analysis of 25 school-based randomized control trials was completed to determine effects on violent, aggressive behavior (Park-Higgerson, Perumean-Chaney, Bartolucci, Grimley, & Singh, 2008). Interventions with a single approach had a mild effect. Interventions focusing on at-risk older students reduced aggression. Non-theory-based interventions worked better. Because these results do not fit previous findings, the process of identifying program components that are effective is clearly complex.

SEL Programming Effects on Academics

If SEL programming is to be successfully implemented in schools, it must support the mission of schools. Advocates of SEL programming needed to demonstrate an effect of SEL programming on the academic achievement of students in order to convince school administrators of the value of SEL. There have been critically important reviews and meta-analyses conducted to demonstrate the connection between SEL and academic achievement.

In 2008, Payton and colleagues reported the results of three large-scale reviews of the literature on the impact of SEL programs at the elementary and middle school levels. The three studies involved 324,303 students. Results indicated that SEL programming was effective in school settings, in after-school settings, for children with and without problems, in grades K-8, and for racially and ethnically diverse children. SEL programming was effective in urban, rural, and suburban areas. Improvements were seen in SEL skills, attitudes, connection to school, behavior, and importantly, in academic success. Conduct and emotional problems decreased. When general education teaching staff, or mental health staff, implemented SEL curricula, they were as successful as when programs were implemented by research teams. This set of data indicated that academic performance of students improved by 11–17 percentile points.

Durlak, Weissberg, and Pachan (2010) examined SEL programs that occurred in part of a school year or after school hours and were supervised by adults. In all the programs examined, at least one goal was the development of personal or social skills. They found that programs had positive and statistically significant effect on the students who participated. Problem behaviors were reduced, self-perceptions improved, school bonding increased, attitudes and feelings improved, and prosocial behaviors increased. Not every program was successful. The successful programs were sequenced, used active interactive strategies, were focused, and teaching was explicit (S.A.F.E.). Test-scores improved by 12 percentile points.

A large-scale analysis of 213 school-based universal SEL programs showed that students participating in SEL programs demonstrated significantly better skills. This review focused on *multiple* outcomes as compared to single outcome studies. Improved attitudes and behaviors were demonstrated. A subset of studies showed an 11-percentile point gain in achievement (Durlack, Weissberg, Dymnicki, Taylor, & Schellinger, 2011, p. 405). When students function better socially and emotionally, and exhibit appropriate SEL skills, they are better adjusted in terms of attitudes about themselves and others. They exhibit increased prosocial behaviors and are less stressed. Unfortunately many studies reviewed did not collect follow-up data. Those studies that did collect outcome data determined that improvements were retained for 6 months or more, although gains were not as strong as immediately post-intervention. The largest effect sizes were for the specific SEL skills taught, i.e., ability to recognize emotions in oneself and others, stress-management, empathy for others, and problem-solving skills. Researchers found that either classroom teachers or school-based mental health staff could successfully implement programs without the outside help of university trainers. SEL programs were successful at elementary, middle, and high school levels, although more research is needed at the high school level. Programs were successful in urban areas, in rural schools, and in suburban schools. More research is needed in rural schools. This study did not find an advantage to multicomponent programs possibly because multicomponent programs are very complex and challenging to implement.

Durlack et al. (2011) suggested that programs must be well designed and well conducted. Implementation is a critical variable. In general, more successful youth programs are interactive in nature, use coaching and role-playing, and employ a set of structured activities to guide youth toward achievement of specific goals. This was the case in a meta-analysis of mentoring programs (DuBois, Holloway, Valentine, & Cooper, 2002), and also in the case of drug prevention programs (Tobler et al., 2000).

Team Considerations in SEL Programming

There are a number of issues that need to be considered when locating and selecting SEL programming for a given school system. It is critical to know the local system very well and the needs of the students and families within that system. It is critically important to look at what is being done already, what is working, and what is not working.

Once a school system determines that SEL programming would be relevant to the mission of the school, once a prevention team in a school has determined that the system is ready to make such a significant change, once a needs assessment clearly identifies the issues to be addressed and a baseline has been established, and once the administration and school staff members are onboard and willing to make the changes needed, a prevention team would be assigned the task of developing an overarching comprehensive plan. One aspect of this plan would involve the selection of a SEL program, or programs that could be combined, to address the needs of all students in the system, K-12. Addressing the needs of all students would involve establishing a school-wide or system-wide plan to include programming for students at the universal level, the targeted level, and the intensive level. Considerations when reviewing SEL programming include the developmental level addressed by programs, the evidence-base for programs, and whether or not the programming identified actually fits a given school system.

Program fit is extremely important (Small, Cooney, Eastman, & O'Connor, 2007). The program must match the values and culture of the student population and the local community. The goals and objectives of a program must match the goals of the school team. The school team will need to locate efficacy studies to determine whether or not the program has been successful with diverse populations of students. The evidence-base for the program and also the rigor of the program are critical because the program needs to be strong enough to address the risk factors identified in the student population. It is important to make sure that sufficient staff resources are available for implementing programming. Funding also needs to be addressed, i.e., grants, local funds and the proportion of special education monies that can be used for prevention. Different priorities and trade-offs may be necessary.

An interesting study was conducted to see if researchers could determine which *specific SEL* skills were related to social success. Both typical and clinic-referred multicultural elementary-level students from urban public schools participated in this study (McKown, Gumbiner, Russo, & Lipton, 2009). One important skill had to do with teaching students to "read" nonverbal behavior. Another had to do with the ability to share personal experiences and to interpret social information. Important skills for team members included the ability to describe problems, set social goals, generate various solutions, and decide what to do. Three domains of SEL skills, the ability to read social cues, to decide social situations, and to exhibit empathy along with the ability to self-regulate, predicted success. Because a range of SEL skills are needed, school teams want to look for programs teaching a variety of skills.

As the school prevention teams review various programs, they need to determine if positive outcomes have been found in similar communities. They need to determine if the risk factors are similar and need to match the local population in regard to age, race, ethnicity, socioeconomic status, and type of location with the efficacy study participants. They need to determine if the program fits the capacity of the school system including space, staff, and resources. They want to determine if the program goals and objectives match the values and practices of the local school system. Staffing requirements must be considered. Importantly, will the identified programs offer something different and better than what is already in place in the

Table 8.1 Program features which make implementation easier

- Programs need a clear framework of objectives and a clear sequence of activities
- Clear instructions for implementing strategies that actively involve students are critical
- A methodology for teachers or other staff to apply skills learned to other subject areas and physical areas of the school will help integrate learning throughout the school
- Easy-to-follow lesson plans make a huge difference to teachers and encourage implementation fidelity
- When assessment and monitoring tools are provided, this saves time
- Strategies for family involvement and developing school–community partnerships are extremely helpful
- Training for staff that will implement the programming makes a difference
- Training for staff beyond classroom teachers generalizes learning
- Availability of technical support is important
- Tools for outcome evaluation save time

Source: Payton et al. (2000)

local school system? The reason that these considerations are important is to prevent school teams from simply picking off agency lists of curricula or programs. Program selection requires hard work and responsible decision-making (Table 8.1).

A rating scale is available for school teams when reviewing programs (CASEL, 2003, p. 36). Because some evaluations of interventions have not shown treatment effects when programs are implemented in schools, it is important to choose programming that is empirically validated (Schoenfeld, Rutherford, Gable, & Rock, 2008). School teams should look for the strongest data available, keeping in mind:

- Research to determine the efficacy of SEL programs is ongoing
- It is necessary to stay on top of the research; and unfortunately
- The strongest program to address a particular issue may not fit a given school

A recent meta-analysis of 75 studies examined the effects of universal SEL and/ or behavior programs (Sklad, Diekstra, Ritter, Ben, & Gravesteijn, 2012). Some of the interventions examined could not be considered programs in that they did not have a manual, did not describe a sequence of components, did not train those implementing programs, and did not monitor or evaluate implementation. Studies of universal programs evaluated using experimental or quasi-experimental studies had positive effects, with the largest effects on social–emotional skills, attitudes toward self, and prosocial behavior. Researchers recommended that schools select SEL programs that have manuals, use a connected set of activities, use active learning strategies, and teach skills focused on SEL versus generally positive development. Programs with the right design and the right mix of variables will most likely be successful and produce good results. Programs can also be successful because of a particular target population, the approach, and the characteristics of the individuals implementing a program (Olds, 2003).

There are several tools that can be utilized when implementing SEL curricula in schools; the Beliefs in SEL Teacher Scale (Brackett, Reyes, Rivers, & Elbertson, 2009; Brackett, Reyes, Rivers, Elbertson, & Salovey, 2012) measuring comfort and commitment; and, the SEL Integration Scale (Collie, Shapka, & Perry, 2011, 2012), which helps school teams determine the degree to which SEL is integrated in the general program and the school.

There are huge differences in SEL curricula and programs. The various curricula have different constructs and different outcomes (Olds, 2003). The ways in which outcomes are measured differ as well, and some measures used for various programs are not of the same quality as others. This does not make a team's work easy. In order to get the best outcomes for the effort that it takes to put SEL programming in place it will be necessary to think of preventive work from preschool through grade 12 and to determine how the programs will fit, one with the others, so that a comprehensive school-wide or district-wide effort can be made to meet the needs of all children. To demonstrate the range of SEL curricula, a list of the various curricula mentioned in this textbook can be generated. This list does not cover all of the curricula that might be considered by a given school. For a more comprehensive list, the various rating agencies should be explored (Table 8.2).

SEL Programming at the Preschool Level

There are key social and emotional competencies needed at each developmental level, and programs that a school or school team might consider for implementation would need to address those competencies. Kindergarten teachers say that about half of their students have difficulty working in a group and about one-fifth of students have social skills weaknesses (Whitted, 2011). Teacher's response to behavior problems of children can be punitive, with particular consequences for African American children. SES and ethnicity influence teacher ratings of student behavior when these are compared to behavior ratings by observers who are not teaching in the classroom (Humphries, Keenan, & Wakschlag, 2012). For this reason, different raters should be used when evaluating the behavior of African American children. Humphries et al. did not find that urban African American preschool aged children exhibited different social–emotional behaviors than their peers. Recognizing this, and trying to correct it, is important for school-based mental health workers in that a strong student–teacher relationship is related to behavior problems.

Important aspects of SEL for young children if they are to successfully negotiate interactions with children their own age involves mastering developmental tasks associated with each stage of development (Denham & Weissberg, 2004). For example, preschoolers need to be able to interact positively as they move from their homes to playgroups, playgrounds, or preschool classrooms. Young children's social–emotional skills and their ability to self-regulate prepare them for public schooling (Liew & McTigue, 2010). When young children are able to do something they need to do, overcoming any urge to do something they might want to do or prefer to do, they are exhibiting *effortful control*. Effortful control is an important component of self-regulation. Early problems with self-regulation can be observed in aggressive behaviors, impulsivity, poor attention, or social reticence.

Table 8.2 SEL curricula and programs

- *The following list of SEL curricula and programs represent some of the wide range of curricula from which a school team might choose for responding to local needs*
- *Aban Aya Youth Project* (Flay et al., 2004)
- *Adolescent Coping with Stress Course* (Schultz & Mueller, 2007)
- *Adolescent Depression Awareness Program* (ADAP) (Swartz, 2011)
- *ALAS* (Rumberger & Larson, 1994)
- *All Stars* programs (Hansen, 1996)
- *Al's Pals* (Geller, 1999)
- *Beyondblue* (Spence et al., 2005)
- *Caring School Community* (http://www.devstu.org)
- *Check and Connect* (Lehrt, Johnson, Bremer, Cosio, & Thompson, 2004)
- *Check, Connect, and Expect* (CCE) program (Cheney et al., 2010)
- *Check-in, Check-out* (Crone, Horner, & Hawken, 2004)
- *Coca-Cola Valued Youth Program* (http://www.idra.org)
- *Cognitive Behavioral Intervention for Trauma in Schools* program (CBITS) (Jaycox, 2004)
- *Communities that Care* (Hawkins et al., 2009)
- *Coping Cat Program* (Kendall, 1994)
- *Coping Power Program* (Lochman, 2000)
- *Dina Dinosaur* (Webster-Stratton, 1990)
- *Early Risers* (August, Realmuto, Hektner, & Bloomquist, 2001)
- *Early Risers Skills for Success* (http://www.psychiatry.umn.edu)
- *Facing History and Ourselves* (http://www.facing.org)
- *Families and Schools Together* (FAST) (Kratochwill, McDonald, Levin, Bear-Tibbetts, & Demaray, 2004)
- *FAST Track* (CPPRG, 2011)
- *First Steps to Success* (Walker et al., 1997)
- *Friend to Friend* (Leff et al., 2007; Leff, Kupersmidt, & Power, 2003)
- *FRIENDS* program (Barrett, Lowry-Webster, & Holmes, 1999)
- *Giraffe Heroes Program* (Graham, 1999)
- *Good Behavior Game* (Embry, Staatemeier, Richardson, Lauger, & Mitich, 2003)
- *I Can Problem Solve* (Shure & Spivack, 1980, 1982)
- *Incredible Years* (Webster-Stratton, 1982)
- *Interpersonal Cognitive Problem Solving* (ICPS) (Shure & Spivack, 1988)
- *KidsMatter* (Dix, Slee, Lawson, & Keeves, 2012)
- *LifeSkills Training* (*LST*) (Botvin, 1996; Botvin, Baker, Botvin, Filazzola, & Millman, 1984)
- *Lions Quest* (http://www.lions-quest.org)
- New Hope Project (http://www.mdrc.org)
- *Not On Tobacco* (*NOT*) *Program* (Dino et al., 2001)
- *Open Circle* (Seigle, 2001)
- *PATHS* (Greenberg & Kusche, 1998)
- *PATHS to PAX* (Domitrovich, Bradshaw, et al., 2010)
- *Peacemaking Skills for Little Kids* (Schmidt & Friedman, 1988)
- *Penn Resiliency Program* (Gillham & Reivich, 2004)
- *Positive Action* (Flay & Slagel, 2006)
- *Preschool PATHS* (Domitrovich, Cortes, & Greenberg, 2001)
- *Problem Solving for Life* (Spence, Sheffield, & Donovan, 2003)
- *Project ALERT* (Ellickson, Bell, Thomas, Robyn, & Zellman, 1988)

(continued)

Table 8.2 (continued)

- *Project FLAVOR* (Johnson et al., 2007)
- *Planet Health* (http://www.planet-health.org)
- *Project Northland* (Komor et al., 2004)
- *Project Toward No Drug Abuse* (Sussman, Dent, & Stacy, 2002)
- *Promoting Alternative Thinking Strategies* (Kam, Greenberg, & Kusché, 2004; Riggs, Greenberg, Kusché, & Pentz, 2006)
- *Project Towards No Tobacco* (TNT) (Sussman, Dent, Stacy, Hodgson, et al., 1993)
- *Resolving Conflict Creatively Program* (DeJong, 1994)
- *Resourceful Adolescent Program* (RAP-A) (Shochet et al., 2001)
- *Responsive Classroom* (http://www.responsiveclassroom.org/)
- *Seattle Social Development Project* (SSDP) (David, von Cleve, & Catalano, 1991)
- *Second Step* (http://www.cfchildren.org)
- *Second Step Preschool/Kindergarten* (McMahon, Washburn, Felix, Yakin, & Childrey, 2000)
- *Strengthening Families Program* (SFP) (Kumpfer, Pinyuchon, de Melo, & Whiteside, 2008)
- *SDM/SPS* (Elias & Bruene-Butler, 2005a)
- *Steps to Respect* (Committee for Children, 2001)
- *Strong Kids* (Merrell, Carrizales, Feuerborn, Gueldner, & Tran, 2007a; Merrell, Carrizales, Feurborn, Gueldner, & Tran, 2007)
- *Strong Start* (Merrell, Whitcomb, & Parisi, 2009)
- *Strong Teens* (Merrell, Carrizales, Feuerborn, Gueldner, & Tran, 2007b)
- *Talking with TJ* (Dilworth, Mokrue, & Elias, 2002)
- *Too Good for Violence* (Bacon, 2001; Dilworth et al., 2002)
- *Tools of the Mind* (PreK-K) (Bodrova & Leong, 1995, 1996)

Children who enter schools with positive SEL skills and competencies are more likely to be successful (Denham & Weissberg, 2004). The skills at the preschool level that are considered particularly important include self-awareness, self-management, and emotional expressiveness. These skills operate together to help young children develop successful relationships. SEL skills can be fostered when children become attached to caring adults and when adults guide them in regard to the rules for behavior in dyadic and group situations. Rules, limits, and supervision by adults are important in this process. In addition, specific socialization techniques are helpful. Directly teaching young children about emotions, modeling expressions and positive behaviors, reacting with encouragement to children who show their emotions, talking about emotions, and helping children know that emotions are "okay" is critical. Emotion "coaching" and proactive discipline that attends to cultural values and variations can facilitate successful SEL programming at the early childhood level.

SEL Programs at the Preschool Level

Reviews of research conducted on prevention programs suggest that an investment in well-conducted preschool interventions would be a good investment (Durlak, 2003; Westhues, Nelson, & MacLeod, 2003). Nelson, Westhues, and MacLeod

(2003) conducted a meta-analysis on the effectiveness of preschool prevention programs available at the time of their study. They looked at cognitive, social–emotional, and parent–family outcomes for disadvantaged children. Social–emotional outcomes were found to be moderate while children were in various programs. The longer the intervention, the greater the impact on social–emotional outcomes but only *if* the program lasted at least 1 year. Outcomes were modest, but some advantage continued through eighth grade (Olds, 2003).

Denham and Burton (2003) looked at a number of programs and determined that four programs were effective for the SEL functioning of preschool students. *At-risk 4-year-olds* (Denham & Burton, 1996), *Second Step Preschool/Kindergarten* (McMahon et al., 2000), *Preschool PATHS-Promoting Alternative Thinking Strategies* (Domitrovich et al., 2001; Domitrovich, Cortes, & Greenberg, 2007), and the *Incredible Years* program (Webster-Stratton, Reid, & Hammond, 2001) were effective. Izard et al. (2008) added *Al's Pals* (Geller, 1999) to this list. These programs have some interesting features. Each of the programs addresses emotion development, social skills, problem solving, and conflict resolution. Denham and Burton (1996) implemented a social–emotional intervention for at-risk 4-year-olds at 7 day-care sites. Students participating in the intervention demonstrated decreased negative emotions, were more involved in learning, and exhibited more prosocial behaviors according to their teachers.

SEL Programming at the Elementary and Middle School Level

Early elementary students are developing skills which involve expressing and managing basic emotions, learning the differences between positive and negative emotions, considering the feelings of others, tying emotions to contexts, generating alternative possibilities, and using language to express differences in emotion. At this age, children tend to continue to use behavior rather than cognitive approaches to deal with stress (Kress & Elias, 2006). Children are also developing peer interaction competencies, learning to express empathy toward others, and they are learning about their own strengths. By the middle elementary level, students "feeling" vocabularies are expanding. They have some strategies to cope with strong emotional contexts (can calm down) and coping strategies expand. Students at this level can set goals, understand their own strengths and weaknesses, and can handle failures. Skills for making friends, dealing with rejection, and completing projects are important. They are developing the ability to anticipate others reactions and to manage conversations. There are many SEL programs available for this age group. School teams need to determine which risk factors that they want to address using needs assessment data.

When in middle school, early adolescents are quite self-critical. They understand the many sides of arguments, they are sensitive to social norms, and are aware of self-talk. They can set goals but cannot always carry them through. Feelings of belonging to groups are important at this stage of development as is social problem solving (Kress & Elias, 2006). Early adolescents are interested in personal accomplishment, decision-making, and peer relations. Balancing independence and interdependence is a key skill. Again, for each developmental level appropriate SEL programming needs to fit the needs of students at that level. There are an ever-increasing number of SEL programs for middle school level students.

Sample SEL Programs/Curricula at the Elementary and Middle School Levels

Kress and Elias (2006) recommended various SEL programs based on the developmental needs of children and adolescents at each developmental level. Using this approach for early elementary level students, they recommended *Interpersonal Cognitive Problem Solving* (ICPS) (Shure & Spivack, 1988), *Second Step* (http://www.cfchildren.org), and *Responsive Classroom* programs (http://www.responsiveclassroom.org/). For students at the middle elementary school level, they recommended *Providing Alternative Thinking Strategies* (PATHS; Greenberg & Kusche, 1998), *SDM/SPS* (Elias & Bruene-Butler, 2005a, 2005b, 2005c), and *Open Circle* (Seigle, 2001).

CASEL (2012) has recommended a list of stronger SEL programs associated with specific elements and desired outcomes. This list would be helpful to school teams who had identified either specific goals or specific desired outcomes. The guide rated 19 programs as of 2012, according to design, implementation supports, and impact on students (http://casel.org/guide/). These programs are only a very small sample of the many SEL programs available at the elementary and middle school levels. If violence prevention or creating a safe school environment were needs, and increasing attachment to school were the goal, programs that would meet those criteria would include *Steps to Respect* (Committee for Children, 2001), *Responsive Classroom* (http://www.responsiveclassroom.org), and *Caring School Community* (http://www.devstu.org/). If drug prevention were the goal, programs such as *Lions Quest* (http://www.lions-quest.org), and *Caring School Community* could be considered. If there were behavioral, social, and emotional needs in the student population, and teachers wanted to reduce disruptive and aggressive behaviors, *PATHS* (PATHS, Greenberg & Kusche, 1998), would be a strong program a school team might consider for implementation.

Hughes and Barrois (2010) examined programs designed to improve the SEL school climate and/or to improve social interactions in class. The studies in this group had to meet specific criteria. They needed to be implemented by the classroom teacher, have a control group, and have at least one efficacy study published in a peer-reviewed journal. They identified seven different programs that met the parameters, only two of which could be considered efficacious given the stated criteria: *PATHS* and *Second Step*. These programs serve as good examples of SEL programming at the elementary school level.

Promoting Alternative Thinking Strategies (PATHS) is designed to promote social and emotional thinking in elementary school students (Curtis & Norgate, 2007). *PATHS* at the elementary level focuses on the development of emotional understanding and expression, prosocial behaviors, friendship skills, emotion regulation, and problem solving (Domitrovich et al., 2009). Lessons are taught two times a week and school staff use strategies to enhance students' self-control and interpersonal problem solving in the general school environment. Outcomes have included increased emotional understanding and decreased behavior problems. A study of intervention schools and control schools using pre- and post-assessment showed significant improvements for student groups using the program (Curtis & Norgate, 2007). When interviewed, teachers thought that *PATHS* helped students acquire a better understanding of emotions. Teachers also reported that students were more empathetic and demonstrated improved self-control.

Bierman et al. (2010) conducted a clustered, randomized controlled trial involving sets of schools in three locations. Multiethnic students were involved over three grade levels in early elementary school. Teachers in grades 1, 2, and 3 implemented the *PATHS* curriculum. Teachers and peers rated students who remained in the program over time more prosocial and less aggressive. Teachers reported improved academic functioning. Interestingly, significant effects according to *peer* reports were found only for boys. Effects were stronger in schools with fewer disadvantaged children. More aggressive students at baseline benefitted more over time than more typical children. This larger longitudinal study produced significant preventive outcomes and demonstrated the efficacy of the *PATHS* program.

Second Step is a primary prevention program for students as early as preschool through grade 9. The curriculum deals with three social–emotional competencies. These involve developing empathy, social problem solving, and anger management (Frey, Hirschstein, & Guzzo, 2000). The objectives include reducing aggressive behaviors and increasing students' social competency. The Centers for Disease Control and Prevention provided the funding for an experimental effectiveness study of the *Second Step* curriculum for second- and third-grade students (Grossman et al., 1997). Although parents and teachers did not observe change, the observers reported changes in a positive direction in regard to both decreases in aggressive behaviors and increases in prosocial behaviors. Another efficacy study of the *Second Step* program determined that students who received the preventive intervention required less adult management, were less aggressive, and preferred prosocial goals (Frey, Nolen, Van Schoiack, & Hirschstein, 2005). Additionally, the girls who received the intervention were more cooperative. Teachers felt that social behaviors of intervention students improved with more experience with the program. A quasi-experimental evaluation of the *Second Step* curriculum was conducted with third- through fifth-grade students in a rural elementary school (Taub, 2002). Students were followed for a year post-intervention. There were multiple raters of the same students. Teachers rated students in the intervention group higher than students in a comparison school at the end of the intervention year, but rating scales indicated an increase in disruption in the spring of that year. However, 1 year later, students at the intervention school were rated less antisocial than at baseline. Prosocial behavior improved first, changes in disruptive behaviors decreased slowly. Independent observers identified positive changes in following classroom directions and engaging appropriately with peers. The impact of the curriculum was modest and positive.

Students who received the *Second Step* program in another study showed significant gains in knowledge about empathy, anger management, impulse control, and bully-proofing (Edwards, Hunt, Meyers, Grogg, & Jarrett, 2005). There were significant positive changes seen on rating scales and positive changes were seen on report card items around respectful and cooperative behaviors. Teachers reported modest gains in prosocial behavior. In a study in an urban area, *Second Step* was implemented in six schools with third- to fifth-grade students. More than half of the students were racial and ethnic minority students (Cooke et al., 2007). There was no control group in this study. Almost two-thirds of students showed positive changes on survey measures in attitudes and prosocial behaviors, although there was no significant decrease in aggressive behaviors over 1 year's time. Participating students were less likely to self-report an increase in negative behaviors. Using measures from fall to spring in any given school year in the USA tend to show an increase in aggressive behavior. *Second Step* developers point out there is typically an increase in prosocial behavior before there are any decreases in negative behavior. Finally, Neace and Munoz (2012) implemented the *Second Step* curriculum in an urban school system. This study was part of a 3-year project using two large groups of students. There were improvements in students' attitudes and in addition, there were improvements in behavior.

SEL Programming at the High School Level

There are fewer choices of programs to enhance social competency for high school students, and implementation at this level is particularly challenging. It is far more common to find prevention programs targeting specific problem behaviors of adolescents at the high school level, and there are many evidence-based prevention programs from which to choose that target-specific problems such as teen pregnancy prevention (Office of Adolescent Health: http://www.hhs.gov), dropout prevention (National Dropout Prevention Center: http://www.dropoutprevention.org), and violence prevention and substance abuse NREPP (http://www.colorado.edu). There are also more general sites including programs for a variety of teen risky behaviors. The U.S. Department of Justice: Office of Justice Programs (http://www.ojjdp.gov) is a good example. This is not to say that there are no programs that target social competency in adolescents, but perhaps due to the difficulty of fitting a program into the secondary school general curricula, and the perception that adolescents do not need this service, most research-based preventive programs are for students at-risk needing secondary prevention.

Intensive social competency interventions and programs are far more likely to target middle school students at the universal level than they are to target high school students although some efforts to develop universal preventive interventions are under development such as the *Strong Teens* program (Merrell et al., 2007b). A pilot study to evaluate the Strong Teens curriculum was published by Merrell, Juskelis, Tran, and Buchanan (2008). In a study with a *very small* number of students, the 12-week program was implemented using self-report pre- and post-test measures of student knowledge of the concepts presented and negative symptoms. Significant improvements were noted for this group of students. The *Strong Teens* curriculum was adapted for a group of immigrant Latino teens in another small study (Castro-Olivo & Merrell, 2012). Students who participated demonstrated increased knowledge and positively rated the adaptations.

Kress and Elias (2006) recommended programs for adolescents based on the developmental tasks for student in this age group. Effective programs at the secondary level include *Lions-Quest*, and especially their *Skills for Action*, service learning program (www.lions-quest.org), the *Giraffe Heroes Program* (www.giraffe.org; Graham, 1999), *Facing History and Ourselves* (www.facing.org), and the *Resolving Conflict Creatively Program* (DeJong, 1994).

As an example of a high school program that targets risky student behaviors, *LifeSkills Training* (*LST*) is a school-based prevention program (Botvin, 1996). The program provides information using culturally and developmentally relevant content and language. The active teaching strategies include discussions, structured group activities, and role-playing. There are three program levels (elementary, middle, and high school). This is a significant advantage in selecting SEL programming. *LST* teaches drug resistance skills along with additional social skills (Botvin & Griffin, 2004). It has been shown to be effective in a series of randomized controlled efficacy trials. Students who participated in this multicomponent program reduced use of drugs up to 50 % more so than students in control groups. The program works as a preventive effort with students from a wide variety of backgrounds and types of communities. Content includes self-management skills, general social skills, resistance skills, and changing attitudes. The program focuses on risk and protective factors connected with beginning to use drugs and also on resistance skills.

Disadvantaged sixth-grade students in 41 city schools participated in the *LST* program (Botvin, Griffin, & Nichols, 2006). Students in the 20 experimental schools who received the program were significantly less likely to engage in delinquent behaviors, verbal or physical aggression, or fighting. They were less likely to start using drugs. The randomized controlled study design was a key strength of this study, in addition to a predominantly minority school population, and a large sample. This study demonstrated the wide-ranging outcomes of the *LST* program.

Prevention in Action Challenge: Evaluate a SEL Curriculum

Locate a social–emotional learning curriculum that has potential for meeting the needs of students in a particular school with which you have some familiarity.

Complete the template below:

Name of the SEL Prevention Curriculum: _____

Description of the Program:

(*Note: You can find descriptions of each program on its respective program website; however, do **NOT cut and paste** the description. Write a description of the program in your own words and include a citation. You may want to emphasize the important assets of the program.*)

Grade Levels and School Type (for which the program would be appropriate):

(*Note: School type refers to urban, suburban, or rural, small versus large, public versus private, etc.*)

Evidence Base:

(*You will need to **locate** the efficacy studies that have provided data to support the program and determine how strong that evidence may be (randomized controlled study by independent researchers on one extreme, to a single study in one area of the country by the person(s) who designed the program at the other extreme). Describe the methodology of the efficacy study sufficiently so that the rigor will be clear. Include references to the specific studies written in correct APA style.*)

Ratings:

(*This refers to agencies which have rated the program using one of the many labels evidence-based, promising, etc.). First, indicate the agency or agencies that have rated the program, the label given to the program, what that label means. Find the interpretation of the label on the agency's website. In cases where no agency has rated the program, indicate that the program has not been rated, and why it might be chosen over other programs.*)

Overall Determination:

(*Indicate whether or not the program should not be considered by a school prevention team and why this is the case.*)

Chapter 9
Evidence-Based Prevention of Internalizing Disorders

The Word Health Organization has determined that depression and anxiety are the most prevalent chronic disorders (Magalhaes et al., 2010). Anxiety and depression are internalizing disorders. Children and adolescents with internalizing disorders experience worry, fears, shyness, decreased self-esteem, feelings of sadness, and depressive symptoms. Interestingly these feelings and experiences are interrelated in clinical populations, and factor analytic research makes it clear they are closely associated with one another (Ollendick, Shortt, & Sander, 2008). Anxiety disorders often, but not always, precede depressive disorders when a child or teenager experiences both disorders.

The consequences of internalizing disorders are considerable including serious consequences for health and costs during young adulthood (Keenan-Miller, Hammen, & Brennan, 2007). Adolescent depression, for example, has consequences during teen years affecting peer, school, and family functioning (Jaycox et al., 2009). Adolescents with symptoms of depression also exhibit coexisting emotional and behavioral complications. Adolescents at risk for depression find that negative mood interferes with ability to perform in class, complete homework, concentrate, and interact with classmates (Humensky et al., 2010). Subthreshold anxiety can interfere with social interaction, with feeling "okay," performing in class, and developing social skills. Anxiety symptoms affect memory and thinking skills (Mazzone et al., 2007). Anxiety is associated with school failure in girls. Although behavioral problems are more likely to affect school success in boys, anxiety does so as well.

There are important cultural differences in the prevalence of internalizing symptoms and disorders in young people, as well as in the presentation of internalizing symptoms (Anderson & Mayes, 2010). When African American students experience anxiety, they also experience concurrent and long-term academic, social, and psychological problems. A study of low-income African American first grade students, who were highly anxious, tended to score lower on achievement tests and lower in peer acceptance (Grover, Ginsburg, & Ialongo, 2006). Depressive symptoms are strongly connected to substance use in middle school students particularly for Hispanic students, as some student may try to self-medicate feelings of depression and stress (Kelder et al., 2001).

G.L. Macklem, *Preventive Mental Health at School: Evidence-Based Services for Students*,
DOI 10.1007/978-1-4614-8609-1_9, © Springer Science+Business Media New York 2014

Depression appears to be increasing in the United States population possibly because of better identification and screening tools and/or because individuals are increasingly willing to admit to symptoms (Ingram & Smith, 2008). Several studies have found similar associations with sexual risk behaviors (Lehrer, Shrier, Gortmaker, & Buka, 2006). Kosunen, Kaltiala-Heino, Rimpelä, and Laippala (2003) found that for both boys and girls, self-reported depression was related to increased numbers of sexual partners and lack of use of contraception.

Anxiety and Depression: One Disorder or Two?

Gorman (1996) reported research indicating that there are genetic and neurobiologic similarities between the disorders of anxiety and disorders of depression. About 85 % of individuals diagnosed with depression report significant anxiety. The association between panic disorder, generalized anxiety disorder, social phobia, other anxiety disorders, and depression is strong. Hale, Raaijmakers, Muris, van Hoof, and Meeus (2009) report that 25–50 % of teens with depression also have comorbid anxiety. Additionally, 10–15 % of teens with anxiety disorders have comorbid depression. The two internalizing disorders have strong effects on one another. The presence of one of the two disorders predicts that the youngster will experience symptoms of the other disorder. It is more likely that a depressed child or adolescent will also exhibit an anxiety disorder, than for a child with an anxious disorder to also have a depressive disorder (Ollendick et al., 2008).

Anxiety and depression are frequently comorbid and in fact, comorbidity is the rule (Aina & Susman, 2006). There have been questions raised in the literature whether or not there are two disorders or only one disorder. Practitioners in the UK describe a syndrome called mixed anxiety and depressive disorder, or cothymia, for patients in whom the two disorders have equal functional significance (Tyrer, 2001). Das-Munshi et al. (2008) feel that mixed presentation of anxiety and depression is so common that it is the norm. After studying early and middle adolescents for 5 years, the self-report data that Hale et al. (2009) collected on the other hand led them to feel that in spite of the strong relationship between the two disorders, they are best considered distinct.

Following 1,580 children over a 14-year period, researchers concluded that anxiety disorders start in childhood or early adolescence, whereas mood disorders begin and increase sharply in adolescence (Roza, Hofstra, van der Ende, & Verhulst, 2003). Another group of researchers wondered whether anxiety would be the best predictor of later depression (Keenan, Feng, Hipwell, & Klostermann, 2009). They collected data from 2,451 girls from age 6 to 12 years. They determined that 8 years of age was the earliest that researchers could relate early symptoms of generalized social anxiety to depression appearing in early adolescence. Symptoms of depression early on had the strongest relationship with depression in middle school.

One theory to explain the strong relationship between anxiety and depression has to do with cognitive style. Negative affectivity has been implicated in this relationship (Axelson & Birmaher, 2001; Ollendick et al., 2008). Children with this particular cognitive style exhibit a negative bias in information processing. This bias is a characteristic of both depression and anxiety. Others feel that anxiety and depression are related to three temperaments: high negative affect, low positive affect, and physiological hyperarousal. Combinations of these three temperaments have different outcomes. High negative affectivity with low positive affectivity results in poor outcomes for depression but not anxiety (De Bolle, De Clercq, Decuyper, & De Fruyt, 2011).

Anxiety Disorders in Children and Adolescents

Anxiety disorders are common worldwide and are among the most common disorders in children and adolescents. A child with anxiety symptoms would be diagnosed with an anxiety disorder if his or her anxiety was occurring frequently, was very intense, or if it lasted a long time and resulted in notable functional impairment (Ollendick et al., 2008). Some researchers report the prevalence rate between 8 and 27 % (Bienvenu & Ginsburg, 2007) while others report 7–12 % (Ollendick et al., 2008). When early and middle adolescents were followed for a 5-year period, panic disorder, school anxiety, and separation disorder symptoms decreased a little but social phobia remained stable. Girls demonstrated a small increase in generalized anxiety disorder as they proceeded through adolescence (Hale, Raaijmakers, Muris, van Hoof, & Meeus, 2008).

Anxiety disorders are often comorbid with one another and with mood disorders. A second anxiety disorder is the most frequent comorbid disorder. Children with an anxiety disorder are at risk for dysthymic disorders (Ollendick et al., 2008). Kendall, Brady, and Verduin (2001) report a study showing 79 % of the diagnosed children had at least one comorbid diagnosis. Muris, Steerneman, Merckelbach, Holdrinet, and Meesters (1998) found 84.1 % of their sample of children with pervasive developmental disorders had at least one anxiety disorder. The median age of onset of an anxiety disorder was 11 years of age. Phobias and separation disorder were seen as early as age 7 years, and social phobia appeared around 13 years of age (Bienvenu & Ginsburg, 2007). Children of anxious parents are seven times more likely to develop anxiety symptoms and disorders. When anxiety disorders are not treated, they tend to increase in severity. Cognitive theory suggests that underlying beliefs and processes may fit specific anxiety disorders. Starcevic and Berle (2006) suggest that in panic disorder, anxiety sensitivity is particularly strong. In generalized anxiety, pathological worry stands out along with intolerance of uncertainty. Thought–action fusion fits obsessive–compulsive disorder, along with intolerance of uncertainty.

A group of researchers followed 1,420 children, aged 9–13 years until they were 16 years old (Costello, Mustillo, Erkanli, Keeler, & Anbgold, 2003). They found that during this period of time, 36.7 % of the children in the study had at least one psychiatric disorder. Risk of a new diagnosis, based on a previous diagnosis, was significantly higher for girls than boys. The risk of having at least one mental health disorder by age 16 years was much higher than estimates. Young people in the study with subsyndromal anxiety symptoms demonstrated impaired functioning even when they did not show sufficient symptoms for a diagnosis. This makes both universal and targeted prevention important. The students who developed an anxiety disorder had an average of two symptoms of anxiety the year before they were diagnosed. When examining social withdrawal specifically, researchers find that 85 % of children who were withdrawn remained withdrawn, while about 8 % experienced decreased symptoms and 7 % experienced increased symptoms. It is important for practitioners to understand that there are several patterns of anxiety progression in middle school children (Oh et al., 2008).

Parents of children with anxiety disorders have been intensely studied. They tend to be more controlling than other parents, they tend to be overinvolved with their children, and they tend to overprotect them. They have also been described as less accepting and less warm (Ollendick et al., 2008). Fathers appear to influence the development of social confidence in anxious children. Mothers tend to model or teach social wariness to their children (Bögels, Stevens, & Majdandžić, 2011). Some mothers of children with anxiety disorders exhibit other behaviors as well. They talk less often to their children and they tend not to use many positive emotion words. They discourage their children from talking about emotions (Suveg, Zeman, Flannery-Schroeder, & Cassano, 2005). Parents with social phobia have children at high risk of developing social phobia (Knappe et al., 2009).

Somatic symptoms are common in anxious children (Kingery, Ginsburg, & Alfano, 2007). When a child experiences physical symptoms, which cannot be explained medically, this child is said to be experiencing "functional somatic symptoms" (FSS) (Campo, 2012; Janssens, Rosmalen, Ormel, Van Oort, & Oldehinkel, 2010). Campo (2012) reports that FSS are consistently connected to internalizing symptoms in school-aged children. There appears to be a two-way relationship involved. When a youngster experiences one or more FSS, anxious–depressive symptoms develop later on. Anxious and depressive symptoms are significantly associated with FSS in childhood and adolescence. It may be that these share common risk factors, and treating either anxious symptoms, depressive symptoms, or FSS improves all three. In African American children, one study found that 83 % of the adolescents experienced one or more somatic symptoms some or most of the time. These symptoms were positively correlated with the severity of anxiety symptoms and perceived competence, and may serve as one of many risk factors for anxiety among African American students (Kingery et al., 2007).

Risks for Anxiety Symptoms and Disorders

The risk factors for anxiety disorders include behavioral inhibition, a stressful environment, parenting that is not helpful, and negative peer relationships (Degnan, Almas, & Fox, 2010). Behavioral inhibition is a temperament associated with social reticence, fearfulness, avoidance in new situations, and avoidance of people with whom the child is not familiar (Hirshfeld-Becker et al., 2008; White, McDermott, Degnan, Henderson, & Fox, 2011). Behavioral inhibition can be identified as early as preschool and is associated with risk for social anxiety. In behaviorally inhibited children, difficulty shifting attention increases the risk for anxiety problems. Adolescents who were behaviorally inhibited when they were very young exhibited an attentional bias to threatening stimuli in the environment (Pérez-Edgar et al., 2010).

The TRAILS study was designed to identify risk factors for anxiety through the adolescent period (Van Oort, Greaves-Lord, Ormel, Verhulst, & Huizink, 2011; Van Oort, Greaves-Lord, Verhulst, Ormel, & Huizink, 2009). A community sample of 2,220 children was evaluated at three periods over 5 years. Girls showed more anxiety than boys, and this remained stable during adolescence. Anxiety symptoms decreased during early adolescence and then increased again from middle to late adolescence. Rejecting parenting was found to be a risk factor for anxiety in early adolescence. Peer victimization was related to long-term anxiety.

Weissman et al. (2006) found the risk for anxiety disorders was three times as high in the children of parents who were depressed. These children were also at risk for major depression and substance dependence. Children of parents with depression, who also had panic disorder or agoraphobia, had an additional risk of anxiety and/or depressive disorders. The study demonstrated the association of depression and several of the anxiety disorders. It also demonstrated the transmission of anxiety disorders from parents to youth.

Ethno-cultural Differences in Anxiety

There are some ethno-cultural differences in the diagnosis of anxiety disorders when White American, Hispanic American, and African Americans are compared in regard to lifetime prevalence rates for anxiety (Asnaani, Richey, Dimaite, Hinton, & Hofmann, 2010). White Americans are more likely to be diagnosed with generalized anxiety disorder, social anxiety disorder, and panic disorder. African Americans are more frequently diagnosed with post-traumatic stress disorder than individuals in any other category. Asian Americans are less likely to be diagnosed with various anxiety disorders than Hispanic Americans, or White Americans. Asian Americans tend not to endorse anxiety symptoms in self-reports, even when studies were conducted in their respective languages. It is important to consider race and ethnicity when working with students in multicultural schools or schools in general. Practitioners need to be aware of the fact that urban and low-income Latino youth, in grades 5 through 7, report more intense symptoms of anxiety than children in other groups (Martinez, Polo, & Carter, 2012).

Even though African American students may demonstrate a lower prevalence for most anxiety disorders, when an African American child has a parent who is anxious, that child is four times more likely to meet criteria for an anxiety disorder or other mental health disorder (Chapman, Petrie, Vines, & Durrett, 2012). The most common diagnosis for children of parents with anxiety is phobia, social phobia in particular. Practitioners need to be aware of the risks for African American children, because African American families are less likely to seek or agree to treatment due to stigma. Some parents may not trust professionals.

American Indian adolescents have been found to have higher rates of distress than the overall US population possibly due to higher rates of exposure to trauma (Goodkind, Lanoue, & Milford, 2010). Some researchers have found a high risk for social anxiety in American Indian adolescents along with risk for other types of anxiety (West & Newman, 2007). Behavioral inhibition in childhood predicting later social anxiety has been found in some groups of adolescents.

Depressive Disorders in Children and Adolescents

Depression is a serious problem among children, young adolescents, and adolescents. It is significant and yet has been ignored (Saluja et al., 2004). In a study of schoolchildren in grades 6, 8, and 10, as many as 18 % of students reported that they experienced symptoms of depression. Twenty-five percent of girls reported symptoms and 10 % of boys in this age group reported symptoms of depression. The older students reported more symptoms than the youngest students. American Indian teens reported the highest prevalence followed by Hispanic, then White, Asian Americans, and African American students in that order.

One complication of depression is that youngsters who are depressed do not always report feeling sad or depressed (Ollendick et al., 2008). Younger children say they feel that activities aren't fun anymore, or they exhibit irritability and argumentativeness. Depression is cyclic. Students tend to recover from a major depressive episode within 2 years, but sadly, as many as half or more of these students will reexperience another depressive episode at some time in their lives.

Risk Factors for Depressive Symptoms and Disorders in Adolescence

Depression is a complex illness with a multifactorial causal structure (Garber, 2006). There are both psychological and physiological aspects of depression. It is not likely that researchers will find a single cause for depressive disorders, and so it is not likely that reducing one risk variable would be sufficient to prevent depressive disorders. Risk factors described in the literature include physiological changes at puberty, stress, unhealthy adaptations to stress, interpersonal interaction differences between girls and boys, and socialization differences in families and among peers.

There are many risk factors for depression in adolescence. An important study by Mazza, Fleming, Abbott, Haggerty, and Catalano (2010) has helped to identify many early predictors of adolescent depression. They examined the relationship between early predictors and depression 7 years later collecting data on 1,239 children in ten

Table 9.1 Risk factors for depression

Anxiety disorders (Silk, Davis, McMakin, Dahl, & Forbes, 2012)
Personality issues (Kushner, Tackett, & Bagby, 2012)
Body objectification and inauthenticity in peer relationships (Tolman, Impett, Tracy, & Michael, 2006)
Negative life events (Hankin & Abramson, 2001)
Bullying and use of substances (Saluja et al., 2004)
Parental rejection and lack of support (Hutcherson & Epkins, 2009)
Parental depression (Ollendick et al., 2008)
Maternal anxiety and depression (Spence, Najman, Bor, O'Callaghan, & Williams, 2002)
Perceived social acceptance and loneliness (Hutcherson & Epkins, 2009)
High levels of disengagement (Calvete, Camara, Estevez, & Villardón, 2011)
Early antisocial behavior (Kiesner, 2002)
Decreased social status (Albertine et al., 2007)
Need for approval and success (Calvete & Cardenoso, 2005)
Early maturing girls (Koinson, Heron, Lewis, Croudace, & Araya, 2011)
Perceived stress (Yarcheski & Mahon, 2000)
Maternal conflict and lack of paternal closeness (Vazsonyi & Belliston, 2006)
General parental discord and family conflict (Hammen, 2009; Mazza et al., 2009)
Antisocial behavior for boys (Mazza et al., 2009)
Low school achievement for both boys and girls (Mazza et al., 2009)
Stress during adolescence for girls (Mazza et al., 2009)
Early maturation (Koinson et al., 2011)
Perceived stress (Yarcheski & Mahon, 2000)
Conflict between parents (Mazza et al., 2009)
Maternal depression for girls (Mazza et al., 2009)

schools in the Pacific Northwest. Anxiety was a significant predictor of depression 7 years later as was early antisocial behavior. Mazza et al. found that early antisocial behavior of girls in grades 1 and 2 was significantly related to intensity of depression 7 years later. This suggested a "turning in" of problems as a result of societal pressure. Depression itself was a risk factor for other emotional disorders. Preschool oppositional and aggressive behaviors predict internalization at 10 years of age for girls, whereas social problems at school entry predict internalizing difficulties for boys at 11 years. The list of risk factors for adolescent depression is lengthy (Table 9.1).

Boys, experiencing anxiety symptoms in sixth grade, were 1.5 times more likely to experience depressive symptoms during high school than boys who had not experienced anxiety symptoms (Gallerani, Garber, & Martin, 2010). Girls experienced high rates of depressive symptoms whether or not they had experienced anxiety in middle school. Young girls who are more physically mature than their peers are especially concerned about their weight. When these girls are exposed to relational bullying, they experience depressive symptoms (Compian, Gowen, & Hayward, 2009). Social victimization or bullying is associated with rejection, exclusion, loneliness, decreased self-esteem, and important for this discussion, depression (Poteat & Espelage, 2007). Gay and lesbian schoolchildren experience considerable victimization. Many feel that they are not safe at school (Poteat & Espelage, 2007). Verbal abuse causes a high amount of stress for these students. Homophobic victimization causes more stress for boys than girls along with anxiety and depression. Girls tend to respond to verbal abuse by withdrawing.

An important study of urban Hispanic adolescents determined that children who had been retained had lower self-concepts and both past and present depressive symptomatology (Robles-Piña, Defrance, & Cox, 2008). Yet another group of researchers found that self-criticism interacted with symptoms of depression to predict decreased grade point averages mostly in boys (Shahar et al., 2006). Students who have less skill in obtaining reinforcement in their environments tend to exhibit greater depression (Ryba & Hopko, 2012). Also to consider are factors which exacerbate anxiety and depression such as insufficient sleep. Interestingly, Gangwisch et al. (2010) found the association between short sleep and depression strong enough to hypothesize that lack of sleep could be associated with the etiology of depression.

Gender Differences in Depression

The rate of depressive symptoms and clinical depression in girls increases in early adolescence so that it reaches a prevalence of 2–3 times that of boys (Clarke et al., 2001; Garber, 2006; Keenan & Hipwell, 2005). The gender difference in depression begins between the ages of 11 and 13 years (Cyranowski, Frank, Young, & Shear, 2000; Hankin & Abramson, 2001). The gender difference in anxiety begins even earlier. By age 6 years, girls are twice as likely to have had an anxiety disorder than boys (Lewinsohn, Gotlib, Lewinsohn, Seeley, & Allen, 1998). The rate of depression is fairly equal in boys and girls before early adolescence. Several researchers have suggested that the rate of depression is even higher in boys than girls during elementary school (Merry, McDowell, Wild, Bir, & Cunliffe, 2004; Pattison & Lynd-Stevenson, 2001). Girls also experience more severe depression than boys (Ryba & Hopko, 2012). The gender difference persists into adulthood.

Among middle school girls, anxiety, worry, and oversensitivity predict symptoms of depression (Chaplin, Gillham, & Seligman, 2009). Interestingly, when mothers are depressed, their daughters tend to maintain depressive symptoms that they experience themselves. Boys do not continue to demonstrate depressive symptoms in relation to their mothers' symptoms (Cortes, Fleming, Catalano, & Brown, 2006). Grabe, Hyde, and Lindberg (2007) found that body shame is related to depression in 11 and 13 year old girls. Keenan and Hipwell (2005) found that excessive empathy and compliance predicted depression in girls. In addition, they found that poor regulation of negative emotions was implicated as well.

The relationship between risk factors and later depression in preadolescent girls is complex. Preadolescent girls who do not experience much positive emotion will have more depression if parents are controlling. Preadolescent girls with weak sadness regulation will experience more intense depression than peers if their parents are not very accepting (Feng et al., 2009). Ryba and Hopko (2012) point out that many factors explain more frequent depression in girls including genetics, hormones, adrenal functioning, neurotransmitter systems, more frequent victimization and trauma, role restrictions, interpersonal orientation, increased vulnerability to others' pain, rumination, attributional styles, greater reactivity to stress, lower self-concept, and a higher prevalence of anxiety disorders.

Ethno-cultural Differences in Depression

Although the gender difference is quite clear and there is much agreement around gender differences in depression, the question of ethno-cultural differences in depression is less clear. The data available is somewhat variable (Liu, Chen, & Lewis, 2011). Disorders and syndromes vary across cultures in prevalence, in risk factors, in protective factors, in diagnosis, and the meaning of emotion as it is expressed (Canino & Alegria, 2008). Culture colors every aspect of emotional health and illness. Culture determines how a student will express psychological upset. Both gender and nationality determines whether or not a child will seek help (López & Guarnaccia, 2008). The National Comorbidity Survey Replication (Breslau et al., 2006) indicates that race and ethnic differences in regard to mood and anxiety disorders in minority groups emerge in childhood.

The risk of symptoms of depression appears to be twice as high among Latinos, as compared to other ethnic groups. A study exploring the risk factors of depression among Latinos determined that the key risk factors for this group included low support in school, low acculturation, and coming from a one-parent household. Factors unique to girls in this ethnic group included low household income. The highest risk was for girls at age 14 and 15 years. Interestingly this age period was not as high risk for boys; in fact, this age period was the lowest risk period for Latino boys (Mikolajczyk, Bredehorst, Khelaifat, Maier, & Maxwell, 2007). Another study found that neighborhood risks were significantly associated with boys' symptoms of depression (Behnke, Plunkett, Sands, & Bámaca-Colbert, 2011).

The Latino population is diverse. The Latino groups for which we seem to have more data are Mexican American students and children from Puerto Rico. The Mexican American population is growing at a fast rate in the United States. Mexican Americans experience more mental health difficulties than other ethnic groups including anxiety and depression and are the most underserved (Pate, 2010). They tend not to seek help, and when they do, they tend to stop treatment early. Immigrant Mexican American students report higher social anxiety than young people born in the United States from Mexico. Polo and López (2009) explain this difference as due to differences in stress, related to both low proficiency in English and also to acculturation stress. Bauman (2008) found that Spanish-speaking Mexican American students in grades 3 through 5 exhibited more symptoms of depression than their English-speaking peers. Mexican American students in a primarily minority school did not experience more victimization in this study and acculturation did not explain differences in depressive symptoms. However, for those students who were relationally bullied, symptoms of depression were evident. Practitioners need to be aware of the peer culture and pay attention to the demographics of their schools.

In a study of urban Hispanic adolescents, Robles-Piña et al. (2008) identified more depression, and more intense depression, along with lower self-esteem in Hispanic students than other students. Hispanic girls had more negative feelings about their bodies and experienced more marginalization. In this urban sample, 42 % of students had been retained in kindergarten, first grade, eighth grade, or ninth grade. The urban Hispanic students who had been retained had lower self-concepts, more past and current depression, and lower grade point averages than their peers. The majority of students were retained in kindergarten. This presents a challenge for school psychologists in that there are clear alternatives to retention. In addition there are a variety of preventive interventions which could address the self-concepts of those students who have been retained.

Puerto Rican children express stress somatically. Anxiety disorders and acculturative stress are associated with abdominal pain and headaches in this group (Duarte et al., 2008). Cultural stress was more significant than acculturation. However, López and Guarnaccia (2008) did not find that acculturation was significant for Puerto Ricans and Cubans in regard to mood and anxiety disorders.

An interesting cultural syndrome among some Puerto Rican children and adolescents is nerve attack or ataques de nervios (Canino & Alegria, 2008). Ataques de nervios describes distress or upsets including crying and screaming, with verbal or even physical aggression (López & Guarnaccia, 2008). These behaviors occur when there has been a very stressful event that involved significant others. Ataques are more prevalent in women and in lower SES populations. Between 4 and 5 % of children have been reported to have a lifetime prevalence of ataques. These ataques are associated with a number of disorders on the anxiety and depression spectrum and are associated with exposure to violence and stress in daily life (López et al., 2009). Guarnaccia, Martinez, Ramirez, and Canino (2005) found a slightly higher incidence of 9 % in a community sample of children. They found that there were more adolescent girls than boys with a family history of ataques de nervios.

When exploring depression and depressive symptoms in the Asian American population, it is important to be reminded of the diversity among Asian Americans which include Chinese, Japanese, Korean, Vietnamese, Hmong, Cambodian, and Laotian students. In the US populations, data suggests that the prevalence of depression is lower among Asian Americans than in other ethnic/racial groups. Asian Americans who are depressed receive treatment less often than other groups (Kalibatseva & Leong, 2011). Some researchers have found that Asian high school students actually had a higher prevalence of depression than others and the risks were similar to those affecting Caucasians students (Song, Ziegler, Arsenault, Fried, & Hacker, 2011). Being foreign born was found to be a risk specific to Asian adolescents. One point of confusion in thinking about depression among Asian Americans is the difference in the experience of depression in Eastern cultures versus Western cultures. Recent views of the multidimensionality of depression suggest that Westerners may psychologize depression while Asians somatize depression. Westerners consider the body and mind as separate, whereas Easterners see the body and mind as integrated. The key symptoms of depression in the West are sadness or a depressed mood. The key symptoms among many other cultures are body symptoms such as changes in appetite, headaches, backaches and stomachaches, difficulty sleeping, or exhaustion. Asian American rates of depression are higher than their peers who live in their first countries. Not only is the experience of depression different but also there are cultural differences in reporting, in the criteria used to make diagnoses, and in the tools used to diagnose depression in these groups once they are in the United States.

When we consider Asian American children and adolescents, we must acknowledge that our data is not yet very good. For example, the significant predictors of depressive symptomatology in Korean students in middle school in Korea were low family support, low satisfaction of friendships, weak problem-solving abilities, and poor body image (Jee, Haejung, Hwa, & Eunyoung, 2010). Whether or not this would be similar in Korean children in the United States is not known. Our tools for diagnosis have limited cultural validity. It is difficult finding adequate samples that are homogenous enough to provide the information needed. Children may respond to inquiries about their emotional life from their own cultural perspectives. Recent studies indicate that physicians are missing emotional problems in Asian Americans (Kalibatseva & Leong, 2011). School professionals may be having the same difficulty.

African American boys tend to avoid seeking help for depression because of the stigma associated with depression. Frequently African American families do not trust professionals (Lindsey, Joe, & Nebbitt, 2010). There is some data available to suggest the African American girls do not experience adolescence in the same way as European American students. African American girls reach puberty earlier than Caucasian girls. African American girls do not seem to exhibit the decrease in self-esteem at adolescence that girls in other groups experience (Adams, 2005, 2010). In African American university students, higher depressive symptoms are related to lower self-esteem (Munford, 1994). Yet, Granberg, Simons, Gibbons, and Melby (2008) argue that African American school-aged girls are typically more satisfied with their bodies, which they theorize would make them less vulnerable to depression at least around weight concerns.

In some situations African American girls are more likely to experience depression. When African American girls attend schools in which they are not the majority, they experience increased symptoms of depression and report more somatic symptoms (Walsemann, Bell, & Maitra, 2011). Predominantly minority schools may protect African American students from discrimination and improve their attachment to school. This in turn would affect whether or not they would experience symptoms of depression. It is important to look at subgroups when exploring racial and cultural differences in mental health and illness. A study of African American students in grade 8 in another school indicated that both racial discrimination and gender discrimination were related to depressive symptoms (Cogburn, Chavous, & Griffin, 2011). When researchers looked at African American students in urban areas characterized by low income, they found life event stress was significantly associated with symptoms of depression. Living in a dangerous area of a city places children at risk because they have little control over their worlds. These children might benefit from learning what they can control and how to adapt to situations in which they have no control. This approach may reduce depressive symptoms. Hall, Cassidy, and Stevenson (2008) found that fear of lethal events was related to expressions of anger, whereas fear of harmful events that were not lethal was related to depression in African American adolescents. These findings may help school-based mental health professionals determine need for preventive activities.

Roberts, Roberts, and Chen (1997) studied ethnically diverse middle school boys and girls in grades 6–8. African American students and Mexican American students reported more depression without impairment than other groups. Mexican American students had elevated depression both with and without impairment. Girls reported more depression as did students who believed that they were worse off than their classmates. A study that examined different ethnic groups and depressive symptoms among high school students determined that ethnic differences disappeared when parent educational level was used as a control (Kennard, Stewart, Hughes, Patel, & Emslie, 2006).

Treatment of Internalizing Disorders

There is considerable data available in regard to the *treatment* of internalizing disorders. Federal funds have supported two large studies. One study focused on anxiety and the other on depression in an effort to determine the most efficacious treatment for the two disorders. The Treatment for Adolescents with Depression Study (TADS) was a multisite research study which compared the short- and long-term effectiveness of treatments for 327 adolescents from age 12 to 17 years of age diagnosed with major depression to medication alone, combined CBT and medication, and placebo (March et al., 2007). Best results were found for the combined treatment. The Child/Adolescent Anxiety Multimodal Study (CAMS) was a multisite, randomized placebo-controlled trial that compared the efficacy of cognitive-behavioral therapy (CBT) with antianxiety medication, and combinations of these treatments over a 6-year period, involving 488 students aged 7–17 years of age, were involved in the study (Compton et al., 2010). All students in the treatment conditions had been diagnosed with one of three anxiety disorders in the moderate to severe range. This study used the best available experimental designs and data analysis. Kendall's *Coping Cat*, a CBT (Kendall, 1994; Kendall et al., 1997), and the *C.A.T. Project* (Kendall, Choudhury, Hudson, & Webb, 2002), a version of the *Coping Cat* Program for adolescents, were compared against medication alone and against CBT combined with mediation. All three interventions were equivalent in reducing symptoms and were superior to treatment with a placebo. Combined CBT and medication worked best.

When school-based prevention or intervention programs are examined, CBT is the approach most frequently used for both anxiety prevention for prevention of depression and for preventive efforts to address both anxiety and depression with the strongest support (Cuijpers, van Straten, Smit, Mihalopoulos, & Beekman, 2008; Dobson et al., 2010).

There is considerable data available for the treatment of clinical levels of anxiety and depression. A recent meta-analytic review of treatment for anxiety disorders in children indicates that there are moderate effect sizes for the use of CBT with children (Reynolds, Wilson, Austin, & Hooper, 2012).

Neil and Christensen (2009) evaluated 27 outcome trials from 20 programs designed to reduce anxiety symptoms in school-aged children. They determined that most anxiety prevention programs were effective in reducing symptoms. Most of the programs that they located were for adolescents, targeted nonspecific anxiety symptoms, and used CBT. A meta-analysis of 63 studies of school-based interventions with 8,225 anxious and depressed students treated with CBT and 6,986 students in comparison conditions determined the appropriately focused CBT was moderately effective for anxious students and mildly effective for depressed students in reducing symptoms (Mychailyszyn, Brodman, Read, & Kendall, 2012).

Reynolds et al. (2012) concluded that interventions for anxiety in students were moderately effective using a meta-analytic review. Involving parents did not make a difference, but interventions targeted at specific anxiety disorders, and work with older children and adolescents were more effective. A study of 88 students averaging age 10 years, half of whom were Latino students, found that anxiety symptoms were reduced with greater effects when parents were also involved (Pina, Zerr, Villalta, & Gonzales, 2012). Latino ethnicity and the Spanish language did not change program effects suggesting that CBT strategies can be effective for Hispanic/Latino children if the intervention is delivered in a culturally responsive manner.

Prevention of Internalizing Disorders

There is a considerable need for effective *prevention* programs for children and adolescents around issues of anxiety and depression. Prevention of anxiety is still a relatively new research interest according to Lau and Rapee (2011). A review of available studies indicated that universal anxiety prevention programs show modest but promising results while targeted, secondary prevention programs show somewhat larger effects. Unfortunately, in the case of prevention of depression, our knowledge is still rudimentary (Pössel, 2005). Some researchers feel that it is too soon to implement prevention programs because those prevention trials that have been conducted are small, and results have not been replicated in schools on a large-scale basis in the United States (Garber et al., 2009). It may be too soon to recommend a single prevention program for internalizing disorders (Nehmy, 2010).

Merry and Spence (2007) point out that prevention of internalizing disorders is compromised when addressed in only one setting, i.e., at school. When prevention is considered, there are not a large number of programs that address internalizing disorders from which to choose. Practitioners will need to carefully research the several programs that are accumulating data to support their implementation, in order to find a program that may be helpful.

A major impediment in regard to prevention of internalizing disorders has to do with identification of need. Teachers in schools are the primary referral agents for students who need services. Students with internalizing disorders are under-identified and under-referred (Walker, Nishioka, Zeller, Severson, & Feil, 2000). Kleftaras and Didaskalou (2006) found that 30 % of students self-reported a high level of symptoms, but their teachers felt the students had behavior problems, or teachers felt their students' problems were not relevant to school.

There are a number of reasons for under-referral by teachers to include the fact that symptoms are hard to observe in class. Internalizing problems are less disruptive to teachers and therefore considered less concerning. Teachers do not feel capable of detecting internalizing problems and are not trained to do so. Teachers may also feel that there isn't support for internalizing problems available at the school level, or, teachers may feel that mental health is family business. Teachers need training to identify internalizing problems because even those students who may not meet the criteria for clinical depression or clinical anxiety are struggling and need support. It may be important to advocate for screening for internalizing problems as another way to identify students who need services. However, screening for mental health problems can be contentious.

Universal prevention programs for depression have not been around very long. Prevention programs for anxiety have been around longer and there is more data to support them. Anxiety prevention needs to be put in place early. Currently, program developers are working to develop anxiety prevention programs as early as the pre-school level (Cuthbert, 2010; Rapee, Kennedy, Ingram, Edwards, & Sweeney, 2010). The need for preventive efforts for depression at the middle school level is a common call to action (Keenan-Miller et al., 2007; Kelder et al., 2001; McCabe, Ricciardelli, & Banfield, 2011; McCarty, Violette, & McCauley, 2011; Saluja et al., 2004). Depression prevention is most likely best established at middle school. There have been several reviews of depression prevention/intervention programs specifically for the school setting (Hilt-Panahon, Kern, Divatia, & Gresham, 2007; Schultz & Mueller, 2007). Unfortunately, there are few evaluation studies of prevention programs specifically for preventing depression middle school girls in spite of the need for programs for this age and gender group (Schultz & Mueller, 2007).

School-Based Secondary Prevention

The literature on secondary prevention (Tier 2) is more encouraging than the literature on primary prevention for internalizing disorders. Preventive interventions appear to be more successful if students are selected based on multiple indices of risk. A key group would consist of students with a family history of depression who are already demonstrating symptoms (Kovacs & Lopez-Duran, 2010). School-based CBT specifically is the intervention of choice in that it has been determined to be effective for both girls and boys, in childhood, and for adolescents. It is effective across ethnic groups and for students with comorbid complications (Shirk, Kaplinski,

& Gudmundsen, 2009). Although there is also some support for interpersonal psychotherapy to prevent the onset of depressive disorders for children and adolescents (Cuijpers et al., 2008), CBT has the strongest empirical support. In the case of prevention of anxiety, a meta-analysis has demonstrated that the active condition for helping children with anxiety is cognitive-behavioral (In-Albon & Schneider, 2007). In the case of depression prevention, the components used most often are cognitive restructuring, scheduling pleasant activities, and problem solving, although additional components are used in some variations of CBT (Hilt-Panahon et al., 2007). All have been shown to be effective.

The best-known selective program for anxiety is the *Coping Cat* Program (Kendall, 1994). Although this program typically is used for treatment of anxiety in children, it can be used for prevention as well and can be delivered in groups. The *Coping Cat* Program is a CBT intervention for school-aged children ages 6–17 years. The program was reviewed by NREPP in October 2006. The "quality to research ratings" were 3.4–3.7 out of 4.0. Several efficacy trials of the *Coping Cat* Program determined that anxiety decreased, and importantly, depressive symptoms decreased as well (Kendall, 1994; Kendall et al., 1997). Benefits held for 12-months post-intervention. The *Coping Cat* Program uses relaxation, cognitive restructuring, problem solving, and exposure tasks to help student learn to control anxiety symptoms. Video components and case vignettes are included (Podell, Mychailyszyn, Edmunds, Puleo, & Kendall, 2010). The therapeutic relationship, games, activities, and discussion of problems have been shown to be important in gaining effects (Kendall & Southam-Gerow, 1996). The efficacy of the *Coping Cat* intervention for use in small groups has been established as well (Flannery-Schroeder, Choudhury, & Kendall, 2005).

Selective prevention programs for depression target students who have some indicator(s) of risk for depression such as being female, having experienced the death of a parent, parental divorce, placement in a juvenile detention facility, living in dysfunctional families, a family history of depression, atypical affectivity, negative cognitive schemata, a depressogenic attributional (negative thinking) style, depressive rumination, or negative self-perception (Kovacs & Lopez-Duran, 2010). Students with low positive affectivity, difficulty repairing negative moods, and physical symptoms as well as family risk would constitute a group of risk factors to target in secondary prevention. These are developmentally relevant, easy to assess, and can be changed. The content of the intervention needs to match the several identified vulnerabilities among small groups of students.

Research suggests that targeted prevention for depression is more effective than universal preventive intervention. There seems to be more evidence for targeted prevention, although multilevel prevention work is most strongly recommended. There have not been very positive effects associated with attempting to involve parents when working with adolescents with depressive symptoms. This may simply mean that effective ways of involving parents have not as yet been designed. If targeted prevention is planned, it is important to build in controls to avoid stigma. Be careful about the time of day that programming is offered. Be thoughtful in regard to *where* in the school the program is offered. Avoid promising tremendous change, and make sure that implementation fidelity is excellent (Schultz & Mueller, 2007). Use of components of CBT to address more than one cause of depression, building strengths instead of focusing on weaknesses, including strategies to deal with thoughts and behaviors that are not helpful, strong adherence to protocols, and including booster sessions have been found to be effective in reducing symptoms of depression (Hilt-Panahon et al., 2007).

There are several specific programs to consider. The *Penn Resiliency Program* developed in 1990 to reduce symptoms of depression and to build resilience includes teaching problem-solving skills and coping skills (Gillham, 1994; Jaycox, Reivich, Gillham, & Seligman, 1994). This prevention program was designed for students aged 10–14 in small groups. There are two major components, cognitive-behavioral techniques and social problem solving. Booster sessions and a parent component are available. The program has been used as a universal prevention program and as a targeted program. School professionals have implemented the program with training. There have been a number of evaluations of the program with positive results. The program reduces symptoms of depression and anxiety, and the effects last for 2 years in some studies. The program has been effective for girls and boys although it may take time after program completion for the effects to be seen (Schultz & Mueller, 2007).

A meta-analysis of 17 controlled evaluations of the *Penn Resiliency Program* showed that positive effects resulted whether the intervention was targeted or universal, when leaders were research team members or school providers, whether symptoms were low or high, and with both girls and boys. Effects lasted at least 1 year (Brunwasser, Gillham, & Kim, 2009). All girl groups appear to be beneficial for reducing feelings of hopelessness (Chaplin et al., 2006). Low-income Latino middle school students have been shown to benefit from this program but interestingly, African American students did not (Cardemil, Reivich, Beevers, Seligman, & James, 2007). Gillham et al. (2007) trained teachers and counselors to implement the *Penn Resiliency Program* in three middle schools. In two schools students' symptoms of depression decreased, indicating that when implemented well, this program can be successful in a school setting.

The *Adolescent Coping with Stress Course* is an abbreviated version of the Adolescent Coping with Depression Course delivered in a group setting to adolescents at risk for depression. There are 15 one-hour sessions. The program has been evaluated several times with very positive results by program developers (Schultz & Mueller, 2007). The *Problem Solving for Life* program is a universal prevention program for adolescents aged 12–14 developed in Australia and is designed to be implemented by teachers. The program combines cognitive restructuring and problem-solving skills training. It is best for students with elevated symptoms. Evaluations indicate that there are short-term effects.

The *Resourceful Adolescent Program* (RAP-A) was also designed in Australia and is delivered by teachers or school mental health staff to groups of students 12–15 years (Shochet et al., 2001). The program lasts one school semester and is delivered once per week. The content of the program includes stress management, problem solving, building support networks, managing conflict, taking perspectives, and cognitive restructuring. There is a companion program for parents. There have been several efficacy studies showing some positive effects lasting 18 months (Wolfe, Dozois, Fisman, & DePace, 2008). Two versions of RAP-A have been developed for teens in ninth grade. *RAP-A* is a school-based group program. *RAP-A* consists of 11 sessions intended to help students develop resilience and support. An evaluation of the program resulted in short-term improvements with mixed improvement at 18-months post-implementation (Pössel, 2005).

A review of school-based anxiety and depression prevention interventions completed in 2011 determined that 65 % of 28 programs were effective for depression and 73 % were effective for anxiety prevention, although the effects were small (Corrieri et al., 2013).

School-Based Primary Prevention

An effort to increase awareness of depression has been attempted using a curriculum called the *Adolescent Depression Awareness Program* (ADAP) for high schools (Swartz, 2011). The goal is depression literacy, i.e., changing students' knowledge and encouraging help seeking for depression. It has been implemented in four states and in Washington, DC schools and is expanding nationally. An Australian initiative, *beyondblue*, is also a depression literacy effort with a curriculum for high schools (Pirkis et al., 2005; Spence et al., 2005). However, this program has been challenging to implement. A 3-year study of 25 pairs of secondary schools matched according to SES was randomly assigned to implement *beyondblue* or to a control group (Sawyer et al., 2010). Researchers did not obtain significant differences in depressive symptom reduction between the intervention and control groups. Problems encountered included inadequate teacher training to implement the intervention with fidelity, difficulties engaging students, and the lengthy time frame needed to effect change in whole-school interventions.

A more successful effort has been the *FRIENDS* program (Barrett, Lowry-Webster, & Holmes, 1999). This program is a well-established *universal* program for anxiety prevention using CBT techniques. The FRIENDS program was developed from the *Coping Koala Group Program*, the Australian version of Kendall's *Coping Cat Program* (Bernstein, Layne, Egan, & Tennison, 2005). It involves 10–12 sessions with an additional four sessions for parents. The program teaches an acronym:

- F = feeling worried
- R = relax and feel good
- I = inner helpful thoughts
- E = explore and plan
- N = nice work, reward yourself
- D = don't forget to practice
- S = stay calm for life

Evaluation studies indicate that the program is best for younger children, for girls, and for those with more symptoms of anxiety. Studies with children of mixed race backgrounds have been successful (Bienvenu & Ginsburg, 2007). The *FRIENDS* program (Australian developed) is evidence-based and targets both children and early adolescents (Barrett & Pahl, 2006; Farrell & Barrett, 2007). It is the *only* evidence-based prevention program that has been endorsed by the World Health Organization. A randomized clinical trial of the *FRIENDS* intervention was conducted with 71 children aged 6–10 years old with anxiety disorders and compared to a wait-list group (Shortt, Barrett, & Fox, 2001). Sixty-nine percent of children were diagnosis-free at post-intervention and 68 % were diagnosis-free at 12-months follow-up. Parental involvement was helpful as parents encouraged consistent use of strategies.

Fisak, Richard, and Mann (2011) conducted a meta-analytic review of anxiety prevention programs and determined that immediate effects were positive but long-term effects were mixed. Programs that used the *FRIENDS* program were stronger than other interventions. Effectiveness depended on whether or not mental health professionals ran the intervention as compared to laypersons. Variables such as the duration of the program, age of participants, gender, or universal versus targeted programs were not important in that they did not reduce effects. The fact that program type (universal versus targeted programs) did not matter is significant in that most studies have shown that targeted programs for prevention of internalizing symptoms and disorders have stronger effect sizes. Children seem to benefit from the *FRIENDS* program regardless of prior risks.

Barrett, Lock, and Farrell (2005) evaluated the effects of the FRIENDS program in sixth and ninth grade students as compared to participation in a monitoring group. Students at high and moderate risk experienced significant decreases in both anxiety and depression immediately post-intervention and also at 12-months follow-up. The program was more effective immediately post-intervention for sixth grade students in regard to anxiety reduction, although both groups showed equal effects at 12 months. The earlier intervention had the most positive effects.

There have been a series of studies determining the effectiveness of the FRIENDS intervention worldwide and also in the United States, although international studies comprise the bulk of the literature to date. For example, 638 children from 14 schools in Germany were divided into treatment and control groups (Essau, Conradt, Sasagawa, & Ollendick, 2012). Children participating in the FRIENDS program experienced significant reductions in symptoms of anxiety and depression. Younger children benefitted early on, 11- and 12-year-old students did not show gains until 12-months post-intervention. When parents were involved, effects were greater.

Bernstein et al. (2005) conducted one of the several published studies of the *FRIENDS* program in the United States. This group compared nine weekly sessions of school-based group CBT and group CBT plus expanded parents training, with a no-treatment control. The CBT treatments were more effective in comparison to no treatment, and adding the parent component resulted in significantly more improvement. Although the control group also made gains during the study period, the treatment group made gains in *both* reading and math achievement scores. The treatment group also experienced decreased stress and reduced victimization.

A study involved 98 third through fifth grade predominantly African American children in the United States. Students attended 13 biweekly 1-h sessions and were exposed to a modified version of *FRIENDS* (Cooley-Strickland, Griffin, Darney, Otte, & Ko, 2011). Although all students made gains during the study period, the students participating in the *FRIENDS* program experienced decreased stress and victimization. Students also showed improved reading and math achievement scores. Not every study of the *FRIENDS* program has had positive results, a study of fourth to sixth grade students with anxiety symptoms looked at the effectiveness of *FRIENDS* as compared to story-reading in two longitudinal studies (Miller, Yang, Farrell, & Lin, 2011). This study did not find intervention effects. Prevention work is not easy.

Anxiety management and relaxation training have been shown to be promising for students who exhibit symptoms of both anxiety and depression in a few studies (Hilt-Panahon et al., 2007). Adolescents with symptoms of both internalizing problems experience decreased symptoms of depression with CBT alone (Garber, 2006). Children with anxiety should be targeted as well as children with depressive symptoms for depression prevention programs (Garber, 2006).

Currently there is considerable interest in subsyndromal symptoms or subthreshold disorders, as this is important when we think about preventing internalizing disorders (Mazzone et al., 2007). More students present with elevated symptoms of depression than those that meet the formal criteria for a depressive disorder (McCabe et al., 2011). Students at risk also report heightened negative feelings, reduced positive feelings, reduced self-concepts, and psychosocial issues. At-risk students may be the most disadvantaged because they will not receive services nor will they be identified.

School-based mental health professionals also need to address behaviors such as smoking in girls who experience depressive symptoms (Galambos, Leadbeater, & Barker, 2004). Smoking is highly correlated with depression. As smoking behavior increases in girls, depressive symptoms increase as well. Smoking predicts depression among younger students. Preventive efforts need to address smoking as depressive symptoms are addressed. Early diagnosis and family-based education are important in the prevention of depression and anxiety in adolescents. Children from families with a history of anxiety or depression need early preventive efforts. Preventive programs to strengthen preadolescents' sense of competence are critical. Ability to identify depressive symptoms in themselves and strategies to cope with sad, irritable, and lonely feelings must be included in prevention efforts in schools.

When students feel that they can control situations, events, or tasks, anxiety decreases (Williams, 2008). A student's belief about his or her ability influences avoidance behavior. Because avoidance behaviors prevent corrective learning, it is important to deal with them in prevention efforts. Mastering avoidance behavior by itself can decrease anxiety. Of note, increasing environmental rewards has been of benefit to depressed adults (Ryba & Hopko, 2012). This may be helpful in preventing depression in preadolescents as well.

Clearly it is important to identify students *before* they develop symptoms of internalizing illness. Children demonstrating a combination of symptoms that would not warrant a diagnosis are at risk of progressing to a first episode of major depressive disorder. The complication is that because many of these children will not develop a diagnosable depressive disorder, school teams may avoid preventive programming (Kovacs & Lopez-Duran, 2010). This explains why the effect sizes of prevention programs are modest and perhaps this fact contributes to hesitancy to implement prevention programs in school as well.

Prevention in Action Challenge: Create an Outline for an In-service Presentation or Workshop for Teachers or Parents to Identify Internalizing Disorders

Prepare an outline of an in-service presentation or workshop to train teachers (and/or parents) to identify internalizing disorders in children or adolescents. Include the following:

- Incidence/prevalence of internalizing disorders
- Signs, symptoms, and causes of anxiety and depression
- The fact that internalizing disorders are common and treatable
- What internalizing symptoms might look like in school
- Strategies for supporting students with internalizing issues in class
- Importance of personal connections
- The importance of referral of students at risk

Resources:

1. Huberty, T. J. (2004). *Depression: Helping students in the classroom.* National Association of School Psychologists (http://www.nasponline. org)
2. School and classroom strategies: Depression (http://studentsfirstproject. org)
3. Teen depression: A guide for parents and teachers (http://www.icpt.co)
4. *Teen depression.* MN ADOPT (http://www.mnadopt.org)

Chapter 10
Fidelity Versus Adaptation

Implementation science is an emerging field of study (Kilbourne, Williams, Bauer, & Arean, 2012). NIMH defines implementation as "use of strategies to adopt and integrate evidence-based health interventions and change practice patterns within specific settings." Implementing evidence-based preventive programming in schools includes selecting effective preventive interventions and implementing them in the same way they were designed by the researchers who originally developed the program (Sanetti, Gritter, & Dobey, 2011). When a prevention program is implemented in a school, past practice indicates that it may or may not be successful. It is only when practitioners determine whether or not a program or preventive intervention has been implemented very much as the developers of the program intended can they have any confidence at all in whether or not they will get the same results as the original studies which determined that the program was effective in the first place.

There are many aspects of implementation that need to be explored, the most critical of which may well be treatment integrity. Treatment integrity has many names. In some cases it is referred to as treatment fidelity, in others it is called implementation fidelity, or intervention integrity. It is also referred to by the terms procedural reliability, treatment compliance, or treatment adherence (Gresham, 2009; Sanetti & Kratochwill, 2009; Schulte, Easton, & Parker, 2009). The terms treatment integrity and treatment fidelity are used interchangeably (Margulis, 2012). No matter which term is used, this concept relates to whether or not a preventive program was delivered as intended (Carroll et al., 2007). The integrity with which the preventive effort is implemented will determine whether or not "it works." Unfortunately, treatment integrity isn't typically measured in schools (Sanetti, Fallon, & Collier-Meeka, 2011). This is not surprising in that, sadly, the majority of researchers do not report treatment integrity data either (Sanetti, Dobey, & Gritter, 2012).

The four general dimensions of treatment integrity include content, quality, quantity, and process (Sanetti & Kratochwill, 2009). *Content* has to do with which steps of the interventions process were actually put in place. *Quality* refers to how well the steps were implemented. *Quantity* has to do with how much of the

G.L. Macklem, *Preventive Mental Health at School: Evidence-Based Services for Students*,
DOI 10.1007/978-1-4614-8609-1_10, © Springer Science+Business Media New York 2014

intervention was delivered. *Process* has to do with how the content and steps were actually delivered. When intervention fidelity is measured, the two most commonly measured aspects are dosage and quality (Ransford, Greenberg, Domitrovich, Small, & Jacobson, 2009).

There are actually many dimensions of treatment integrity to consider when preventive interventions and programs take place in schools. These include:

- *Adherence* (number of elements delivered)
- *Exposure* (number and length of sessions)
- *Quality* (implementer's skills delivering the preventive intervention)
- *Program differentiation* (when one program is compared with another)
- *Dosage* (the amount of treatment delivered)
- *Participant comprehension and responsiveness* (engagement or enthusiasm)
- *Mastery* in both the training situation and in the setting in which the skills are intended to be used (Dusenbury, Brannigan, Falco, & Hansen, 2003; Sanetti, Gritter, & Dobey, 2011; Schulte et al., 2009)

Students must actually use the skills they are taught and so it is critical to know whether or not skills were taught in the first place. It is also critical to know whether or not students learned the skills, whether students use the skills in situations in which they are needed, and whether or not this makes a difference. When evaluating how a particular preventive intervention was *delivered*, modeling, role-playing, rehearsal, and feedback have been shown to be effective. For targeted prevention programs, quality of delivery, exposure, and responsiveness of those participating in the program are particularly important.

In school prevention work, when exposure and adherence are measured, school intervention teams know how many hours of the curriculum or program, and how many steps of skills development, were taught (Sanetti & Kratochwill, 2009). There are additional considerations. For example, not all program components may be equally critical. Programs that are more flexible, and can be adapted to fit the local school, may be implemented better. There could even be a threshold that once reached will result in the same outcomes as if every aspect of a program were implemented perfectly. This knowledge is not readily available, although there have some attempts to identify a threshold. In some cases, and for some prevention programs, less than perfect implementation may be "good enough." Durlak and DuPre (2008) note that when some programs are implemented with 60 % integrity, it may be possible to obtain positive outcomes. The often-quoted ideal is to deliver a program with 80 % integrity. Not very many programs are able to achieve 80 % implementation. And there is not a great deal of data to support the goal of "at or above 80 %" treatment integrity (Sanetti, Fallon, & Collier-Meeka, 2011).

Durlak and DuPre (2008) reviewed 30 years of data to determine what might affect outcomes. They identified 23 contextual factors that influenced implementation. Of 542 interventions examined, no studies had documented perfect implementation. Programs implemented better had better results in terms of knowledge, attitudes, and/or behavior change. Durlak and Dupre's analysis of 500 of the studies determined clearly that *level* of implementation matters. Empirical support for the effect of implementation on outcomes was strong. Additionally, they determined that some programs were implemented successfully when between 60 and 80 % of the program was implemented. Of the factors that influenced the degree to which prevention programs were implemented with fidelity level of funding, implementers who appreciated the need for the program, implementers who believed the program would work, and programs with at least some flexibility made a difference. Not only does the implementation of the core components determine outcomes but also efficient monitoring is a key to success.

Studies indicate that a higher level of treatment integrity has the effect of better outcomes in most cases (Sanetti & Kratochwill, 2009). Practitioners must always watch for "intervention drift" and be very much aware of the likelihood of implementers' adaptations that may or may not affect outcomes. Intervention drift has to do with the small changes made by those implementing programs either without being aware of the fact that they are making changes or when they make changes with good intentions. In either case the changes were neither planned nor condoned by program designers. At the same time, it is likely that not all intervention components are absolutely vital to achieve outcomes. We also know that when program elements are implemented exactly as written, they may not meet local needs. The core elements of preventive programs always need to be retained.

Extent of Problems Involving Treatment Integrity

Schulte et al. (2009) point out that there is a good deal of data to indicate that treatment integrity has not been the central focus in research studies and in practice. Treatment integrity has been neglected. The rate of incorporation of treatment integrity is low. Implementation that is perfect in all dimensions is not likely to occur. Although "best practices" would indicate that practitioners must pay attention to implementation and measure fidelity of implementation when preventive programs are implemented; unfortunately, fidelity of this aspect of practice is often ignored. Surveys show that only 11.3 % of school psychologists measure fidelity of practice when consulting with teachers about a student, and only 1.9 % of school psychologists collect this type of data when consulting with a team of teachers and other staff (Keller-Margulis, 2012, p. 343). Experts suggest that a "high level" of integrity exists when 80 % or more of an intervention or program is implemented. When less than 50 % of an intervention or program is implemented, this would be considered to be a "low level" of implementation. Hopson and Steiker (2008) suggested that strict implementation is "rare."

There have been a number of studies examining the degree to which preventive programs have been implemented in schools. When 1,905 teachers were surveyed regarding their implementation of substance use prevention programs, researchers determined that only 15 % followed the curricula closely (Ringwalt et al., 2003). Twenty percent of teachers implementing the curricula did not use the curriculum guide. Teachers' use of the curricula was affected by whether or not they felt that the training they received was effective and whether or not they felt supported by the school administration. Other researchers indicate that the degree to which teachers implement preventive interventions can be described as low to moderate (Sanetti, Fallon, & Collier-Meeka, 2011, p. 87). Teachers who work with minority students tend to adapt the curricula so that it will better fit their students (Botvin, 2004). Some of the reasons they make changes include students' limited English proficiency and the fact that students have been exposed to violence (Ringwalt, Vincus, Ennett, Johnson, & Rohrbach, 2004). Ringwalt et al. (2003) feel that at least some changes to the curricula may be inevitable when prevention programs are implemented. Teacher training is clearly important to avoid making adaptations that would affect outcomes of preventive programming.

In a sample of schools implementing substance use preventive programs during the 1998–1999 school year, Ennett et al. (2003) found that 62.25 % of teachers taught the content but only 17.44 % used the recommended teaching strategies, and only 14.23 % used both the content and teaching strategies described by program designers. Well-researched interventions are not always used in schools but when evidence-based preventive programs are used, implementers were more likely to use both the content and the teaching strategies prescribed. A study of elementary schools using substance use prevention curricula determined that 72 % of districts used a curriculum in this category at the elementary level, but only 14 % used one that was evidence-based (Hanley et al., 2010).

In a study published in 2002, Halifors and Godette determined that only 19 % of 104 school districts in their study implemented a research-based curriculum as it was originally designed. Implementation was clearly poor. The problems that Halifors and Godette (2002) identified included lack of training for teachers, insufficient materials, and teachers' dropping some lessons for various reasons. Teachers used teaching strategies with which they were comfortable instead of strategies associated with the curriculum or programs. They used the curriculum with students of different ages/grades than those for which the intervention was designed. Systems-level issues affect implementation. Inadequate funding or infrastructure, ineffective decision-making, and lack of support affected implementation. Schools tend to use programs that are heavily marketed rather than using research-based programs that would take some time to find and to determine whether or not they fit the particular district. Halifors and Godette found that only 19 % of schools in more than 1,500 districts were implementing curricula with fidelity. By 2005, only nine universal curricula for elementary substance abuse prevention were even considered evidence-based (Hanley et al., 2010).

Although by 2003 there had not been much research on fidelity of implementation, already the research on drug abuse prevention was indicating that when programming was not implemented well, there was a loss of effectiveness of programs (Dusenbury et al., 2003). Researchers found that most teachers did not teach entire curricula, and over time they tended to teach less and less of a given curricula. Training alone has not been found to be sufficient to guarantee full implementation of a program. The key components of strong fidelity of implementation appear to be stronger teacher training, the characteristics of the program, the particular teachers implementing the program, and the organization or school itself. Since teachers are likely to make changes in a program that they are implementing, the more flexible the program, the more likely that it will meet student needs and the less likely that effectiveness will be diminished. It is important when schools are selecting preventive programming that they collaborate with program developers to make sure that programs are sufficiently flexible so that they can be implemented well in a different setting.

Unfortunately, even when schools carefully train school staff in evidence-based prevention there is no guarantee that implementation of a program will be successful (Bohanon & Wu, 2011). Beyond the support of all stakeholders involved, there is need for explicit, shared, and measurable goals. An effective process for identifying students at risk is needed (p. 37). Layers of prevention that are well integrated may in fact provide more support for students than a single preventive program or intervention alone and provide more support for teachers as well. When schools collect data and develop systems to support change and sustainability, practices can be kept in place over time.

Challenges and Barriers

Durlak (1997) found that less than 5 % of 1,200 studies reviewed shared information on implementation. Implementation of universal prevention programs faces strong challenges including getting schools to even consider them in the first place when schools are so stressed by other priorities involving academics and policy (Committee on the Prevention of Mental Disorder and Substance Abuse, 2009). In order for a program to be approved so that it can be implemented, multiple stakeholders must agree. Administrators may question the effectiveness and efficiency of universal preventive efforts because the dose may be too low for students at high risk, or outcomes may not be immediate enough. Many prevention program outcomes are stronger when implemented over time. The effects at the end of the second year are typically stronger than at the end of the first year of implementation (Schroeder et al., 2011). Yet, universal preventive efforts can be successful when implemented long enough. They can be successful when delivered at a sufficient intensity. They can be successful when the program is aimed at enhancing resilience to protect students from multiple disorders or when the program is aimed at problems that are found in large numbers of students. Bullying prevention is an example of a preventive effort reaching large numbers of students. The Safe and Drug-Free Act of 1999 and NCLB provided an impetus for schools to select stronger prevention programs.

Evidence-based programs are not as likely to be as effective in the local school community as they were in controlled clinical research trials (Lochman, 2003). The school context is a dynamic and complex system (Masten, 2003). The school context itself influences practice (Short, 2003). Change is never easy. It is common for stakeholders in any organization to resist change (Elliott, Kratochwill, & Roach, 2003).

Table 10.1 Barriers to implementing preventive programs with integrity

---

- Poor to no training for those implementing the program (Hopson & Steiker, 2008)
- Few resources available (Gresham, 2009; Hopson & Steiker, 2008; Langley et al., 2010)
- Large class sizes (Hopson & Steiker, 2008)
- Low morale among staff (Hopson & Steiker, 2008)
- Lack of time due to other responsibilities (Gresham, 2009; Hopson & Steiker, 2008; Mihalic & Irwin, 2003)
- Difficulty finding time in the school schedule (Mihalic et al., 2008)
- Lack of support from school administrators (Hopson & Steiker, 2008; Langley et al., 2010; Mihalic et al., 2008)
- Difficulty getting teacher and administrator support (Langley et al., 2010; Mihalic et al., 2008)
- Classroom management challenges (Mihalic et al., 2008)
- Complex teaching strategies needed (Gresham, 2009)
- Too many competing responsibilities for mental health professional (Langley et al., 2010)
- Conflict in professional networks (Langley et al., 2010)
- Materials or manuals that were not useful (Langley et al., 2010)
- Lack of relevance of the program to participants (Langley et al., 2010)
- Challenges around parental engagement (Langley et al., 2010)
- Difficulty getting teacher buy-in (Langley et al., 2010)
- Poor compatibility with the school culture (Langley et al., 2010)
- Teacher burnout (Ransford et al., 2009)
- A negative school climate (Ransford et al., 2009)
- School disorganization (Ransford et al., 2009)

When addressing change, stakeholders need to engage in a dialogue about school climate. There must be an awareness developed about the need for change among school staff members, students, and the community. It is necessary to encourage expressions of concerns and frustrations of individuals involved in school change.

When considering SEL programming, for example, the likelihood of accountability around high stakes testing may build a barrier of resistance to anything new or innovative. Work needs to proceed carefully or failure will interfere with future school change attempts. New programming must fit into the contextual reality of the school environment. Elliott et al. (2003) indicate that 80 % or more of the school staff must commit to the change if it is to be successful. The actions and outcomes of the new programming must be continually evaluated over time. The school culture itself can influence whether or not a new program will be successful. The behavior of students is critical because misbehavior can affect teacher willingness to use interactive exercises or can take away time so that the curriculum is not covered (Mihalic, Fagan, & Argamaso, 2008).

Major barriers exist at the systems and organizational levels because of competing responsibilities. This is a particularly strong barrier in school settings (Langley, Nadeem, Kataoka, Stein, & Jacox, 2010) (Table 10.1).

Although some school mental health workers have been trained to select evidence-based preventive interventions, the training does not always result in fidelity of implementation even for this group (Langley et al., 2010). When trainers are knowledgeable and enthusiastic, training is more successful. Manuals with carefully described activities that are easy to use facilitate adoption. When the entire staff and stakeholders see the need for change, implementation will be more successful. Resources that help include time, money, materials, and space (Langley et al., 2010). Interviews with implementers of the *Cognitive Behavioral Intervention for Trauma in Schools* program (CBITS) (Jaycox, 2004) determined that there were significant barriers to success. The primary barriers were at the systems level. Teachers had issues about taking students from class. Finding a place to work with students in the school was challenging. Partnerships with mental health agencies for consultation improved the likelihood of successful implementation in this study, along with administrative support within the school.

In addition to numerous barriers to implementing preventive programming with integrity, maintaining implementation fidelity is a challenge. Although an intervention may be initially delivered with treatment integrity, over time, this effort may decrease. When school professionals implement a program as compared to bringing in experts from outside schools, they are better able to deal with scheduling and calendar conflicts. Teachers who are hesitant to allow students to be pulled out of class and may respond better to in-house mental health professionals they know, than to outside the school collaborators. Professionals within schools such as school psychologists, or other mental health workers, may also have too many competing responsibilities to help teachers with preventive programs, unless their role is redefined. Outside the school mental health workers who come into schools to implement programming may have decreased competing priorities, but they have difficulty with the politics of the school. The importance of getting teacher, administrator, and parent buy-in *before* attempting to implement a program is paramount. Raising awareness of the targeted problem through in-services, parent meetings, and stakeholder focus groups can help. Parent engagement in school activities has long been a recognized barrier to providing services for all children. Obtaining parent permission for a student to participate may be an obstacle. It is unfortunate when needy students cannot be included because parental permission cannot be obtained.

Every program has an explicit or implicit idea about how students learn which can be seen in the design of lessons, in the sequence of lessons, and in the way staff are trained (Elias, Zins, Graczyk, & Weissberg, 2003). Schools must be "ready" to deal with new programming. In order to be ready, school staff must be willing to collaborate with one another and take ownership of the programs. This takes time. It is hard to give up what you have worked on and accept something new. Resources may have to be freed up and redistributed. Supports must be visible and staff members need time to get fully onboard. Unfortunately programs can't just be dropped into a school schedule; they must be integrated with other programming and the rest of the school day.

When preventive interventions are implemented in disorganized schools, programming is not typically implemented well and outcomes are compromised (Ransford et al., 2009). On the other hand, when teachers receive demonstrations, corrective and encouraging feedback, and opportunities to practice, they are more likely to implement program with integrity. When solid administrative support is added to good training, implementation improves even more. Beyond this, lessons with familiar formats and familiar instructional materials are easier to implement. A study of ten elementary schools demonstrated the importance of teacher beliefs about the program. Administrative support and perceptions of school connectedness influenced the number of lessons taught, use of program materials, and participation in activities (Beets et al., 2008).

Halifors and Godette (2002) found that when programs were implemented, they were adapted to a significant degree by teachers. Reed (2004) studied the implementation of *Second Step: A Violence Prevention Curriculum* (Committee for Children, 1992). Reed found that most teachers did not implement the curriculum with integrity. Although teachers were aware of components that they skipped, they tended to overemphasize aspects of curricula they preferred (e.g., role-plays). Teachers reported a lack of time to teach all of the components and their concerns were that lessons were not always relevant for the students that they were teaching. When researchers review program implementation, they find that adaptation is not unusual; in fact, "interventionist drift," which refers to unintended changes made by those implementing programs occurs in the *majority* of cases (Sanetti & Kratochwill, 2009, p. 452). Even some implementers of the better programs do not monitor whether or not programs are being implemented with integrity (Steiker, 2008).

Adaptations to Curricula

Prevention curricula may not engage students for a variety of reasons such as when the group is unique in some way or when the group of students is different from the population in the efficacy studies in age or risk status (Mihalic et al., 2008). Ozer, Wanis, and Bazell (2010) gathered data to determine adaptations made to curricula when two empirically supported programs were implemented in urban schools with highly diverse student populations. Interviews, classroom observations, and consultation with program developers showed that *all* teachers made adaptations to their programs. The most frequent adaptations involved changing the format, adding real-life examples, and changing the wording of lessons. The majority of changes were acceptable to program developers although some of the teachers' proposed adaptations were not scientific. Implementers also asked students to give their opinions of the curricula. Students made suggestions for changes in content, but these were not acceptable. When students participated in adapting elements of programs such as changing the language or the videos, there was some evidence that this action, by itself changed students' attitudes (Steiker, 2008). In any program adaptation, implementers should be very careful not to move too far from the core of the program. Yet, some adaptations are quite acceptable. For example, it is important to match the scenarios, and visuals depicted in the programs to the life experiences of the students participating in the program.

Content and Teaching Strategies

Research studies that address implementation of prevention programs have looked carefully at program delivery and whether or not the manner in which a program is delivered determines program success (Botvin & Griffin, 2003). The most challenging aspect of implementing prevention programs has to do with the use of *active teaching* strategies. There is considerable interest in active learning among program developers and implementers. Interactive teaching strategies are most often written about in connection with prevention programs that address drug abuse. In this group of programs, interactive strategies are considered critical elements (Sussman, Rohrbach, Patel, & Holiday, 2003). In a study of the *Project Towards No Drug Abuse* program (Dent et al., 1998), Sussman, Dent, and Stacy (2002) determined that outcomes were closely tied to interactive teaching strategies. In fact, the effects of the program were considered to be "strong" only when the curriculum was taught using interactive strategies. The particular teaching approach that seemed to be particularly effective involved students talking with one another and asking each other questions.

When researchers compared programs that used didactic lectures to those using interactive teaching approaches, they have found that lectures were less effective (Steiker, 2008). In traditional didactic approaches to teaching, the program effects focus on knowledge and attitudes (Ennett et al., 2003). Interactive strategies tend to involve skills such as refusal or competency skills. Cuijpers (2002) looked at the effective ingredients of prevention programs and determined that interactive teaching methods were "superior." Use of lectures and videotapes did not result in outcomes that were as strong as when teachers used discussion, role-playing, and interactive games to teach and practice new behavior (Botvin, 2004). The differences were considerable. Studies suggest that interactive approaches are particularly important when working with adolescents. Sandhu, Afifi, and Amara (2012) compared a program's effect on retaining, synthesizing, and elaborating knowledge and also on satisfying students. The interactive strategies they looked at included open discussion, technology-assisted lessons, case reports, and problem-based strategies. Comparing these strategies with lectures resulted in stronger student satisfaction, improved learning outcomes, better retention, and deeper learning.

Interactive teaching strategies are critical whether students are very young, school-aged, or are adolescents. Researchers examining three Head Start programs implementing evidence-based and comprehensive programs (the PATHS curriculum) determined that implementation quality improved across the school year for some aspects of the program (Domitrovich, Gest, Jones, Gill, & DeRousie, 2010). Gains in student engagement were determined by whether or not teachers could find attractive activities. Variations in engaging students affected the quality of students' ability to problem-solve as well as teachers' ratings of positive and negative student behaviors. Teachers, who generalized the *PATHS curriculum* using activities, affected students' problem solving positively. When working with late adolescents, interactive teaching strategies have resulted in better attendance (Ernst & Colthorpe, 2007), greater attraction (program more popular), and better retention (Costa, van Rensburg, & Rushton, 2007).

In a large study of drug prevention programs, Tobler and Stratton (1997) conducted a meta-analysis of 120 programs conducted in schools. On the basis of their study they were able to group the programs into interactive and not interactive programs. They determined that not only were the interactive programs statistically more effective than programs that were noninteractive, but they were clinically more effective as well. Smaller interactive programs were more effective than larger programs because they tended to be better implemented. Flay (2009) looked at smoking prevention programs conducted in schools. Flay determined that smoking prevention programs that used interactive teaching strategies involving social influence (making a commitment not to use), or teaching social skills (practice in use of refusal behaviors and life skills) had long-term effects. Additional programming strategies that made a difference included having 15 or more sessions and using peer leaders in addition to adult trainers. More classes and continuing the program over several grades were significant as well.

Teachers Implementing Preventive Programming

In a study of the *LifeSkills* program in 432 schools at 105 sites, researchers evaluated adherence to the curriculum, the quality of delivery, and the responsiveness of the student participants (Mihalic et al., 2008). The more highly the characteristics of the program were rated, and the better the students behaved, the more of the program that was taught. Student behavior and quality of delivery were related as teachers who managed students better used more interactive teaching strategies. Teachers with highly positive attitudes toward the program tended to teach all of the lessons. Seventy-one percent of those implementing the program taught all of the lessons and used 86 % of the activities. Student responsiveness did not relate to any of the variables measured. Researchers recommended that schools choose programs that are not too complex, that are flexible, and that fit the time available in the classroom. The availability of consultation and effective monitoring made a difference as well.

Ennett et al. (2011) evaluated fidelity of substance use prevention program implementation in 342 middle schools from a national random sample of schools, during the 2004–2005 school year. In these particular schools there was high quality of program delivery and student responsiveness. Quality of program delivery was determined by whether or not the implementers felt confident to teach the program and whether or not they encouraged student participation. Encouragement of student participation was more significant in regard to delivering a curriculum with integrity than previously thought. Those delivering the curricula tended to teach the lessons, but did not as often follow the delivery methods required by the curriculum. Only about one-third of school staff taught the entire curriculum on the schedule recommended by program designers. One-quarter of the school staff delivered both the content and teaching strategies as designed. Researchers felt that more attention was needed to support interactive delivery strategies because only a third of implementers used the interactive strategies as frequently as the curriculum demanded. This was actually a good result when the study was compared to earlier studies, but challenges remain.

Some programs are more successful than others (Ennett et al., 2011). Schools using *Project ALERT* (Ellickson, Bell, Thomas, Robyn, & Zellman, 1988), *LifeSKills* Training (LST), and the *All Stars* (Hansen, 1996) programs delivered a greater percentage of lessons. Unfortunately, the more successful implementers tended to use nonevidence-based curricula and materials that they developed themselves. This could dilute an evidence-based program. Of note, class discussions were not considered interactive teaching approaches in this study as they have been in other research studies. The rationale here was that rather than being discussion among peers, the discussions tended to take place between teachers and students. This lowered adherence estimates. Ennett et al. warn that until schools can demonstrate higher levels of adherence to curricula content and teaching strategies, outcomes will continue to be diluted.

Success in Implementing Prevention Programs

In reviewing what works in regard to implementation, Schulte et al. (2009) reported that when school principals were asked to encourage and monitor implementation, teachers implemented more lessons. When those who implemented programs had supervised practice, along with a manual and seminar, they implement programs better than teachers given only a manual. When schools use a tool to help them predict whether or not implementation will be successful, treatment integrity improves.

School personnel must also be "ready" to accept new programming if it is going to be successfully implemented. Direct training is important (Sanetti & Kratochwill, 2009). Training techniques such as role-play, rehearsal, demonstrations, and feedback tend to have considerable success in the intervention mastery of adults. Importantly, more experienced teachers tend to implement a program with greater fidelity as do teachers who work at lower grade levels (Ransford et al., 2009). Strong leadership in a school made a difference. Teachers who believe that they can influence all students' achievement can make a positive difference. And, when they believe that administrators support their efforts, they work harder on generalization. Teachers do better when the format of the prevention program is familiar, when teaching requires less technical expertise, and when coaching continues throughout the year.

When treatment integrity data is provided to schools by prevention program designers, school staff members will be better able to judge whether or not an intervention can be adapted to their school (Sanetti, Gritter, & Dobey, 2011). Paying attention to the fidelity with which a preventive program is implemented is considered "best practice" (Margulis, 2012). The types of data that a school psychologist or a school team would collect around implementation should reflect what is needed in order to make decisions.

Poor implementation fidelity can result in little or no behavioral change in students. Higher dosages, and implementing a prevention program well, can lead to strong effects (Webster-Stratton, Reinke, Herman, & Newcomer, 2011). Studies indicate that when the program goals are clearly relayed to school staff, when progress made and success of programs are shared with school staff, when teachers received refresher training, when their work was observed in the classroom, and when teachers had a chance to talk with one another, implementation was more likely to be effective (Ringeisen, Henderson, & Hoagwood, 2003).

Many studies and literature reviews indicate that programs do not incorporate safeguards against violations of treatment integrity when programs are implemented (Schulte et al., 2009). Complex programs and interventions are difficult to implement and the quality with which they are implemented may be compromised. Features of implementation that influence whether or not a program will be *sustained* include how consistently the program is implemented. Also important is whether or not parents, teachers, and students are involved. Whether or not a program is integrated into the general curricula and whether or not a program is developmentally appropriate for the students who participate are variables of influence (Ringeisen et al., 2003).

Schools need to concentrate on more than academics alone. Schools will be more successful if they promote social and emotional learning in conjunction with academics (Dix, Slee, Lawson, & Keeves, 2012). There is evidence of a relationship between the academic achievement of students and their mental health. In Australia, *KidsMatter* is a social–emotional learning program that has been developed for universal implementation. Schools that implemented the *KidsMatter* program with fidelity had a practical payoff. Students in those schools demonstrated improved learning outcomes, equivalent to 6 months more schooling…over and above any influence of socioeconomic background (Dix et al., 2012, p. 50).

Improving Implementation Fidelity

Leadership is a critical factor in whether or not any change effort will be successful in a school (O'Connor & Freeman, 2012). Surveys of school professionals indicate that although a clear majority of them feel leadership has a substantial effect on implementation of new programs, only 11 % agree strongly that such strong leadership is in fact taking place. Important questions for change agents to explore include: How are decisions made in this district? And what percentage of staff believes that all children can function well? If school staff members were asked to record the percentage of students that they believed could function well in their school, this would provide food for discussion, which might eliminate or decrease biases among staff. This might be helpful in deciding what would need to be done before a program was implemented. Discussions of resource allocation would help. In order to convince a school that a new program is worth the effort, change agents must make a connection between the effects of prevention programs, interventions, and outcomes for which schools are accountable (DuPaul, 2003). Connections must be made between short-term improvements in students' emotional functions in and long-term improvement in academics. New programs take time and have costs. Schedules may need to change, and some programs and activities may be discarded so that others can take their place. This is a good deal of change with which to contend.

A supportive environment reflected in perceptions of school climate is critical when a new program is implemented (Beets et al., 2008). A study found that both principal leadership and teacher support predict implementation success. Principal leadership has been demonstrated to be three times as large as teacher support. Teachers' perceptions of the principal's leadership and communication were critical. Schools with a majority of minority students taught by African American teachers were more effective in regard to implementation in this study.

Teacher training makes a difference in fidelity of implementation. An interesting example of teacher training takes place as part of The *Incredible Years* (*IY*) series of programs. The *IY* program is used in kindergarten through grade three in some public schools. The *IY* programs are a series of three prevention programs for high-risk students aged 3–8 years. The programs involve children, teachers, and parents. The *Teacher Classroom Management* (TCM) components include 6 days of training over one school year by group leaders chosen from the school faculty. Skills are modeled through consultation with a coach. Teachers choose their own goals and self-monitor their own progress. Video vignettes with actors representing the local culture, role-play, small group work involving discussions, creating behavior plans, and completing practical assignments are part of the teacher training. Social networks are built among teachers. Adaptations are built in to include increased training sessions for teachers who need a higher dosage, increased practice scripts, increased educational support, and parent workshops. Weekly coaching for particular populations with less experienced teachers is available as well. Sterling-Turner and Watson (2002) point out that direct modeling of how to implement a curriculum is more likely to ensure that the teacher really understands the process. Direct training works better than indirect training in regard to treatment integrity. When teachers are involved in choosing the curriculum or intervention, they are more likely to accept it and implement it well.

Teachers who are cynical about change are less likely to implement new interventions with integrity (Lochman, 2003). Teachers are more likely to implement interventions that fit with their own teaching style, their beliefs, their skills, and their expectations (Hunter, 2003). They prefer positive interventions generally and interventions that take less time. Performance feedback has been frequently discussed in regard to increasing on task behaviors of students and in regard to wholeclass interventions, peer tutoring, and other interventions in schools (Solomon, Klein, & Politylo, 2012). A meta-analysis of studies involving consultation when teachers were implementing interventions showed that performance feedback had a significant effect on student behavior change at all levels of schooling, in general and special education, whether it occurred daily or weekly. When feedback is offered a number of times rather than once, the effect is stronger. The implications of the study are interesting in that performance feedback is both easy to accomplish, is acceptable to teachers, and has a great enough effect on implementation integrity to be worth any time that it might take.

When a school climate is positive, teachers are more committed to their work and their schools. Collaboration with other teachers and beliefs in social–emotional learning were related to teacher commitment (Collie, Shapka, & Perry, 2011).

When teachers have good relations with their students and feel that students behave well and want to learn, teachers are less stressed, more satisfied with their work, and feel more competent. Teacher training with follow-up and ongoing support makes a difference. Supervision and/or coaching are very important, as is data collection (Kutash, Duchnowski, & Lynn, 2006). Keeping records of progress and what is affecting implementation is helpful. Hahn, Noland, Rayens, and Christie (2002) evaluated a model for implementing the *LifeSkills* (LST) Program (Botvin, Baker, Botvin, Filazzola, & Millman, 1984). When program trainers and teachers completed questionnaires, researchers found that teachers were less likely to implement the elements of the program with which they were less confident and which were different from standard classroom practice (were more innovative).

Programs can be implemented well of course. Rosenblatt and Elias (2008) found that whereas students typically manifest a drop in their grade point averages as they transition to middle school, a transition program *Talking with TJ* (Dilworth, Mokrue, & Elias, 2002) implemented over fifth and sixth grades in a city low-income district did not show as large a drop when teachers taught higher doses of the program sessions.

The Work of a Resource Team

When a new program is seriously considered for implementation, a resource coordinating team may be an excellent mechanism for making things move along. A resource team can use resource mapping, analysis, priority- setting, and redeployment strategies to facilitate change (Adelman & Taylor, 2003). Kovaleski and Pedersen (2008) described the responsibilities and activities of a resource team. Determining the duration and frequency of the strategies to be used, determining when the strategies would be used during the school day, determining how the classroom routine will change so the new program can fit in, and determining the supports needed would be part of the responsibilities of the team. Reteaching or coaching and modeling strategies that teachers have not as yet learned and holding discussions with teachers giving supportive individual feedback on the level of implementation achieved could be involved as well. The school principal's role would involve checking lesson plans and making sure that strategies are used. Students who do not respond well to the prevention intervention would need to be identified and referred to a problem-solving team. Meeting individual student needs would not be part of this teams' responsibility. The resource team deals with systems-level issues. The resource team would be responsible for designing, collecting, analyzing, and recording data. Progress monitoring would be used to make sure that approximately 80 % of students reach proficiency levels in regard to skills taught.

Teacher training may be part of the responsibility of the resource team or the team may be responsible for arranging for training. Components of professional development include working with teacher networks and study groups (Kratochwill, Volpiansky, Clements, & Ball, 2007). The amount of time involved in professional development, the time over which professional development is spread out, and working with groups of teachers who in practice work closely together make professional development more effective. Learning must be active (role-play, group discussion, case studies, demonstrations, problem solving) and focused. Early on when a program is being implemented, co-teaching, mentoring and coaching are important. Specific strategies are needed to make sure that there are changes in practice (Bero et al., 1998). Informal practices will not be effective. Only when strategies are in place can the resource team be sure that change is due to interventions and not to contextual factors. When implementers use manuals in training, they stick to the protocol much better although individual differences may still be seen in how well treatments are delivered (Meehan, Wood, Hughes, Cowley, & Thompson, 2004).

Kovaleski (2007) wrote that the ability of public schools to implement NCLB might be determined by the quality of intense and ongoing staff training, building collaborative support, and the leadership ability of administrators. This may also be the case in regard to program implementation and in regard to the use of evidence-based preventive interventions. Initially reluctant teachers tend to be more accepting of new prevention programming when they see that it actually works.

Data Collection and Data-Based Decision-Making

When implementation fidelity is measured, schools have a better idea of whether outcomes are due to implementation problems or are due to a model of change that doesn't work in a particular situation (Century, Rudnick, & Freeman, 2010). When measuring treatment integrity, it is important to know that the core or critical elements of a program are implemented. These core structural and procedural elements (what to do) may be obtained from the program developers. In addition, there are core or critical elements of the instructional approach (how to do it) for many preventive programs.

Currently we lack sound treatment integrity measures, so school teams must explore how they can measure whether or not a program or preventive intervention is being implemented well (Sanetti, Fallon, & Collier-Meeka, 2011). Possible ways to measure implementation include direct observation, permanent product review, or self-reports. Multiple measurement approaches would work best because self-reports can overestimate integrity. The frequency of collecting treatment integrity data should match the intensity of the preventive intervention. If integrity is unsatisfactory, performance feedback and negative reinforcement have been recommended to improve the situation.

Monitoring can be accomplished using a checklist of steps for implementing a preventive intervention (Keller-Margulis, 2012). Procedural checklists are also helpful (Greenwood, 2009). Checklists help implementers avoid mistakes. Using ongoing monitoring protocols is important, and available of technical assistance should be accessed (Elias et al., 2003). Lane, Kalberg, Bruhn, Mahoney, and Driscoll (2008) measured implementation fidelity using self-report and direct observation but found that the data varied by both the rater and the method that was used to measure fidelity. Lawson et al. (2009) developed an implementation index (the KidsMatter Implementation Index). The index involves measures of fidelity, dosage, and quality of delivery. Questions were developed to measure the three categories. The final tool contains 37 items, which are scored. Cut scores determine highest and lowest levels of implementation. Scores on teacher, parent, and project director responses were combined to determine a total index score. Schools with scores above +1 SD were determined to be high implementers. High implementing schools developed and implemented plans and reviewed and adjusted those plans (p. 9). They invested time in planning and implementing the initiative and sent information home to parents. Parents did not feel that the quality of delivery differed between high or low implementing schools, but teachers felt that professional development differed, and the project directors rated the high implementing schools as involving more staff planning.

At best, program delivery requires that the content or skills generalize beyond the classroom (Domitrovich, Gest, et al., 2010). Generalization is difficult to measure using self-reports of implementers. Observations of teachers in practice along with collections of student behavior and other outcomes are needed. In practice, observations help determine how well a teacher is implementing the lessons of a program (Ransford et al., 2009). In order to sustain programs that have been successfully implemented, schools need to be familiar with additional resources and tools that can help (George & Kincaid, 2008).

An Example of Program Implementation Monitoring

The Blueprints project staff evaluated the *LifeSkills Training* initiative which was implemented in 432 schools in urban, suburban, and rural areas serving students of various socioeconomic status and racial/ethnic backgrounds, over a 3-year period (Mihalic et al., 2008). The *LifeSkills Training* initiative teaches self-management skills, decision-making, communication, assertiveness, and coping with anxiety. It also teaches drug resistance skills and knowledge of the consequences of drug use. Teachers implement the universal curriculum using direct instruction, discussion, skill rehearsal, and demonstrations. Students receive 15 lessons in the sixth and seventh grade the first year, 10 booster sessions the second year, and 5 sessions the third year as part of the 3-year program. A few violence prevention lessons are available, but these were optional and not included in the study. Technical assistance was provided via telephone. Self-report data was collected from staff and trainers, yearly teacher surveys, and classroom observers collected data. A variety of additional pieces of data were collected such as program and school characteristics.

On average, 86 % of the program objectives and activities were implemented and 71 % of teachers taught all required lessons over the 3-year period meeting dosage requirements (Mihalic et al., 2008). Teachers used all of the teaching practices recommended, and 89 % of students were observed to participate in the lessons.

Teachers who adhered to the program requirements and met the dosage criteria rated the program favorably. Importantly, when teachers stuck to the program requirements and used interactive teaching techniques, they were rewarded with better student behavior. Strong local coordinators kept teachers motivated and reduced program drift. Teachers reported that the most challenging aspects of implementing the program included finding time in the schedule for the program, gaining full support, and dealing with student behavior problems. The bottom line was technical assistance and implementation monitoring. These were found to be critical for resolving problems.

Implementation is complex and many barriers and challenges must be faced. Staff skills are critical to the success of a prevention program (Mihalic & Irwin, 2003). A key variable in the success of a new prevention introduced to a school has to do with student behavior. Teachers say that their greatest challenge in the classroom is managing students' behavior (Reinke, Stormont, Herman, Puri, & Goel, 2011).

Interventions are seldom delivered as planned particularly in classrooms where children are inattentive, where student behavior is uncontrolled, or when the curriculum doesn't match the group well (Elias et al., 2003). When students misbehave, it is as if teachers are being "punished" for all of their efforts to help them, and teacher intervention fidelity drops (McConnachie & Carr, 1997). Suggestions for helping teachers deal with student behavior include team teaching, coaching teachers, and giving them strategies to deal with misbehavior. When this is accomplished, teachers will have increased control of interactive teaching techniques (Mihalic et al., 2008). Teachers who are not as skilled may need training in classroom management before a new program requiring interactive teaching techniques is implemented.

Teachers must be able to demonstrate skills not only during training but when they are alone in a busy classroom without support. Training can be improved by conducting training in several different environments and under several conditions. Program drift can be addressed through monitoring, observations, and/or booster trainings. Integrity-monitoring records with specific components that must be scored individually by each teacher implementing the program can decrease program drift. Vollmer, Sloman, and Pipkin (2008) describe practice without treatment integrity monitoring, as "potentially dangerous."

Models for Improving Implementation

Baker (2002) developed a model for implementation of prevention programs consisting of seven steps. Bershad and Blaber (2011) also developed a model consisting of seven sequential steps or phases (pp. 22–23) (Table 10.2).

Bradshad and Blaber emphasize that a whole-school approach encompasses several critical components to include a positive and responsive school environment, evidence-based curricula and instruction, and a comprehensive continuum of mental health programs and services.

Table 10.2 Implementation models

Baker (2002)	Bershad and Blaber (2011)
• Needs assessment	Convene a school and community coalition
• Readiness assessment	Assess mental health problems, needs, and resources
• Program assessment through change theory or a logic model	Develop and implementation plan
• Core components analysis and developer consultation	Secure financial resources
• Implementation balancing fidelity and adaptation and following a process that takes the student population and larger context into consideration	Monitor and address challenges
• Process and outcome evaluation attending to implementation fidelity	Create and carry out a communication plan
• Sustainability by revisiting implementation fidelity adaptations and making the program routine in the school	Build sustainability

Sanetti, Fallon, and Collier-Meeka (2011) outline phases of intervention as follows:

(a) Designing and implementing an intervention
(b) Designing treatment integrity assessment and evaluation plan
(c) Using treatment integrity and student outcome data, to make implementation decisions

The complexity of a program, whether or not it is viewed as effective and whether or not it is compatible with programs already in place, affects treatment integrity. Treatment integrity allows schools and practitioners in schools to say with confidence that changes in students' behavior(s) resulted from preventive efforts involving implementation of a preventive curriculum, preventive service, or preventive program (Sanetti et al., 2012).

Sustainability

Programs are most likely sustainable when there have been systemic changes so the larger system supports teachers' efforts. A prevention program must be linked with a school's mission and it must be considered a priority. This policy commitment along with sufficient resources is critical but not sufficient.

Principal support, belief in the program on the part of the teachers who will implement it, and belief that the program will be effective are also critical. Teachers must additionally believe that they are capable of implementing the program, and that the program will not take too much effort and time to implement. Teachers must be comfortable with the teaching method contained in the program. Teacher training must be provided along with ongoing consultation. Han and Weiss (2005) feel that in order to be sustainable, a prevention program must be acceptable to teachers.

To be effective, it must be possible to implement the program without an excessive need for resources, and the program must be flexible so that it can be safely adapted to conform to changing circumstances. The program must have clear goals, a clear structure, be easy to use, and be integrated into the general programming of the school (Mihalic et al., 2008). These characteristics added to systemic changes and supports would increase the likelihood that the program would be self-sustaining.

Forman, Olin, Hoagwood, Crowe, and Saka (2009) reviewed interventions to determine factors that would facilitate implementation and sustainability of strong prevention programs. They found that teacher support, administrative support, and good training were critical. Lack of funding was a major challenge along with finding time partly due to the competing priority of academics and other competing priorities. Visibility of the program contributed to sustainability along with positive outcomes data. Staff turnover worked against sustainability. For schools interested in implementing a prevention program, the major issues to address include obtaining administrator and teacher support before beginning, making sure that there are long-term financial resources, determining the availability of long-term consultation and training, matching the program to the school mission, publishing outcomes and program impact, and providing for training and engagement of staff when there is teacher turnover. Another important suggestion was to encourage school psychologists and counselors to take on the role of program champion given their training in mental health.

Weist (2003b) reminds us that there is little research on strategies to maintain stakeholder involvement. We additionally don't know to what degree stakeholder involvement affects the school's commitment to change or how this might affect the outcomes that school hopes to get. When implementing programs, schools dance along a line of adherence to treatment fidelity and reinventing the very program they are trying to implement. Implementation fidelity can be a major challenge, but it can no longer be ignored.

Prevention in Action Challenge: Determining Implementation Fidelity Using Goal Attainment Scaling

Common approaches to monitoring implementation include completing a checklist, using a log of activities, completing a survey, or using a focus group to discuss problems and successes (James Bell Associates, 2009). Some of the data that is needed includes an assessment of the content that is delivered, the activities that were used and the time spent on the various activities, how lessons were delivered, whether or not students were engaged, and satisfaction of both the implementer and the students. Another tool to consider is goal attainment scaling. Kiresuk and Sherman (1968) developed goal attainment scaling (GAS) to determine the effect of service delivery on individual outcomes. Goal attainment scaling is a criterion-referenced tool that can be used

(continued)

(continued)

for individuals, groups, or whole systems (Coffee & Ray-Subramanian, 2009). It is a flexible tool that can be used quantitatively or qualitatively. The person implementing the curriculum and/or a coach can complete the tool.

Revise this tool to fit the implementation of mental health curriculum or program at a school with which you are familiar.

Monitoring tool:

	Adherence	Exposure	Mastery and satisfaction
+2 (much more than expected)	100 % of lessons and 100 % of the lesson elements were delivered	The required number of hours was spent this week on the lessons plus many generalization efforts	Both students and the teacher felt engaged plus skills were learned and used beyond the classroom
+1 (somewhat more than expected)	90 % of lessons and 90 % of the lesson elements were delivered	The required number of hours was spent this week on the lessons plus one generalization effort	Both students and the teacher felt involved in the lessons
0 (as expected)	85 % of lessons and 85 % of the lesson elements were delivered	The required number of hours was spent this week on the lessons	Both students and the teacher felt lessons went well
−1 (somewhat less than expected)	75 % of lessons and 75 % of the lesson elements were delivered	The required number of hours was cut by 25 % this week due to test preparation/assemblies/ days off	Students or the teacher (one or the other) felt the lessons went well
−2 (much less than expected)	50 % of lessons and 50 % of the lesson elements were delivered	The required number of hours was cut by half this week for structural (tests, etc.) or personal reasons	Neither the students nor the teacher were satisfied with the lessons this week

Baseline mean for each goal weeks 1 and 2= _____ Mean for each goal weeks 6–9= _____

Mean for each goal weeks 3–6=_____   Mean for each goal weeks 9–12=_____

Chapter 11
Adapting Programs for Various Racial and Ethnic Populations

We are all the same in many ways and we are all different in many ways. Seventeen categories of difference between people have been identified including sex, race, color, ethnicity, language, religion/beliefs, features determined by genes, minority membership, birth, disability, age, sexual orientation, and property/poverty (Charter of Fundamental Rights of the European Union 2000, reported in Bartolo, 2010). Here we are interested in the impact of race and class on mental health, which are strongly interrelated in the United States (Winstead & Sanchez-Hucles, 2008). Race and class interact with all of the other dimensions of diversity to make subgroups and individuals unique and perceived by others as "different." Unfortunately, minority status and poverty/low income can be barriers to mental health services. Add discrimination, no insurance, lack of childcare, no transportation, and conflicting work schedules to issues associated with poverty, and the unequal access to mental health care is clear. The values and belief systems of subgroups differ and coping strategies differ according to race and culture. There is considerable understanding that differences in how people from a given culture experience health symptoms are due to cultural differences (Bernal & Sáez-Santiago, 2006). However, the majority of prevention programs are universal programs based on White, middle-class American values (Corneille, Ashcraft, & Belgrave, 2005).

At present there is considerable interest in racial and ethnic differences in mental health and in cross-cultural issues (Winstead & Sanchez-Hucles, 2008). Researchers have either assumed that most populations are similar although their circumstances and environments may differ, or researchers have attributed differences to oppression and discrimination (Roosa & Gonzales, 2000). If we assume that all groups are the same, we would be able to implement an evidence-based program and expect that it would work for all children and adolescents. If we assume that cultures vary, we would need to develop prevention programs that target every single cultural group. The first model is the "cultural equivalence" model and the second is the "cultural variance" model (Cauce, Coronado, & Watson, 1998).

Of course cultural adaptations are simply one type of adaptation to which we might want to apply evidence-based interventions or prevention programs (Barrera & Castro, 2006). The original research around a given prevention program is made up

G.L. Macklem, *Preventive Mental Health at School: Evidence-Based Services for Students,*   213
DOI 10.1007/978-1-4614-8609-1_11, © Springer Science+Business Media New York 2014

of efficacy studies. Efficacy studies determine whether or not a particular prevention program or intervention actually works (Miranda et al., 2005). The participants in an *efficacy* study must be carefully described while complications, or interfering variables, need to be eliminated. The risk factors need to be just about the same for all participants in a study, and comorbid factors cannot be present. "Effectiveness" studies are designed to determine whether or not the prevention program will work in the "real world." In the "real world" the population may be somewhat dissimilar. The location in which practitioners implement the program may differ. The population involved may be larger. In addition, there may be different questions asked when a program is implemented in school.

- How long does the program need to be implemented to get results?
- What real-world issues affect outcomes?
- How adequate is the content?
- Is the program cost-effective?

Minorities and ethnic/cultural concerns have been underrepresented in prevention research (Castro, Barrera, & Holleran Steiker, 2010; Roosa & Gonzales, 2000). Minorities tend to be missing in efficacy studies (Miranda et al., 2005). This does not mean that we totally lack evidence-based interventions for ethnic minority populations. We do in fact have some effective interventions for minority population (Kataoka, Novins, & DeCarlo, 2010). Huey and Polo (2008) reviewed the literature and found no well-established treatments for ethnic minority students, although there were "probably" or "possibly" efficacious interventions for ethnic minority children and adolescents with internalizing or externalizing problems. Less acculturated young people have not been represented in efficacy studies. And, there have not been many evaluations of cultural adaptation effects (Huey & Polo, 2010).

Children have become the most diverse population in the United States. This is the case both racially and ethnically related to immigration (Passel, 2011). Immigrant youth comprise one group that is particularly diverse. Immigrant children are those children and adolescents who either were born somewhere other than the United States or are children of immigrant parents. The numbers of first- and second-generation immigrant children are growing at a rapid rate and represent a significant proportion of school-age children in the United States (Pumariega & Rothe, 2010). Long-term stressors for this group of children include discrimination, possible marginalization, and economic issues. Acculturation is a key issue for this group of children who may experience acculturation stress. Acculturation stress can result from intergenerational conflict between home and school or between school and community norms and values. Acculturation stressors include language learning, learning new social norms, interacting with people who are diverse, and lack of cultural diversity in particular communities (Miller, Yang, Farrell, & Lin, 2011). Acculturation stress does not apply to all racial or ethnic groups, but it is one additional complication of providing prevention services to diverse groups of children and adolescents.

Schools *must* be concerned about prevention, given the fact that unless we become concerned about prevention, we cannot meet widespread needs of students in the area of mental health. School professionals must be aware of race–ethnic–cultural issues because minorities are rapidly becoming the majority population, and this societal change is coming most rapidly among children (Hernandez, Denton, & Blanchard, 2011). Additionally, as we develop a deeper understanding of the fact that culture provides the context for child development and we learn to appreciate the principles of social justice, school psychologists and other mental health practitioners must promote prevention and whole-school health for *all* children (Bartolo, Borg, Cefai, & Martinelli, 2010).

Points of View

In recent years there has been an interesting discussion about whether or not prevention programs should or should not be adapted for minority children and adolescents. The top-down view is that no changes should ever be made once a program or intervention has been shown to work (Steiker et al., 2008). The bottom-up view is that the original program may not be relevant for a particular group. In fact the subgroup or minority group's needs may never have even been considered when the original program was designed. Adaptation from this point of view is needed in order to make the program relevant and responsive. If a program is not adapted, the program may not work. The top-down and bottom-up approaches (Backer, 2002) are two major views that often clash. Another way to look at this is that the two approaches represent equally important professional values (Castro et al., 2010).

A more specific variant of the "no changes" viewpoint is the *Therapy Ingredient Model* (La Roche, Batista, & D'Angelo, 2011). This view suggests that each psychological problem is addressed by a very specific set of activities that work for everyone. Those in favor of this view argue that once the essential factors that result in change are identified and implemented, problems will be ameliorated. Additionally, this view suggests that there are some interventions that are as effective for one problem as they are for most psychological problems or disorders.

In order to deal with both concerns, researchers could determine the efficacy of the program and build in an adaptation variant before publishing the program. Once adaptations have been tested and demonstrated to work, only then would they be implemented carefully following the program manual with fidelity. This is an expensive approach in that it would require identifying the core elements of each program that could not be changed in order to obtain the same outcomes that the original program studies produced. An even more extreme suggestion is the ideal that every evidence-based program would need an adapted version for every major ethnic group. This would present a challenge in recruiting and retaining low-income multicultural populations for study. It would be very expensive. Yet another point of view suggests that evidence-based treatments and programs that are implemented by culturally aware school staff are sufficient and no further adaptation is needed (De Arellano et al., 2005). Whatever point of view takes precedence, the bottom line for an evidence-based program is whether or not implementing the program results in the desired outcomes (Muñoz & Mendelson, 2005).

Cardemil (2010) points out that the majority of well-established interventions have limited generalizability. The top-down or "make no changes" approach was clearly articulated by Elliott and Mihalic (2004). They argued that our knowledge of core components of scientifically demonstrated programs was inadequate. For this reason implementers were not able to determine what to delete, or modify, and therefore adaptation was not a viable option. Elliot and Mihalic used findings from the Blueprint Replication Initiative to show that local environments were very different one from another, but it was possible to get "buy in" if program implementers built local capacity by conducting a needs assessment, carefully selected an evidence-based program, identified local practitioners to "champion" the program, and developed links between agencies. Elliot and Mihalic argued that local staff could implement a program with fidelity. Research did not support the need for adaptations, and changes were often exaggerated. They cited several programs that were equally effective for minority students and White adolescents and questioned the assumption that there are always differences in outcomes between populations. They described the current youth culture as "blended" and "bargaining away of fidelity would most likely decrease program effectiveness" (p. 51). Others agreed that there was mixed evidence around the need for and success of making adaptations to efficacious programs (Lee, Altschul, & Mowbray, 2008).

The bottom-up or culturalistic approach takes a different stand on adaptation. This group argues that cultural mismatch can undermine the success of a program. The key sources of mismatch include the characteristics of the particular target group, large differences between the participants and those delivering the program, and administrative and community variables (Castro, Barrera, & Martinez, 2004). A longer list of mismatched variables would include the language of participants versus the language of those implementing the program, or the language of the materials. It would include the challenge of implementing a program designed for the city in a rural area. Differences in risk factors, poor staff cultural competency, and trying to implement a program when a community isn't ready to do so would affect program outcomes.

Lau (2006) described to components of interventions to include engagement, or the ability of individuals to become successfully involved; and outcomes, or the ability of the program to change whatever is targeted for change. Individuals need to be recruited to participate in a prevention program. They need to attend sessions and must be satisfied with the content and activities if the program is going to work. Cultural appeal by itself is not sufficient to make a program effective (Castro et al., 2004). The bottom-up view argues engagement is critical.

Castro et al. (2010) feel that the argument in favor of cultural adaptation will strengthen as our schools become more and more diverse and as schools select more evidence-based programs and interventions. If a program is not relevant to the needs and preference of participants and they have the option of dropping out, they will do so. Of course students in schools may not be able to drop out of a program, but the program can lose its effectiveness if students do not feel that it is relevant. Students may disrupt programs if they do not become engaged. This may be the case even when the program is implemented with integrity. A program that students find interesting and important will be motivating and participants can be expected to engage and benefit.

Backer (2002) argues that it is necessary to attend to both program fidelity and adaptation, i.e., to *balance* the two. There is data available to indicate that many evidence-based programs can be effective even though adaptations have been made. When adaptations are made, they may involve changing the components of the program, changing the nature of the components, changing the presentation, changing the intensity of the components, and cultural modification of the program. If programs cannot be modified, there may be resistance to implementing the program or the program may not meet local needs. If scientific analysis is used to identify the core components or main ingredients of a program and these are maintained rigorously, the program will most likely meet needs.

There are population differences and environmental differences that make adaptation necessary (Backer, 2002). Resources are commonly limited, and it may be that staff will not implement a program at all unless changes are made. The bottom line may be that making adaptations occurs in spite of implementers' best efforts. The unplanned adaptations are often made by teachers without knowledge of program theory, without consulting program developers, and can involve deleting entire components of a program or involve additions that may not be scientifically valid (Elliott & Mihalic, 2004). These threaten program outcomes or risk effectiveness. The prevention program's theory base must be kept intact.

Unfortunately, adaptations are often made to programs by staff on site without the use of scientific guidelines and without evaluating whether or not the adapted program continues to be as effective as the original efficacy study or studies (Castro & Alarcón, 2002). Some adaptations are inappropriate and will compromise outcomes (Backer, 2002). Additionally those professionals or a resource team implementing the program typically do not consult with the program developers or use focus groups to determine if the program is appropriate for the community in order to get ideas about how to safely make the program more appropriate. St. Pierre (2004) found that teachers were unlikely to implement programs with fidelity and implementation if the prevention theory was not consistent with some school views of curriculum delivery.

Considerations When Contemplating Adaptation

Given the arguments both for, and against, cultural adaptations have merit, and the fact that school professionals will most likely make adaptations to programs, it makes the best sense to plan adaptations before implementing a new preventive intervention. There are four major issues to consider when considering adaptations:

- Practitioners need to determine whether or not adaptations can be justified.
- School professionals need to determine how adaptations might be made, in a manner that does not interfere with program integrity.
- Adaptations must be evaluated to determine their effectiveness.
- Implementers must also deal the fact that not all students in a particular cultural or ethnic group are alike (Castro et al., 2010).

Castro et al. (2010) suggest that when a particular student group has unique risk or resilience factors and particular content or components do not contribute to the outcomes for this particular group, adaptation can be considered (p. 224). Other issues that would justify adaptation include the presence of unique symptoms in the local student population, or the fact that the program simply does not work for a given subgroup. It is critical that implementers do not make adaptations that are so significant that an entirely new program is created. In this case it would be better to locate a different evidence-based program rather than make such significant adaptations.

Another consideration involves examining different process models (Castro et al., 2010). A number of models are available in the literature and the challenge becomes choosing the one that best fits the local expertise and local staff time considerations. There are evidence-based programs available that specify which adaptations were made in research studies and whether or not they affected outcomes. Griner and Smith (2006) conducted a meta-analytic study of 76 studies to determine whether or not outcomes were compromised when cultural adaptations were made. They determined that there was a moderately strong benefit when changes were made. Interventions to engage a particular group were four times more effective. Content delivered in students' first language versus English was twice as effective. When groups were the same race versus mixed race, the effects were four times more effective. This meta-analysis involved interventions for a wide range of age groups.

When Huey and Polo (2008) looked specifically at evidence-based interventions for ethnic minority students, they realized that the question of whether or not interventions are equally beneficial for ethnic minorities is very complex and there may not be sufficient evidence available to answer this question as yet. For this reason Huey and Polo recommend first and foremost that schools use evidence-based interventions that have been identified as "probably" or "possibly" efficacious with the specific minority group. This is particularly valid when interventions use components of cognitive-behavioral therapy, interpersonal therapy, or family systems treatments. When adaptations are considered such as the characteristics of the implementers, procedures, or content, if these have not been tested outcomes would most likely be affected. Huey and Polo recommended that only culturally responsive changes already incorporated into evidence-based protocols should be considered. Resource teams should make changes after determining needs rather than assuming that cultural adaptations are routinely necessary. One group that may be expected to need a cultural adaptation is students who may be described as "low acculturated" (Griner & Smith, 2006). A time saver is that younger students may not need adaptations. "Within group" differences may not present a challenge for school-based practitioners who are accustomed to dealing with individual differences. Castro et al. (2010) suggest different program dosages to address individual differences within diverse groups. Clearly adding additional lessons or additional practice may be warranted, but shortening programs, deleting content, or making significant adaptations may violate core components of programs and should be avoided.

Cultural Adaptation

Program adaptations that are sensitive to a group's traditional world views are considered cultural adaptations (Castro et al., 2004). A number of helpful definitions are available to help us think about culture and cultural adaptations (Resnicow, Soler, Braithwaite, Ahluwalia, & Butler, 2000). Of relevance is the definition of cultural sensitivity. *Cultural sensitivity* includes the extent to which the many characteristics of the students with which one is working is taken into consideration when designing, delivering, and evaluating a mental health prevention program. A similar concept is "cultural tailoring." *Cultural tailoring* is a strategy to make all of the prevention program materials more relevant, so the students participating in the program are more receptive to the goals of the program (Goldstein & Noguera, 2006). Cultural tailoring changes the so-called surface structures or changes that help a program "feel more relevant" to a particular student group. There are many considerations when thinking about cultural sensitivity and cultural tailoring. This can get complicated once you consider experiences, norms, values, behaviors, beliefs, history, social, and environmental variables.

Resnicow et al. (2000) differentiate surface and deep structure. Surface structure has to do with materials and messages. It may also include the media and setting for delivering programs. It has to do with meeting students where they are at the given time. *Surface structure* adaptations establish feasibility and may make a program more easily understood. Surface structure facilitates accepting what the program offers. Examples of surface changes might involve changing the race or ethnicity of characters in scenarios or films (Cardemil, 2010). It may involve delivering the program so that participants feel they are not stigmatized or labeled. Zayas (2010) adds that surface structure adaptations can be thought of as "face validity" issues. They address the acceptability, receptivity, and commitment to benefit from the preventive effort. They encourage students to want to follow-through on what they learn.

Deep structure has to do with cultural, social, psychological, environmental, and historical factors. All of these influence behavior. Deep structure relates to how a particular cultural group may understand the causes of mental health and illness, the course of mental illness, the treatment of problems, and other perceptions. Beliefs and perceptions influence behavior. Preventive activities that deal with deep structure might incorporate various cultural perceptions without refuting them. Deep structure determines impact (Resnicow et al., 2000). Examples of deep structure could include use of cultural metaphors and proverbs (Cardemil, 2010) or appreciating and talking about parents' attitudes around how a child should behave toward adults and authority figures (Zayas, 2010).

Many researchers have proposed strategies for improving and strengthening health promotion program materials and making them better fit various cultures (Kreuter, Lukwago, Bucholtz, Clark, & Sanders-Thompson, 2003; Ringwalt, Ennett, Vincus, & Simons-Rudolph, 2004; Rogler, Malgady, Costantino, & Blumenthal, 1987; Thompson et al., 2008). Peripheral strategies adapt content so that it appears to better fit a subgroup, changing the pictures in the curriculum so the people depicted look like the students participating in lessons, for example. Evidential strategies would involve the addition of data sets such as prevalence statistics that fit a cultural group. Linguistic strategies would include use of the students' native language. Constituent-involving strategies would refer to involving community helpers who are familiar, and trusted, by participants. Sociocultural strategies refer to deep structure and would involve the values and norms with which students and families identify.

Cultural adaptations to program structure may involve use of homework, the order in which skills are presented, or frequent process assessment. An acceptable adaptation might involve adding educational sessions at the beginning of the program or adding family sessions during or at the end of programming. Cultural adaptations in program content might include real-life, relevant, examples or stories to illustrate concepts included in the content. Stories about immigration stresses, or experiences with prejudice and discrimination, might be relevant. Cultural adaptations to delivery of programming might include a friendly and relaxed style of delivery and more collaboration with families. The expertise of participants can be very useful and included in the program. When prevention involves families, the scheduling needs to be flexible and childcare may need to be provided. For any program changes, implementers or the resource team need to collect data to determine whether or not adaptations make a difference. Changes beyond surface structure need to be carefully monitored and measured. Special training may very well be needed for those implementing the program. It cannot be stressed enough, if the underlying theory or core elements of the program are violated, the integrity of the preventive work is compromised and outcomes may not generalize (Cardemil, 2010). Every evidence-based program has active ingredients that result in related outcomes such as a particular dosage, sequence, or intensity that determines effectiveness and should not be changed.

Adaptation Approaches, Guidelines, or Models

It is helpful to have a model to determine whether or not a prevention program is appropriate in the planning stage, after local experts have made some adaptations that they think will not affect program effectiveness. Lopez, Edwards, Teramoto Pedrotti, Ito, and Rasmussen (2002) designed a rubric to help practitioners:

- Understand the cultural context of the problem you want to address.
- Distinguish between the several cultures and between the cultural variables.
- Develop an appropriate delivery system.
- Determine that the evaluation is cultural sensitive.
- Disseminate research findings to all stakeholders.

Although this rubric was designed for researchers, school teams could use aspects of the rubric. An understanding of the problem would include developing a detailed picture of the school community and the broader community. Levels of acculturation and enculturation of participants can be examined perhaps using focus groups. *Enculturation* has to do with the process involved when students identify with their minority culture (Zimmerman, Ramirez-Valles, Washienko, Walter, & Dyer, 1996). Ongoing collaboration to generate and test hypotheses is important, as is frequent contact with stakeholders. Appropriate measurement and data analysis procedures must be planned and used. Findings must be shared with community stakeholders both formally and informally. Zayas (2010) suggests that the issue is more about changing behavior of those implementing preventive programming rather than adapting the program to fit a particular group.

There are a number of adaptation approaches, guidelines, and models for school-based teams to use in planning. Bernal, Bonilla, and Bellido (1995) described a preliminary adaptation model consisting of eight dimensions. The dimensions include language, persons, metaphors, content, concepts, goals, methods, and context. These would each be adapted to the ethno-cultural group with whom practitioners were working. Domenech-Rodríguez and Weiling (2004) proposed three general phases for program adaptation and ten specific areas within each phase along with ongoing evaluation. The model may be most appropriate for program developers and researchers. Hwang (2009) proposed a method for adapting psychotherapy, which involved collaborating with consumers. Although it is more specific, it is an interesting model because it involves reviewing culturally adapted interventions with stakeholders and pretesting it. Barrera and Castro (2006) offer a heuristic framework for cultural adaptation, which includes information gathering, a preliminary adaptation design, preliminary adaptation tests, and adaptations refinement. Finally, Baker (2002) provides the following useful guidelines for schools:

- Identify and understand the program theory.
- Determine the core components of the program under consideration.
- Determine the adaptations necessary for the particular school (funding, politics, diversity).
- Consult with the program developer for technical assistance.
- Develop an implementation plan.

Lee et al. (2008) note that strict adherence to the manuals of prevention programs may not be practical without outside program supervision. Because schools have additional issues to deal with such as financial restrictions, limited capacity, and political climate issues, a planned adaptation approach is recommended. The *Selective Adaptation Model* has four steps:

- Examine the programs theory of change.
- Identify the differences that define your population.
- Adapt the content retaining the core components indicated by program theory.
- Tailor implementation and evaluation to fit the adapted program.

Since both the Baker and the Lee et al. approaches involve program theory, practitioners need to understand the importance of theory. Evidence-based prevention programs depend on theory to determine or explain outcomes. The theory is linked to core components through the activities articulated in program content. Once the school resource team has identified a program of interest, it is critical to determine if the theory is described. If not, it will be necessary to locate meta-analyses or conduct a literature search to determine the program theory (Lee et al., 2008). The core components of the program should link the theory with activities. In some cases it may be necessary to consult with the program developer to understand the program theory. When those who are implementing the program understand the program theory, they will be better able to make adaptations without compromising program fidelity (Lee et al., 2008). Bernal (2009) notes that understanding differences is good for science. When adaptations are made, determined to be helpful, and are documented, they will help other schools as well.

Langford (2010) presented a simplified model that could easily be used by school professionals. Choose a program that is the best initial fit for your local site and population. Understand the program in detail, and adapt it with great care. When choosing a program, it is important to determine which problem or problems you want to address. Identify the factors that contribute to the program. Decide what you want to change, and look for a program that shows that it can make that change. When choosing a program, assess the audience, the community, and the school climate. Determine if it will be possible to sustain the program. Langford points out that it is best to find a program that does not require much change. Understanding the program in detail involves reading and analyzing all of the program materials, talking with the developer, and reading the studies. Identify the core components and the "how" and "why" of program delivery. Finally, think through the adaptations and how they might affect the program. As part of planning, obtain feedback from the participants and the community before implementation begins. Follow "best practices" and what works for the type of program you want to implement. Collect data to track adaptations that are made. This approach is clear, structured, and scientific.

The *What Works Wisconsin* group of researchers has provided a publication to help schools understand what can be adapted and what should not be changed in evidence-based prevention programs (O'Connor, Small, & Cooney, 2007). This is an excellent resource for school teams.

Adaptation Projects Underway and Completed

Leff, Kupersmidt, and Power (2003) have published data on the *Friend-to-Friend* program, a culturally adapted intervention for relationally aggressive urban African American girls (Leff et al., 2003, 2007; Leff, Power, Manz, Costigan, & Nabors, 2001). In adapting this program, researchers worked with students, teachers, parents, and recess staff to design the program. The Alexis Nakota Sioux nation, including community elders, worked with the University of Alberta to adapt an evidence-based program for students at Alexis Nakota Sioux Nation School (Baydala et al., 2009). They utilized focus groups to determine responses to the program. Adaptations incorporated students' cultural beliefs, values, language, and visual images.

An exciting development underway is that some programs currently being used in schools have developed models to make it easier for schools to fit programs to their specific populations. The Resource Center for Adolescent Pregnancy Prevention (ReCAPP) has developed a kit for schools, *General Adaptation Guidance* (http://recapp.etr.org). The website was developed by ETR Associates, a private health education promotion organization in Santa Cruz, California. As of 2013, they had accomplished some impressive work providing adaptation kits for seven different pregnancy and STD/HIV prevention programs.

Adapting Programs for African American Students

School-based preventive work is accessible and affordable. A preventive program can fit into the school schedule and be provided in a less threatening manner than in many other settings. Additionally, manualized evidence-based cognitive-behavioral therapy techniques can be implemented by school psychologists in schools with their current level of training and expertise (Ginsburg, Becker, Kingery, & Nichols, 2008).

Disadvantaged African American children and adolescents receive fewer services than other groups. African American children have a lower prevalence of anxiety disorders than European Americans accord to prevalence studies, but this may be somewhat deceptive given that children rate themselves as more anxious than their African American mothers describe them (Walton, Johnson, & Algina, 1999). Ginsburg et al. (2008) implemented a school-based cognitive-behavioral intervention at the elementary level for anxious African American children. School-based mental health workers implemented this intervention at the Tier 2 level. A modularized approach was utilized to maximize flexibility. Adaptations made included soliciting input from parents and school staff in order to make the protocol ecologically valid and acceptable to stakeholders. Data collection measures were chosen that best fit African American urban populations. Forms were shortened. Complications around missing class, space, and parents work schedules made the work difficult. Adaptations included parent interviews over the phone, shortening sessions to fit into the school schedule, and flexibly accommodating special school activities. In addition, sessions were rotated so students would not miss the same classes too often. Teachers were recruited to help generalize skills and to provide feedback. The use of rewards and positive reinforcement was increased. Feedback from stakeholders, teachers, and parents helped determine that more interactive activities were needed. More culturally relevant materials were needed and homework had to be reduced.

Cooley, Boyd, and Grados (2004) conducted a feasibility study with fifth grade inner-city African American children aged 10 and 11 years who had experienced community violence. The intervention utilized the *FRIENDS* program at the Tier 2 level. The adaptations made to this evidence-based program included connecting the imagery of the program to the real threats that students were encountering, meeting biweekly versus weekly, and deleting the parent component of the program.

Additionally, because these African American children had reading problems, written tasks were handled orally, language was modified, and reading checks were added before activities in sessions. The Australian English of the *FRIENDS* program needed to be changed to American English. It was difficult to engage parents and to get permission for children in spite of several attempts to do so. There were positive and negative aspects of each of the adaptations. More frequent meetings may have helped students invest in the program, but the time to complete homework was condensed. Talking versus writing made the lessons more interactive, but an additional opportunity for reinforcement was lost. Language modifications were necessary due to different concepts of family, i.e., living with grandparents or single mothers as opposed to traditional definitions of family. Modifications were necessary due to lack of knowledge of Australian animals and phrases used in teaching concepts in the original program. Preventive effects were strong and significant, with decreases in physiological symptoms, worrying, and concentration difficulties in spite the adaptations. Test anxiety was decreased in students' classrooms, and behavior improved in school. Children liked the program.

A second, larger study with 98 third to fifth grade students, 8–12 years of age, with 92 % African American and biracial children followed (Cooley-Strickland, Griffin, Darney, Otte, & Ko, 2011). In this study the biweekly sessions were retained. The adaptations made in the feasibility study were used once more, with an additional modification of relaxation exercises. CDs were made for students to take home and an additional activity involving drawing pictures of the violence children had witnessed was added. Implementers received training. The program leader was African American, but not all co-leaders were African American. Three 1-h parent meetings were used for this trial. Extremely disruptive students were excluded. Results showed improved academic achievement in math, improved problem solving, and reduced levels of victimization possibly due to new coping skills. Improved academic skills occurred even though this was not the focus of the program. Significant decreases in self-reported anxiety were found with this short 13-contact-hour program, although there were no significant group differences. It is not unusual for prevention programs not to show differences between intervention and control groups immediately. Low parental consent rates continued to be problematical. The parents' sessions revealed that the parents were too stressed themselves to be helpful to their children.

School programming for urban, low-income African American students are critically important. Disadvantaged urban African American students have often been exposed to community violence. In an effort to understand how community violence and mental health were connected, researchers followed 623 urban children from first grade through adolescence (Lambert, Bradshaw, Cammack, & Ialongo, 2011). Early appearing aggressive and disruptive behaviors and academic readiness for school occurred together and resulted in peer rejection and behavior problems. These in turn led to spending time with deviant peers and exposure to community violence. Another longitudinal study of 175 sixth through eighth grade African American students was conducted over 3 years (Sweeney, Goldner, & Richards, 2011). Students experiencing dysphoric emotions in sixth grade experienced violence in seventh grade. Students in sixth grade who experienced hostile feelings and anxiety experienced violence a year later than the first group, i.e., in eighth grade.

Bell, Anderson, and Grills (2011) suggested that for some African American children, prevention activities must include approaches to change negative images, ideas, and values imposed on them by others. When providing programs for African Americans, Belgrave, Clark, and Nasim (2009) recommend discussions around racism, negative media images, and the condition of African American families. Discussions of the values, traditions, history, and culture specific to African Americans are important. Including information about the historical contributions of specific African Americans is helpful as well. Providing preventive programs in urban schools with low-income children improves attendance, reduces stigma, reaches students who might never receive service, and addresses the constant worries of students which interfere with school performance (Cooley-Strickland et al., 2011).

Racial socialization can be a protective factor in African American families (Cooper & McLoyd, 2011; Rodriguez, McKay, & Bannon, 2008). Parents must make sense out of disparaging views of their group and teach their children how to understand and cope with prejudice and discrimination (Coard, Wallace, Stevenson, & Brotman, 2004). The strategies that parents teach are known as racial socialization. Studies suggest that the more parents use specific racial socialization practices such as talking about racial achievement and preparation for bias and the more parents give messages about racial equality and racial pride, the better their children's social–emotional, behavioral, and academic outcomes. Behavior problems are found less often in African American families when parents use more effective discipline strategies and have moderate to high levels of spiritual or religious coping. These are important when families must deal with racism, discrimination, and other stressors such as poverty and neighborhood disadvantage. Cooper and McLoyd (2011) further determined that racial socialization and adjustment for adolescent African American students was moderated by the quality of their relationships with their mothers. The emotional context in which racial barrier socialization takes place was particularly influential for girls.

Corneille et al. (2005) pointed out significant variability among African Americans. Some groups evidence an *Africentric worldview* that includes strong ethno-racial identity, positive self-regard, positive peer group norms, use of coping strategies, and healthy behaviors. For adolescent girls higher levels of identity are connected to stronger self-esteem, avoidance of risky behavior, and better adjustment. School mental health professionals also need to understand that some African Americans tend to feel that mental illness can be managed without treatment and will look to extended family and community members for help (Ginsburg et al., 2008).

Adapting Programs for Latino/Latinas and Hispanic Americans

The Latino population in the United States comprises the fastest growing group (Furman et al., 2010). Students with Latino/Hispanic backgrounds tend to be economically disadvantaged, experience language barriers, and deal with citizenship problems. Bandy and Moore (2011) conducted a literature review in order to determine what works for Latino/Hispanic children and identified 33 random assignment,

Table 11.1 Principles for making cultural adaptations for Mexican-American students

- Learn as much as possible about each family's cultural practices and beliefs
- Collaborate with teachers and other school staff to locate a staff person who can serve as a liaison to reduce family's apprehension
- Hold an orienting session before implementing a program to address feelings that could interfere with success
- Respect the way in which the family understands the program and understands emotional difficulties
- Establish goals that the family values
- Learn about the cultural norms for parenting practices
- Engage and collaborate with the extended family, involving them as appropriate
- Determine if cultural norms may be the cause when there are problems
- Consult with cultural experts before addressing sensitive issues with the family

Source: Wood et al. (2008)

experimental evaluations of studies. Their determination was that programs targeting families were more likely to be successful. Programs that were adapted to address Latino/Hispanic culture had positive results. When facilitators spoke Spanish, the outcomes were more likely to be positive. Interian, Allen, Gara, and Escobar (2008) suggested some general cultural considerations for Hispanic children. These included providing lessons in Spanish, use of ethno-cultural assessment (determining the number of years in the United States, social supports, etc.), a warm and positive approach, consideration of cultural values, use of phrases and sayings common to the specific group, simplifying concepts, including a variety of activities for practicing skills, and relating appropriately to the family.

Just as studies have explored adapting cognitive-behavioral therapy for African Americans, similar work has been done for Hispanics. For example, Wood, Chiu, Hwang, Jacobs, and Ifekwunigwe (2008) suggested specific adaptations to cognitive-behavioral therapy for elementary-level urban Mexican American children (Table 11.1).

There are not enough culturally competent or Spanish-speaking mental health providers for Latino students (Furman et al., 2010). Latino families may not trust mental health professionals. Those who do may feel that they have been judged unfairly. Services need to be accessible and perceived as credible.

Smokowski, Chapman, and Bacallao (2006) found that Latino adolescents who have a strong investment in Latino culture have more internalizing problems initially. Family conflict, should it occur, deteriorates the protection that family values tend to offer them. For immigrant Latino children, discrimination and parent–adolescent relationships need to be targeted in prevention work.

Adapting Programs for Asian Americans

There are more than 50 subgroups among Asian Americans. These include Cambodians, Chinese, Japanese, Filipinos, Koreans, Laotians, Asian Indians, and Vietnamese. Together individuals in these groups speak over 30 languages (Chu & Sue, 2011). Asian Americans value interdependence and family. Many of these groups must deal with racial prejudice, discrimination, stereotyping, the challenge of learning English, and dealing with adjustment difficulties. Asian Americans in general experience racial discrimination (Gee, Ro, Shariff-Marco, & Chae, 2009). Research involving Chinese, Filipino, and Vietnamese Americans determined that these groups experience psychological stress due in part to discrimination and racism (Mereish, Liu, & Helms, 2012). School-based mental health professionals must understand that Asian American students are more likely to report physical symptoms than psychological symptoms when seeking services.

A major concern is the degree to which adaptations might undermine the outcomes of a prevention program if they affect the core components. Ozer, Wanis, and Bazell (2010) reported on the implementation of school-based preventive programs that are empirically supported. This study explored the question using two substance abuse prevention programs for ethnically diverse high school students. It is an important study for several reasons. First, the predominant group consisted of low-income Asian American students; second, teachers implemented the program and the process of unexpected adaptation of programs was explored.

Prior efforts to address these questions determined that middle school staff do not use interactive teaching techniques or implement programs effectively. Eighty percent of teachers make changes in preventive programs with the goal of making the programs fit student issues (Ringwalt, Ennett, et al., 2004). In the Ozer et al. study (2010), all teachers made adaptations to the prevention programs that they were implementing. Teachers tended to add real-life examples to program content or changed the wording of the lessons. Additionally, they tended to make the programs more interactive. These would be considered to be surface adaptations. However, not all suggestions for adaptations could be supported as scientifically accurate. Although many of the students' suggestions for adaptations were also surface changes, some were less acceptable when shared with program developers. Importantly, involving students in the discussion around cultural fit and checking out the validity of adaptations with program developers is a good model to follow. An example of a program adapted for Hispanic studies is Project Northland (Komor et al., 2004), which was adapted for multiethnic students in Chicago.

Tran and Lee (2010) applied parental ethnic–racial socialization to Asian American adolescents. When adolescents are given "mistrust" messages by parents, the result is diminished competence in social areas. When positive ethnic identity is stressed, social competence is enhanced. Brown and Ling (2012) extended this research and determined that more frequent messages of cultural socialization-pluralism from parents indirectly increased self-esteem.

A Program Designed for Mexican American Students: "Keepin'" it REAL (KLR)

There are few school-based alcohol prevention interventions that have been designed for minority students that have adequate research support. The *keepin' it REAL* intervention (Hecht et al., 2003; Kulis et al., 2005) was designed for

Mexican American students at the middle school level. The prevention intervention was developed focusing on ethnic norms and values. In addition, there is a multicultural version based on Latino, European American, and African American norms and values. This effort would be considered a deeper structure intervention (Stigler, Neusel, & Perry, 2011). The Drug Resistance Strategies Project, which was started in 1991, became the *keepin' it REAL* curriculum for grades 6–9 (Castro et al., 2010). The program teaches four strategies for resisting drug use: R = refuse, E = explain, A = avoid, and L = leave (Hopson & Steiker, 2010). There are ten lessons teaching social skills and antidrug norms with booster activities and a media campaign. Marsiglia (in Steiker et al., 2008) described the development and evaluation of this universal curriculum in terms of "cultural fit." Researchers first identified the norms, values, and behaviors of various subgroups of young people. They created the program/curriculum around these issues. The approach of starting with knowledge of the culture of the population is less expensive, saves time, and allows researchers to implement programming rather than delaying access to prevention efforts until stronger data is obtained. Marsiglia argued that the issue of cultural misfit must be addressed in advance.

Hecht et al. (2003) conducted an evaluation of the *keepin' it REAL* curriculum using three versions of the program in 35 middle schools and 11 control schools. Students were randomly assigned to one of the three versions or to a control group. The three versions were Mexican American, African American/European American combined, and the multicultural version. There were a total of 6,035 students participating in the 2-year study. Outcomes supported the overall effectiveness of the several versions of the program in regard to gateway drug use. In addition, norms, attitudes, and resistance strategies were positively affected.

When the combined three versions were compared to the control group, the increase in use of substances was not as great in the intervention groups because these students tended to use more resistance strategies, and their perceptions had been positively influenced (Hecht et al., 2003). When groups were individually examined, the Mexican American and multicultural versions affected the most outcomes (Hecht et al., 2003). Yet, there were subtle differences between the groups. Students in the Mexican American group evidenced the smallest increase in overall substance use, alcohol use, and marijuana use. They intended to resist offers of drugs, had more realistic perceptions of peer use, evidenced greater self-confidence in ability to resist use, and the change in their attitudes held over time. Students in the multicultural group reported they had learned more resistance strategies, decreased their expectancies for substance use, and they also held on to their changed attitudes. Additionally, this group reported less alcohol, marijuana, and overall substance use (Kulis et al., 2005). Although students in the African American/European American group had the fewest significant outcomes, they reported they had learned more resistance strategies (Hecht et al., 2003). This important study did not find that matching students to a specific cultural treatment group improved outcomes. At the same time, it was determined that culturally grounded efforts were successful.

Research has continued to evaluate the effectiveness of this program. In a study of 2,146 Mexican American students, the *keepin' it REAL* program has been determined to have a greater effect for more acculturated Latinos in middle schools (Marsiglia, Kulis, Wagstaff, Elek, & Dran, 2005). Students who preferred to speak Spanish used substances less than peers both before and after programming. This confirmed previous findings that the Spanish language is a protective factor against drug and alcohol use for middle school students. At the same time, Mexican American students described as English dominant had more positive outcomes in every version of the curriculum. The curriculum has been found to have greater impact on the anti-group norms of boys in seventh grade than on girls (Kulis, Yabikku, Marsiglia, Nieri, & Crossman, 2007). Again, less acculturated boys accrued more benefits.

The *keepin' it REAL* curriculum uses skill building exercises and videos as a primary teaching device. Videos are interesting to young people and help students engage with the program (Steiker, 2008). A pilot project with students in Texas, in high-risk community settings, determined that those implementing the programs did not feel that program materials reflected the life experiences or the culture of their group of students (Holleran, Taylor-Seehafer, Pomeroy, & Neff, 2005). Researchers decided to use students as "experts" in the process of adapting the curriculum workbook and videos. They also extended the curriculum to target 14–19 year olds because students in this age group may start to use hard drugs (Steiker, 2008).

The *keepin' it REAL* adaptation process involved beginning with focus groups and a process evaluation to examine students' actions to adapt the curriculum materials to fit students' culture and the particular setting (Steiker, 2008). The impact of participating in the process on drug use was measured. Students created four new videos, one for each prevention strategy. They rewrote scenarios to reflect their own experiences as witnessed by at least 75 % of the group. They rewrote workbooks in order to reflect their drugs of choice, the settings in which drugs were easily found in their area, how drugs were offered in their local area, local clothing and music, and language styles. Topics were not changed and adaptations were closely supervised. Focus groups were run before and after the videos were created. Participation in this process was very engaging for students. The activity of making changes in the curriculum affected students' attitudes and behaviors regarding alcohol and drugs. A testimonial video was created that had a particularly strong affect on the student designers. The materials were then available to be used with younger students, matching the students who constructed the revisions.

Students in alternative secondary schools have already begun to use alcohol and other substances earlier as compared to students in typical public schools. Data suggests that targeted prevention programs may be more appropriate than universal program for students who are already active users (Hopson & Steiker, 2010). One research study involved four alternative secondary schools. The students in this group also revised the videos and workbook materials to depict the drugs used at their respective schools and revised the language and contexts in which drugs were available and were used. Additional adaptations involved shortening some modules. The effectiveness of the adapted versions showed that younger students experiencing the adapted versions reported significant decreases in alcohol use and in attitudes around accepting alcohol if offered. Older students did not change and so researchers interviewed the students. When interviewed, students indicated that the curriculum evaluated in this study promoted abstinence, which they felt made sense only for younger students. Students wanted to hear stories of people who dropped out of school, which could possibly be integrated into the program without normalizing alcohol use.

REAL Groups, a secondary prevention program for higher-risk students, was developed to accompany the *keepin' it REAL* alcohol prevention program (Marsiglia, Ayers, Gance-Cleveland, Mettler, & Booth, 2012). *REAL Groups* can be implemented along with *keepin' it REAL*. This program attempts to covey deeply held cultural values and norms. Group leaders receive intensive training to deliver the manualized curriculum. Students discuss the norms and values of Mexican American culture to protect them from drug use. They discuss peer relationships and interactions, prosocial behaviors, school and neighborhood adjustment, and group membership. Identified students experience the *keepin' it REAL* curriculum for 10 weeks in the general education classrooms, plus 8 weeks of small group sessions to discuss, rehearse, and apply resistance strategies to real-life situations. The efficacy of the companion secondary prevention program was evaluated with 102 *REAL Groups* students and 102 non-*REAL Groups* students. Because teachers referred students participate in the Tier 2 program, researchers used a *propensity score matching* statistical technique, which used risk factors to form a control group minimizing selection bias. Data collected indicated that *REAL Groups* is efficacious. Significant differences were detected between *REAL Groups* students and nonparticipating adolescents who were matched with these students. Combing a secondary prevention program with the primary prevention program increased the overall effects. Together, these programs form a more comprehensive prevention approach.

Prevention in Action Challenge: Adaptation Sort

Determine whether or not the proposed adaptations to evidence-based programs would be safe to implement, would be implemented only with great care measuring effects, or would be too risky and would negatively affect outcomes.

Adaptation to EBP under consideration	Safe to implement	Only with great care measuring effects	Too risky would negatively affect outcomes
Add celebration of cultural holidays			
Eliminate practice as it takes too much time			
Add role-plays and group problem-solving activities			
Reduce the length of the lessons to fit the school schedule			
Add incentives to make the activities more competitive			
If the program only goes up to grade 6, it is okay to teach it in grade 7 or 8			
Include an adult member of the minority groups as a co-leader			
Add materials that acknowledge social norms and religious beliefs of students			
Change the sequence of lessons so they are easier to teach			
Bring guests into the program who have experienced the behavior you want to change (e.g., drugs)			
Use words and phrases specific to the culture of students			
Add modes of coping common to the target group of students			

Chapter 12
Adapting Programs for Young Children

A summit meeting on young children's mental health held in 2009 emphasized some important issues around the preschool developmental period (Society for Research in Child Development, 2009). One of the key issues was the importance of mental health for normal development. In addition, prevention strategies and evidence-based approaches were emphasized because these can decrease multiple risk factors. Important prevention strategies that were discussed included social and emotional learning programs, resilience, and helping children to recognize and regulate emotion.

The preschool developmental period is a time of rapid physical, emotional, behavioral, and cognitive changes (Egger & Angold, 2006). It is difficult to identify clusters of symptoms in very young children, so errors could be made if professionals identified a child as having an emotional disorder. Equally important, a preschooler's behavior does not typically belong to the child alone. It is more likely the case that not only does the behavior belong to the child but the broader environment is deeply involved as well.

If prevention strategies are going to be effective, there must be better recognition of problems in this age group. Large community studies of preschoolers, that *approximate* the general population, indicate that emotional and behavioral disorders in preschoolers appear to be roughly equal. The overall rate of disorders from four preschool studies demonstrated rates of emotional and behavioral problems are the same as those for older children, although the prevalence rate is somewhat lower if disorders require impairment in order to be identified. Even so, Egger and Angold (2006) concluded that the overall rate of disorders is generally similar across the lifespan, while the pattern of specific disorders has a number of differences as children grow (p. 319). For example, while rates of Attention Deficit Hyperactivity Disorder (ADHD) stay the same, the prevalence of Oppositional Defiant Disorder (ODD) decreases during the preschool period. Rates of specific anxiety disorders and depression increase with age. ADHD is the most common diagnosis given to preschoolers referred for services. Comorbidity is as common in young children as it is in older children. Unfortunately very few young children who meet the criteria for a disorder are referred for an evaluation or receive treatment.

G.L. Macklem, *Preventive Mental Health at School: Evidence-Based Services for Students*, DOI 10.1007/978-1-4614-8609-1_12, © Springer Science+Business Media New York 2014

Investment in Preschool Preventive Programming

Because experiences that affect a child early in life can influence the developing brain and create the foundation for later adjustment and learning, it is critical to invest in programming as early as possible for children at high risk. Programming must involve both high-quality early education programs for children and support for families. To date, there has been no program or service delivery approach that has been demonstrated to be best, so the goal is to look at approaches that have documentation of effectiveness. All efforts to make a difference in the lives of children at high risk require strong programs, implementation fidelity of those programs, monitoring child progress on a routine basis, and high standards. Programmatic support must match needs, and environments must be continuously improved and evaluated.

Research studies do not yet tell us what might constitute the most successful program for young children. Evaluations of strong programs for 3- and 4-year-olds from low-income families have been shown to provide short-term benefits although overall effects are mixed. Programs that are most successful include well-trained and skilled teachers, high adult–child ratios, and a safe language-rich environment with stimulating materials and are consistently attended by the children they are intended to serve.

Early childhood programming varies tremendously across the United States (Center on the Developing Child at Harvard University, 2007). The poor quality of many programs can have negative effects on young children at risk. Programs that do not benefit children tend to be poorly delivered to both the children and their parents. Early childhood programming needs to be strengthened. In addition to developmentally appropriate programs, greater attention to the mental health of young children is needed. There is a high prevalence of depression in mothers of children in low-income families, a high rate of expulsions of disruptive children from programs, a worrisome use of medications with young children, and insufficient professionals available to work with or to consult with families and childcare centers.

A meta-analysis of 123 research studies comparing an early childhood intervention with an alternative program, or to no intervention, examined the effects of both cognitive and affective outcomes. The analysis included both experimental and quasi-experimental research designs and covered the 1960–2000 period. The study showed positive results for preschool programming (Camilli, Vargas, Ryan, & Barnett, 2010). Currently, some states offer preschool for all children. Other states provide programming only for children of the most needy families. Because studies of preschool effects have involved different groups of students, different programs, different time periods, and different selections of studies, a meta-analysis of studies makes more sense when trying to determine the effects of early prevention programming. This analysis provided strong support for positive effects of preschool education on measures of cognition and reading. Outcome studies in the affective domain were more limited. Consistent evidence for the effectiveness of preschool programs, and evidence for long-term prevention effects, was found for the cognitive domain. Positive effect sizes were found for social skills in the social domain, although these effects were less strong. Direct instruction in smaller groups made a difference cognitively for preschoolers.

Difficulties with mental health concerns begin at a young age due to both individual and environmental risks (Stagman & Cooper, 2010). A substantial proportion of psychiatric disorders start in childhood and this suggests that to understand early onset of disorders, the preschool period is the place to begin (Egger & Angold, 2006).

The many risks of mental health difficulties for children aged 3–5 years old include receiving public assistance, having unemployed parents, having teenage parents, being in foster care, being in low-income households, being in the child welfare system, and having a deployed parent (Stagman & Cooper, 2010). When young children have mental health difficulties, they are more likely to miss school due to absences, expulsions, and suspensions.

As of 2010, Barnett reported that over 70 % of children attended a preschool program for 1 year, and about 50 % of children attended preschool for 2 years before entering formal schooling. The major federal programs are Head Start, subsidized programs through grants to states, preschool special education, and tax credits for childcare. States provide additional programming. There are serious problems in that many low-income children are not receiving programming and too many programs are of low quality. If immediate effects of preschool programming are large enough, effects do not totally disappear.

The Value of Preschool Experiences

The skills needed for young children transitioning to public school include self-confidence, the ability to develop adequate relationships with other children and adults, the ability to concentrate and persist on tasks, the ability to communicate emotions, good listening and attention skills, and ability to solve social problems (Ashdown & Bernard, 2012, p. 397). Kindergarten teachers report that social and emotional difficulties affect school readiness and disrupt their classes (National Scientific Council on the Developing Child, 2008). According to the National Academy of Sciences, only 40 % of children enter school with the skills to succeed (http://www.nasonline.org).

Preschool programs of high quality have been found to foster school readiness and predict school success in many studies, especially for minority children in low-income families (Hernandez, Denton, & Blanchard, 2011). Unfortunately the United States ranks near the bottom among many countries in regard to the numbers of children in the 3- to 6-year-old age group who participate in early education programs. There are a number of reasons for this that varies by ethnic and racial group. In the case of Hispanic families, parents may prefer to care for young children at home. Cost can be a huge barrier. Some parents may not be aware of the value of early education. In some neighborhoods there may not be openings, programs may not feel culturally welcoming to parents, and limited English proficiency may keep some families from taking advantage of the services that are available. Socioeconomic and structural factors account for about 50 % of the lower enrollment of minority students in preschool programming.

Nelson, Westhues, and MacLeod (2003) conducted a meta-analytic review, which determined that prevention preschool programs have a small to moderate positive effect on cognitive and social–emotional functioning. The programs also influenced parent–family wellness. Cognitive effects in children lasted up to 9 years of age and social–emotional effects lasted through high school according to researchers. The immediate effects were stronger, but preventive preschool experiences with a direct teaching component and a follow-through component made a difference. The length and intensity of programs for students who live in poor urban areas is particularly important. Effects for African American students in high-quality programs that lasted a year or more and that met regularly appeared to be greater than for children with other backgrounds. A study based on the Early Childhood Longitudinal Study showed that children who attended a center- or school-based preschool program before school entry did better in regard to reading and math skills. The gains children made persisted into first grade (Magnuson, Meyers, Ruhm, & Waldfogel, 2004). Barnett (2008) concluded that well-designed preschool programs can result in improvements in school success later on. Benefits include stronger educational skills, less grade repetition, reduced likelihood of special education services, and in a few studies—reduced delinquency.

In another meta-analytic study, Camilli et al. (2010) reviewed 123 studies in which young children in an intervention group were compared with children who received a different intervention or no intervention. Both experimental and quasi-experimental studies were included in this study. Researchers determined that children attending preschool programs before kindergarten fared better cognitively, had better social skills, and made more progress once in school. Preschool programs using "direct" instruction contributed more to their students' success. Once children entered formal schooling some of the effects diminished, but other effects persisted at about half of the size of the initial effects. Still another recent meta-analysis determined that preschool experiences for an economically disadvantaged child benefited the child cognitively when the preschool was center-based and included a language component. Additional positive factors included early supplements and early interactive reading between parents and their children (before age 4 years). Estimates of positive effects varied with the quality of programs and the rigor of the studies involved. Although collecting data for young children with developmental delays or disabilities is relatively new, 61 % of children who participated in early childhood programs under IDEA completed early services functioning within normal age expectations, i.e., they caught up to their peers. Nearly all children serviced made gains.

A high-quality program develops skills in the content areas and facilitates social/emotional competency along with shaping attitudes (Barnett & Frede, 2010). Although high-quality early childhood programming is far from the norm, it can be found in a variety of childcare programs. Most programs however fall in the "mediocre" category (p. 22). There are issues of teacher qualifications and salary among Head State programs for example. Subsidized childcare programs provide even less in regard to the qualifications of teaching staff. State-funded preschool programs vary in quality although some state-funded programs, such as Oklahoma's universal Pre-K program, have produced larger effects than Head Start programs. One advantage of universal preschool is the finding that disadvantaged young children experience better outcomes when they attend preschools with their more advantaged peers. Most children who start kindergarten with low skill levels are from middle-income families. Interestingly, "the achievement gap between children from middle- and high-income families is as great as the gap between children from low- and middle-income families" (Barnett & Frede, 2010, p. 28). Universal programming benefits all children.

Federal Level Support for Early Childhood Prevention Efforts

The Child Care and Development Block Grant (CCDBG) last revised for FFY 2012–2013 required each state in the United States to submit a plan describing how it would use funds to improve the quality of childcare and help low-income families access childcare (Firgens & Matthews, 2012). The grant provides funding for bilingual caseworkers and translators for parents. It subsidizes space in programs for English Language Learners and calls for bilingual trained staff in addition to other resources. Many states emphasize the need to communicate with children in their home language and to make sure that early childhood environments are culturally aware and sensitive to children and families.

The Foundation for Child Development (FDC) (http://www.icpsr.umich.edu) sponsors a project dedicated to encouraging, building, and disseminating research consisting of longitudinal datasets. The focus is not only on academic competencies but also on the social, self-regulatory, and motivational capabilities of young children. Because education is an accumulative process, the project hopes to foster a longer view than in the past when the focus was on school readiness alone. Children benefit when early childhood education is integrated with early elementary school education. The expectation is that prekindergarten to third grade research studies, with frequent measures and attention to the context of programs, will provide a better prediction of outcomes. It is difficult to get strong effect sizes for specific early childhood programs when the majority of young children attend programs which differ to a great degree. Research studies must determine what children will need beyond preschool programs, how to maximize the short-term gains from early childhood education, and how early elementary school education can support gains made earlier. The FDC recommends ecological thinking to address multiple contexts and multiple time points. Context quality and stability over the Pre-K through third grade period and qualitative research are recommended as well.

Head Start Prevention Programming

In 2006, the federal *Head Start* program enrolled 11 % of 4-year-olds and 8 % of 3-year-olds (http://oig.hhs.gov). State-funded programs served more preschoolers than Head Start. Both types of programs enroll children based on family income, i.e., below the federal poverty level, eligible for public assistance, and some homeless children. There is current debate around the effects of Head Start because studies with different designs and different results have found no effects to positive effects. The strongest, most rigorous studies show immediate and long-term benefits. Head Start's effects are smaller in regard to learning benefits when compared to many state and local preschool programs, with the greatest effects in programs that are the most expensive and have a longer duration of services.

Head Start has been a pioneer in prevention programs for preschool children. Data collection by the Department of Health and Human Services involved a third-grade follow-up study in 2008, although the data was not published until December 2012 (Burke & Muhlhausen, 2013). The study followed 5,000 three- and four-year-old preschoolers from Head Start through third grade. Two cohorts have been followed, a 3-year-old group and a 4-year-old group. The final report examined the impact of Head Start in four domains: cognitive, social–emotional, health, and influence on parenting practices (U.S. Department of Health and Human Services, 2010). Head Start is extremely expensive so the results of government studies on its impact are important.

The long-term results of having attended a Head State program are not encouraging (Burke & Muhlhausen, 2013). Neither the 3-year-old cohort nor the 4-year-old cohort evidenced statistically measurable effects on any of the measures of cognitive ability or academic skills specifically. In regard to social–emotional development, the 3-year-old group results showed no effect on most measures although there was a slight positive effect on social skills and also on positive approaches to learning as measured by parents. Teachers saw no effects. For the 4-year-old cohort, again, most measures showed no effects although parents reported a small decrease in aggressive behavior. Teachers reported measurable evidence of an *unfavorable* impact on emotional symptoms with no effects on other social–emotional measures. When groups of children reached the third grade, they completed self-reports. The 4-year-old cohort reported problems in peer relations. Parents of the 3-year-old cohort reported improved authoritative parenting. Parents of the 4-year-old cohort reported spending more time with their children. The data raises questions around the cost-benefits of the Head Start program. It is important to keep in mind that benefits in the many studies vary according to the site and group served, the length of time the child remained in the program, as well as the quality and type of the evaluation.

There were some positive findings of the government studies, primarily for the 3-year cohort with subgroup benefits in the 4-year cohort. Favorable impacts of moderate size were identified at the end of 1 year, in cognitive areas, health, and in parenting (U.S. Department of Health and Human Services, 2010). The benefits in the social–emotional domain were primarily seen in the 3-year-old cohort where strong evidence was found that Head Start effects child behavior. The 3-year-old cohort demonstrated a decrease in problematic behaviors and hyperactivity, increased social skills, and positive approaches to learning by the end of the age 4 year. This group experienced longer-term positive impacts around relationships with their parents that lasted into kindergarten. Parents of the 3-year-old cohort children used less spanking and a less authoritarian parenting style by the end of the age 4 year. The 3-year-old cohort benefited from participation in Head Start programs, and by first grade the benefits of improved parent–child relationships and parenting practices remained. Head Start benefits for children with special needs lasted into the early elementary school with more significant benefits for children whose parents experienced fewer depressive symptoms. African American children in the 4-year-old cohort and English language learners benefited from Head Start and these benefits lasted through kindergarten.

Racial and Cultural Disparities

Achievement disparities among different groups of children appear long before formal schooling begins (Crosby & Dunbar, 2012). These disparities need to be addressed. Cultural differences that affect mental health include:

- How parents teach their children to interpret and express emotions
- Parental attitudes toward discipline
- Differences in regard to individual achievement versus interdependency
- Attitudes about mental health and emotional problems
- Acceptance or rejection of help from non-family members of the community (National Scientific Council on the Developing Child, 2008/2012)

Much of the work in immigrant families has focused on Hispanic and Asian families although not to the same degree, with much less research on African American families and children.

Research studies show that parents want safe, structured, childcare staffed with trained, warm teachers (Shlay, 2010). This is equally true of African American, Caucasian, and Hispanic families. Differences in use of early childhood programs have a good deal to do with whether or not a family has sufficient information about the value of early childcare experiences, and whether or not they can find and afford care, rather than due to cultural differences. Yesil-Dagli (2011) found that among Hispanic families, use of center-based care was more frequent than parental/extended family care alone or nonrelative care. Variables involved for Hispanic families included poverty, mother's education and work status, acculturation, and household composition. Interestingly, mothers who valued socialization more than other issues for their young children were less likely to use center-based childcare. Some studies suggest that Hispanic families tend to keep the youngest children at home; whereas, African American families are more likely to use center-based care earlier. The difference here was found to relate to economics, work factors, and availability of other Hispanic families in the neighborhood (Fram & Kim, 2008). An earlier study (Currie & Thomas, 1999) determined that when Hispanic children who attended Head Start were compared to siblings who did not have the same opportunity, those children attending Head Start significantly benefited.

All Latino children are not the same. They differ because of national origin, the social class to which they belong, home language, and indicators of acculturation.

A child's socialization takes place in a particular group and community. Socialization is influenced by the surrounding environments in which the children interact outside of their families (Fuller & Coll, 2010). Immigrant children's identity with their culture or ethnic group can strengthen their engagement with schools. Recent research indicates that parenting and general health are strong for immigrants but each declines for second-generation Latino immigrants who live in poor neighborhoods, although this also varies among subgroups. Latino children have been found to benefit more from early childhood education than children from other groups. Unfortunately high-quality preschools are scarce in low-income communities in which many Latinos live. About one-sixth of Latino families whose median incomes fell below the poverty line in 2003 had moved into middle-class neighborhoods. This represents an effort on the part of their parents to provide advantages to their children. It is important to recognize the strengths of families and the efforts they make to help their children use their social assets so their children will be successful in school.

African American immigrant children come to the United States from Africa, the Caribbean, and Latin America for the most part. The assets that these groups may exhibit include support for their children, parent education, parent employment, and English proficiency (Crosby & Dunbar, 2012). These parents are invested in their children's health and education and enroll them in center-based childcare. This group of children exhibits less disruptive behavior than other immigrant or American-born groups. The risk factors for this group include low-income and high rates of obesity. Supportive parent–child relationships make a difference for this group of children. By kindergarten, children of African American immigrants are doing fairly well, outperforming Hispanic children in both immigrant and native families and African American children born in the United States. African American children attending Early Head Start demonstrated the benefits they had gained from parent support and stimulation by the time they were 3 years old (Harden, Sandstrom, & Chazan-Cohen, 2012).

Ogletree and Larke (2010) feel that teachers of young children need to use multicultural education principles because of the changing population of the United States. As of 2009, there were almost 120,000 childcare facilities regulated by state governments. Facilities regulated by the government control training requirements. The National Association of the Education of Young Children (NAEYC) offers a national accreditation program for childcare centers with standards that include culturally, linguistically, and ethnically diverse teaching materials and methods. The *NAEYC Pathways to Cultural Competence Project* (http://www.ecementor.org) urges early learning programs to recruit and retain a diverse teaching staff and ensure that they are trained in cultural competence. Cultural competence is a critical component of a high-quality program. The project has a checklist available, provides recommendations for program directors and teachers, and advocates for a strength-based perspective. The group additionally provides guidance on connecting with diverse families (Table 12.1).

When prejudice and stereotyping occurs, early childhood teachers need to respond quickly, give simple responses, and model respect. They need to immediately clarify misconceptions. Additionally, materials should reflect the cultures and races represented in the population and encourage cooperation.

Table 12.1 Strategies for connecting with diverse families

Cultural awareness
Acknowledgement of different heroes and holidays
Allowing children to share stories about their home and family lives
Adults sharing stories and books with antibias themes
Teaching social problem solving
Offering experiences with real people

Source: NAEYC Pathways to Cultural Competence Project (2010)

Transition to Elementary School

About half of children entering elementary school have difficulty with this transition (Wildenger & McIntyre, 2012). Young children who spent preschool in programs located in public schools exhibit fewer behavioral issues and have better relationships with their kindergarten teachers than do children who attended other types of prekindergarten programs. When preschool is connected to the public school that children will attend, children adapt more easily, are more comfortable when they reach kindergarten, and their parents are more likely to become more involved with schooling in the future. Preschool programs that make a difference use evidence-based practices, teachers are certified, and the programs operate daily for at least 2.5 h a day.

When kindergarten teachers report that children enter school without needed skills, social–emotional and/or behavioral issues stress teachers most (Whitted, 2011). Children with skill deficits in these areas may be rejected not only by peers but also by school staff. They are at risk for school failure. States in which large numbers of preschoolers are expelled from preschool include New Mexico, Maine, Alabama, Delaware, and North Carolina. Aggressive students are likely to continue their inappropriate behaviors throughout their school years if these behaviors are not addressed and ameliorated by third grade (Coie & Dodge, 1998). The more risk factors that young children endure, the more likely that they will fail. Children who attend low-quality childcare are reported to exhibit more aggressive behaviors and general behavior problems. Research has demonstrated over and over again the importance of teachers for poor and minority children. Teachers that have high expectations for these groups of children have a positive influence on the children. High-quality teacher–child relationships reduce behavior problems. Promising and efficacious programs designed to teach young children the skills and competencies they need in the social and emotional areas benefit children by decreasing impulsivity, defiance, and oppositional behaviors. Additionally they improve prosocial behaviors by teaching children empathy skills, how to handle emotions, and how to solve social problems, and they improve self-control. Social and emotional skills are complex and require multilevel interventions starting at the preschool level for all children.

Universal Prevention

Because prevention programs are designed for specific high-risk populations and the fact that this can stigmatize families, universal prevention programs make more sense for young children (Bayer, Hiscock, Morton-Allen, Ukoumunne, & Wake, 2007). Another factor in support of universal programming is that many children with elevated risk are from middle- or upper middle-class families. Just because there are more families in this group, the bulk of children come from this group. Universal programming reaches all children including those at risk.

Significant numbers of young children exhibit serious behaviors that cause considerable concerns, jeopardize their care, disrupt families, and affect their development (Powell, Dunlop, & Fox, 2006). The issue has reached national levels of concern and has led to awareness of the importance of preventive work with the young population of children. Challenging behavior is persistent, intense, and pervasive rather than transitory. When preschoolers exhibit challenging behavior, this behavior can continue, and for some, intensify as they enter public school. Young children with poor social skills and challenging behavior require preventive interventions to get them on track for school success.

Prevention involves formulating and strengthening positive relationships with adults and peers. It involves support for parents to make sure they have the skills and knowledge to interact sensitively with their children. It involves making sure teachers of young children are warm and attentive. Prevention work involves relationship building between teachers and parents (Powell et al., 2006). Classroom prevention focuses on well-designed classrooms, balanced activities, consistent schedules, structure, and contingent interactions between teachers and young children. Social–emotional curricula with a solid evidence base are important as are multicomponent preventive interventions.

Preventing Externalizing Behaviors in Young Children

Persistent and challenging behaviors of preschool-aged children are associated with later difficulties in socialization, adjustment to school, and academic and social problems (Dunlap et al., 2006). A review of the literature by Dunlap and associates determined that behavior problems are long lasting; in fact, behavior problems are as stable as intelligence. Early behavior problems are the single best predictor of later delinquency, early and long-lasting peer rejection, negative interactions with teachers, and disturbing relationships with teachers and parents. Only 1–2 % of families with preschool children access mental health services for their children in a given year. Race and ethnicity complicates underuse of mental health services. Prevention is critical for this group of children, but data supporting preventive efforts are mixed. Programs that offer support for parents and that teach parenting skills have good results.

Preschoolers with emotional and behavioral difficulties are expelled at rates that are three times higher than students of school age. Stagman and Cooper (2010) attribute this to lack of attention to the social and emotional needs of young children. African American preschoolers are 3–5 times more likely to be expelled than other groups. When young children receive mental health services, they demonstrate less disruptive behaviors and are not expelled as often. Carter et al. (2010) examined a cohort of young children at school entry. They determined that approximately 1 in 5 young children (21.6 %) met the DSM-IV criteria for a psychiatric disorder *with impairment* as they entered formal schooling. The risks in this group included persistent family poverty, limited parental education, stress, having been exposed to violence, and low expressiveness of emotions within the family.

Although expelling students was the most severe reaction of a program to challenging behaviors as of 2006, two-thirds of states did not have clear practices for dealing with negative behaviors (Gilliam, 2008). At the preschool level, high rates of expulsion have been identified for boys, for older preschoolers, and for African American students. Expulsions from prekindergarten programs are particularly high in less regulated childcare facilities. Program factors related to the high rates of expulsion include high class size, the number of hours children spend in care (extended day care), and inappropriate student–teacher ratios. Teachers' educational levels, credentials, and experience are not related to rates of expulsion in young children. However, teacher beliefs and job stress do predict elevated rates of expulsion. According to Gilliam (2008), the American Academy of Pediatrics recommends that young children with behaviors that may result in expulsion should be evaluated. Parents need to be involved and if necessary the child should be transitioned to a program that can better meet the child's needs. In addition teachers need breaks. Mental health consultation would be very helpful. Student–teacher ratios need to be fairly low.

Because early childhood teachers say their highest priority is challenging behavior, Hemmeter, Fox, Jack, Broyles, and Doubet (2007) described a program-wide model of positive behavior supports for preschool settings. The major components of the model include establishing a leadership team, developing a plan to include processes for addressing problem behavior, and a PBS Toolkit with resources. When implementing the model, researchers determined that strong leadership was critical. Leaders needed to appreciate that development and implementation takes up to 5 years, and staff recognition makes a huge difference. Behavior consultants were needed for early childhood settings. Behavior consultants focus on building the capacity of the program and make sure that the model remained in place and was used. The Southeast Kansas Community Action Program (SEK-CAP) Head Start adopted a positive behavioral support model in 2001. Fox, Jack, and Broyles (2005) report evidence of reduced referrals, elimination of the time-out practice, improved program quality, increased team planning, improved staff satisfaction, and reduced staff turnover. Importantly there was a shift in attitudes from intervention to prevention.

Preventing Social–Emotional Problems in Young Children

When school adjustment is the goal, researchers feel that social–emotional skills are as critical as academic skills (Perry, Holland, Darling-Kuria, & Nadiv, 2011). Half of all young children with challenging behaviors in kindergarten end up under the special education umbrella by fourth grade. SEL competencies can predict academic skill levels in first grade better than family background or general ability levels (Fox, Dunlap, Hemmetter, Hoseph, & Strain, 2003). Externalizing and internalizing behaviors are first seen in childcare settings. Between 9.5 and 14.2 % of young children below school age experience social and emotional difficulties that have important effects on them both currently and in the future. Yet, less than 1 % of young children with emotional behavioral problems are identified (Cooper, Masi, & Vick, 2009). Many workers in early childhood programs feel that they are not trained to work with children who exhibit problem behaviors or emotional behaviors. Children with difficult temperaments from disadvantaged backgrounds have difficulty with social skills, emotional regulation, and friendship making. Teachers feel children with behavioral and emotional problems comprise their greatest challenges (Fox & Hemmeter, 2009). The goals for universal preschool programs include building positive relationships with children and families, because this is the basis for promoting social competence in young children. The teacher in a preschool program is critically important. Additional practices that are important for all children include a supportive environment and working to engage children in activities and routines. For at-risk children, explicit teaching of social skills and emotion regulation is critical.

The underlying foundation of social–emotional learning (SEL) is that learning occurs in the context of relationships (Elbertson, Brackett, & Weissberg, 2010). Emotional skills are prerequisite to learning skills as emotions drive attentional skills. Attentional skills, in turn, impact learning and memory. Emotions also affect motivation, perception, and behavior. Social skills are related to learning. Attachment, communication, and respect affect learning and positive relationships with teachers. They also enhance motivation and engagement. A sense of belonging is relevant to school success. SEL programs at the preschool level have positive effects in the short term (Ashdown & Bernard, 2012). Importantly, SEL skills can be taught.

The goals of social–emotional curricular programs (SEL) have to do with enhancing protective factors and decreasing risk factors in young children (Joseph & Strain, 2003). When young children are taught skills of cooperation and prosocial behavior, they are in a better position to learn and be successful in a school environment. As with older children, SEL programs that include direct teaching and have a longer duration are more successful. There is also some support for the idea that preventive interventions need to be implemented before children are 8 years of age.

Joseph and Strain (2003) reviewed the literature with the goal of locating SEL curricula that had the support of peer-reviewed efficacy data for the 3–5 year populations. Their goal was to recommend programs that would most likely be successful if implemented locally in a community preschool, or in a preschool attached to a public school. They described eight programs in detail. Their criteria for inclusion involved treatment fidelity, treatment generalization, treatment maintenance, social validity of outcomes, acceptability of interventions, replication across investigators, replication across clinical groups, evidence across ethnicity/ racially diverse groups, and replication across settings. Only two programs came close to meeting their criteria for a "high" level of evidence: The *Incredible Years*: *Dinosaur School* (Webster-Stratton, 1990) and *First Step to Success* (Walker et al., 1997). The *Dinosaur School* curriculum teaches emotional literacy, empathy (perspective taking), how to make friends, how to manage anger, and interpersonal problem solving. *First Step to Success* was designed for at-risk kindergarten students as a secondary prevention program. The *First Step to Success* program involves universal screening of all kindergarten children, parent training, and a curriculum. More recently, Whitted (2011) listed three programs that are effective in the social–emotional domains and in improving behaviors. The three were *Second Step* (Bandura, 1986), *The Incredible Years, and PATHS*: *Promoting Alternative Thinking Strategies* (Kusché & Greenberg, 1994a, 1994b).

Powell and Dunlap (2009) completed a synthesis of curricula and preventive intervention packages for young children to improve social–emotional functioning. The goal was to build and expand on Joseph and Strain's (2003) work. Powell and Dunlop selected programs that were designed to impact SEL skills, were manualized, had been evaluated by at least one study, were published in a peer-reviewed journal, and reported outcomes for the 0–5 age group (preschool through kindergarten). The preventive interventions were evaluated using the same criteria used by Joseph and Strain. The *Dina Dinosaur Child Training Program* met eight of the nine criteria (replication across settings was not demonstrated) as a secondary prevention program. The *Dina Dinosaur* universal classroom curricula for preschool and kindergarten met five of the nine criteria. *Al's Pals* (Dubas, Lynch, Galano, Geller, & Hunt, 1998; Lynch, Geller, & Schmidt, 2004) and the *Preschool I Can Problem Solve* curricula (Feis & Simons, 1985; Shure & Spivack, 1980, 1982; Shure, Spivack, & Jaeger, 1971) each met five of nine criteria. *Al's Pals* is a resiliency-based curriculum that uses developmentally appropriate and active strategies to teach health-promoting concepts and prosocial skills. The *I Can Problem Solve* curriculum emphasizes interpersonal problem-solving skills through generating alternative solutions to problems. Cooper et al. (2009) added the *PATHS Preschool* program, an evidence-based prevention program.

The 2013 CASEL Guide (Domitrovich, Durlak, Goren, & Weissberg, 2013) contains a framework for evaluating universal, well-designed (targeting all five areas of social and emotional competence), and evidence-based programs for both preschool and elementary school programs. Programs included were well designed, outcomes affected social and emotional competence, and programs had training and implementation support. Also included were programs that had at least one carefully conducted evaluation study with a comparison group in addition to pretest and posttest measures to support the program. The programs used explicit instruction for the most part and some also included working with the classroom environment.

Active forms of learning that are sequenced and explicit were identified as more effective. Other effective components included opportunities to practice skills and multiyear duration. The CASEL Guide rated programs according to whether or not the various elements were present in programs and at what level. Information included had to do with study design, evaluation outcomes, the grade range covered, number of sessions, classroom approaches, practice opportunities, the presence of extensions beyond the classroom, and whether or not assessment tools are provided. The preschool programs included in this very helpful document are *Al's Pals* (Pre-K-3), *HighScope Educational Approach for Preschool* (Pre-K), *I Can Problem Solve* (Pre-K-5), *The Incredible Years Series* (Pre-K-2), *PATHS* (Pre-K-6), *Peaceworks: Peacemaking Skills for Little Kids* (Pre-K-2) (Schmidt, 1993; Schmidt & Friedman, 1988), and *Tools of the Mind* (Pre-K-K) (Bodrova & Leong, 1995, 1996).

In selecting a program for the preschool population, resource teams can utilize various compendia of programs. It may be useful to identify which programs are listed by multiple rating agencies. It will be important to look at the criteria the agencies use to evaluate programs, as these may be the same criteria that schools may want to consider in narrowing their search.

An Approach to Strengthening Preschool Programming

Currently, the best approach to dealing with disruptive behaviors is a psychosocial approach (Comer, Chow, Chan, Cooper-Vince, & Wilson, 2013). The largest effect sizes found for early disruptive behaviors used behavioral approaches. Early childhood mental health consultation is a model that builds the capacity of staff, families, programs, and systems through coaching and mentoring (Perry et al., 2011). Program-focused consultation works to improve the quality of programming, specifically the classroom environment. A goal is to build teaching staff members' ability to deal with behaviors that affect that environment. The model appears to be an effective strategy to assist preschools with social–emotional and behavioral challenges, to reduce expulsions, and to improve teacher attitudes and behavior as well as to improve children's behavior.

The state of Maryland has a statewide project providing mental health consultation to childcare providers (Perry et al., 2011). A study based on interviews with consultants, program directors, staff, and parents explored why some preschoolers are expelled and found a variety of reasons rather than a single factor. The expelled children had mental health needs, complicated family situations, problem behaviors, or combinations of these. The preschool environments were a contributing factor as well. The preschool spaces were too open, too noisy, and unstructured. There were insufficient adults present. Routines were not working. Mental health consultants work with childcare staff members to change routines, classroom layout, train staff, and improve behavior management skills. Consultants may model effective practices and help teaching teams communicate with one another and with parents, in an effort to improve classroom climate. Particularly important is the work to engage families with early childhood program staff so relationships are improved and become more collaborative. School-based mental health practitioners could use this consultation model to assist preschool programs that are feeder schools to a local school. The payoff for children, families, the preschool, and the public school system would be well worth the effort.

Long-Term Benefits of Preschool Preventive Programming

The *HighScope Perry Preschool* program was originally implemented in Michigan in the 1960s (Heckman, Moon, Pinto, Savelyev, & Yavitz, 2011). The HighScope Preschool curriculum study randomly assigned 68 poor children to the HighScope model, the Distar model, and a traditional preschool model (Schweinhart, Weikart, & Larner, 1986). The program included a two-and-a-half-hour program implemented daily with weekly home visits from teachers to involve parents. The program involved active learning using open-ended questions and encouraged development of social and emotional skills. There were five cohorts with a total of 123 families. Follow-up interviews were conducted periodically over time. The Stanford–Binet Intelligence Scale scores of children rose dramatically during the first year into the normal range for children in all three high-quality programs. Studies over time, i.e., when children were 15 years of age, showed that cognitive gains tended to hold. However, children who had been in the Distar group had behavioral problems later on (Schweinhart et al., 1986). Ninety-one percent of the original participants were involved in a final interview which occurred when the participants were 40 years old.

The project has received considerable attention from policy makers, academics, and practitioners. The *HighScope Perry Preschool Program* is frequently cited to support the claim of cost-benefits from early childhood education programming (Heckman, Moon, Pinto, Savelyev, & Yavitz, 2010). However, problems with the original randomization process were identified and the data needed to be reanalyzed. Estimated annual social rates of return were generally found to fall between 7 and 10 %, with most estimates substantially lower than those previously reported in the literature (Heckman et al., 2010). Still, the reanalysis confirmed that there were indeed long-term effects for both females and males.

A Closer Look at Several Programs

During the preschool period, children are beginning to be able to differentiate positive and negative emotions. They are learning to regulate thoughts, feelings, and behaviors (Gunter, Caldarella, Korth, & Young, 2012). For these reasons alone, it is important to provide preschoolers with early social and emotional learning experiences. Various curricula should be considered by schools in a position to influence program selection.

Peaceworks: *Peacemaking Skills for Little Kids* (Pre-K-2) (Schmidt, 1993) developed by the Peace Education Foundation in Florida, is a locally funded, skill-building curriculum that provides activities and visual aids. It is somewhat similar to *PATHS*. Pickens (2009) evaluated the curriculum and found that participating children exhibited fewer internalizing and externalizing behaviors than the no-treatment group. The *Tools of the Mind* curriculum uses dramatic play to focus on improving children's academic skills, cognitive skills, and social self-regulation. Bodrova and Leong (1995, 1996) and later Barnett et al. (2008) conducted effectiveness studies of the *Tools of the Mind* program. *Strong Start Pre-K* (Merrell, Whitcomb, & Parisi, 2009) is a curriculum that is part of a series of programs developed to reduce internalizing behavior problems. Faculty and doctoral students at the University of Oregon developed the series of programs, which include *Strong Start Pre-K*, *Strong Start K-2*, *Strong Kids*, and an adolescent version, *Strong Teens* (Whitcomb, 2009). Kramer, Caldarella, Christensen, and Shatzer (2010) looked at the influence of the *Strong Start* curriculum at the kindergarten level. Using a time-series design (with data collected at four points and no control group), they worked with four kindergarten teachers to deliver the curriculum to 67 students. Half of the student population received free lunch. Students gained in prosocial behaviors with moderate and large effect sizes and decreased internalizing behaviors as rated by both teachers and parents. Teachers reported a greater decline in internalizing behaviors than parents reported. Implementers found the program both feasible and acceptable. The *Strong Start Pre-K* version of the series is highly structured and easy to use in that lessons are partially scripted (Gunter et al., 2012). Five additional programs are described next, with a bit more detail.

Al's Pals

Al's Pals is a multiyear program for preschool children through grade three of elementary school (Lynch et al., 2004). The curriculum is implemented over an entire year and has a parent component. Multiple program replications using pre-experimental and experimental research designs indicate that outcomes include an increase in prosocial skills and SEL competencies, along with decreases in aggressive behaviors. Lynch et al. (2004) ran an experimental study of the curriculum in a Head Start program in Michigan, using 17 classrooms with random assignment compared to 16 classrooms making up the control group. Children in the experimental group were rated significantly improved in the social–emotional domain. Improvements were seen in competence, prosocial skills, and positive coping skills. Problem behavior did not change in the experimental group, but it increased in control children. Training of teachers is available.

I Can Problem Solve

The *I Can Problem Solve* curriculum (ICPS) (Shure & Spivack, 1982) involves interpersonal cognitive problem-solving training, which trains children in how to think about problems so that they can solve their own interpersonal challenges (Feis & Simons, 1985). Shure and Spivack implemented the training with 4-year-old urban African American preschool children and compared those receiving the training with children who did not receive training. They determined that the trainings were effective at the preschool level and also at the kindergarten level. The training effects lasted for at least 1-year post-intervention. Trained children were better able to think of alternative solutions to problems; they coped better with frustration, were less aggressive, and were less likely to begin to demonstrate behavioral issues. Feis and Simons (1985) replicated the training in a rural area over 3 years with low-income preschool children. Decreases were reported in both externalizing and internalizing problem behaviors and trained children were less likely to be referred for emotional difficulties. Boyle and Hassett-Walker (2008) conducted an independent 2-year evaluation of the curriculum with 226 kindergarten and first grade students using randomly assigned matched schools. They determined that the *ICPS* prevention program increased prosocial behaviors (stronger effects) while diminishing problem behaviors in children beginning formal schooling. Students receiving 2 years of instruction did better than those receiving only 1 year of instruction. The *ICPS* curriculum is easy to implement and not expensive.

PATHS: Promoting Alternative Thinking Strategies

The Promoting Alternative Thinking Strategies curriculum has been adapted for preschool populations. The efficacy of the preschool version has been evaluated using a randomized trial with a wait-list control group (Domitrovich, Cortes, & Greenberg, 2007). The *PATHS* curriculum is comprehensive in that the goal is to both reduce problematic behaviors and enhance SEL competencies. The *PATHS* curriculum is theory-based. It emphasizes teaching skills and includes opportunities for children to generalize skills. Domitrovich and colleagues studied the implementation of the *PATHS* curriculum over a 3-year period with 246 children. The curriculum was implemented in two regional urban Head Start programs in which 47 % of the children were African American and 10 % were Hispanic. The program consisted of 30 lessons taught by Head Start teachers once a week. The units covered compliments, feelings, a revision of the well-known "Turtle Technique," and social problem solving. Extension activities were included through games, projects, and stories. The program was integrated into the general program.

Implementation fidelity was high. Children's emotion knowledge skills improved, as did their competence according to multiple informants. Receptive emotion vocabulary increased along with recognition of emotional expressions, although social problem solving did not improve. Parents and teachers reported that children experiencing the *PATHS* curriculum were better adjusted in regard to improved social interaction, emotion regulation, and social skills. In comparing *PATHS* to *I Can Problem Solve*, the focus of *PATHS* is wider.

Second Step Early Learning Curriculum

Second Step is most often described as a violence prevention program. It is used frequently in schools. The efficacy of *Second Step* for early elementary school students has been demonstrated. Lillenstein (2001) assigned 184 students in kindergarten, first, and second grade, to one of two groups with 101 students in a wait-list group. The population was White, middle to upper class, and families were intact. The curriculum was implemented once per week for 6 months. Pre- and post-intervention assessments were completed by parents and also by teachers. Measures of social skills and problem behaviors along with observations of children were collected. There was no effect on social skills or problem behaviors, although teachers reported classroom climate improved, and their own management skills improved.

The *Second Step Early Learning* curriculum was designed by the Committee for Children (2010) and is a downward extension of the popular *Second Step K-5* program (Thomas & Gravert, 2011). There are four units involving empathy, emotion management, friendship, and problem solving. The teaching approach is developmentally appropriate using puppet scripts, stories, games, songs, and photos. The teaching approach involves modeling, cueing, and coaching behaviors. Teachers utilize discussion, role-play, and storytelling. There is information to send home, and activities are provided to generalize and reinforce skills and concepts.

Baker, Kupersmidt, Voegler-Lee, Arnold, and Willoughby (2010) trained 49 teachers from 8 Head Start and 22 community childcare centers to implement the 25 lessons along with academic curricula (dialogic reading, preliteracy, math, and communication activities). Teachers implemented 71 % of activities even though weekly consultations were provided and there were ample resources. Researchers noted that teachers slowly decreased the number of components that they implemented. Head Start teachers implemented a smaller number of activities than teachers in community childcare centers. This study points out the importance of implementation and the groundwork needed to insure that a program will be successful.

Wenz-Gross and Upshur (2012) provided teacher training, coaching, and organizational supports to early childhood teachers in improve implementation. Lesson completion and fidelity were measured and were related to teacher attendance during training sessions, teacher turnover, the percentage of children with developmental delays, and both teacher and classroom characteristics. Teachers implemented

88 % of the lessons over 2 years. Researchers recommended attending carefully to teacher morale, teacher skills development, and providing ongoing teacher support to increase implementation fidelity.

The Incredible Years Series

When students exhibit behavior that makes teaching difficult, teachers tend to give those students easier work, reprimand them more, positively reinforce them less often, and actually provide them with less instruction which affects learning. Teacher training may make a difference. The *Incredible Years* (*IY*) Series (Webster-Stratton & Herman, 2010) comprises three curricula designed to prevent behavior problems in multiple settings. The IY Series is built on social learning theories, is timed to specific developmental periods, and targets multiple risk factors. One focus is the transition to elementary school. The IY teacher training programs appear to be promising. There is data to indicate that teacher behavior changes in response to IY training.

Training children to prevent behavior problems is critical. There are several versions of *IY* programs for students designed to prevent the onset of behavior problems. There is a selective prevention version for preschool, kindergarten, and for first and second grade students. The Tier 2 version is a pullout program. Two randomized studies have supported the efficacy of the pullout version. Another successful study was conducted with diverse student populations in elementary schools and Head Start programs. The program worked best for students at highest risk.

Training for parents is also crucial. Webster-Stratton and Herman (2010) recommend universal prevention for all parents and teachers of 3- to 6-year-old children using manuals containing self-learning modules. The *IY* parent programs target parents of children in four age groups. One of these is for parents of children 3–6 years of age (Webster-Stratton & Herman, 2010). The parent programs have been updated for culturally diverse families. The *IY* parent programs have been demonstrated to be effective with Latino, African American, and Asian American populations with few differences in outcomes (Webster-Stratton, 2009). The program has been evaluated in a number of countries with success due its flexibility. Webster-Stratton provides strategies for making sure the program fits a specific group to include:

- Encouraging questions affirming differences
- Collaborating with parents to develop their own group rule and goals
- Asking about cultural experiences and developing relevant cultural metaphors
- Providing modeling representative of the culture of the group
- Increased practice to empower parents
- Directly addressing barriers of resistance to some parenting techniques (Webster-Stratton & Herman, 2010)

A number of studies support the efficacy of the parent programs. The *IY* Series has been researched to such an extent that program developers have information about "optimal" dosage training needs and mentoring to support implementation. For example, the updated preschool program has 14 sessions in the prevention versions. But, when fewer than 14 sessions are delivered effectiveness decreases. The *IY* program works well with other preventive efforts that have similar theoretical bases such as SW-PBIS.

Prevention in Action Challenge: Compare and Contrast Two SEL Curricula

The several programs summarized in the chapter include The Incredible Years Series, Al's Pals, 1 Can Problem Solve, PATHS: Promoting Alternative Thinking Strategies, Tools of the Mind, Peaceworks: Peacemaking Skills for Little Kids (Pre-K2), Strong Start, and the Second Step Early Learning Curriculum. Create a chart comparing and contrasting two of these programs according to:

- Efficacy study designs
- Diversity of populations in the efficacy studies
- Outcomes
- Grade ranges covered
- Number of sessions
- Classroom approaches
- Practice opportunities
- Extensions beyond the classroom
- Tools provided
- Technical support available
- Availability of manuals
- Availability of materials
- Costs

Which program has the strongest support?

Can you think of any reason or reasons why the program might not be best for a given school?

Chapter 13
Tools for Prevention Work in Schools

The first steps of addressing mental health problems in schools include strategic planning (involving goals, objectives, and policies), capacity development, and needs assessment. It is helpful and in most cases necessary to create a team to do the work of addressing student mental health needs in a school. Teams provide multiple perspectives and provide partnerships when addressing problems (Watkins, Meiers, & Visser, 2012).

Formation of a "Prevention" Team

The establishment of a "Resource Coordinating Team" may allow schools to streamline functioning and make mental health services more available and efficient. A resource team is contrasted to a student study team, an eligibility team, or a teacher assistance team. A resource team does not address individual needs, but rather addresses system issues, in particular, resource allocation. The focus is on *all* students, on infrastructure, on collaboration, and on "building a comprehensive, multifaceted, and cohesive, system of supports" (Adelman & Taylor, 2008a, p. 1692). Adelman and Taylor (1999, 2008b) describe the functions of a resource team as:

- Mapping and analyzing resources in order to coordinate them
- Examining and improving the effectiveness of systems
- Working on the process for management of various programs and for communication both within and also outside of the school
- Redeploying and enhancing resources (better uses of resources, eliminating redundancy, adding missing components)
- Mapping, analyzing, and aggregating data to determine school needs
- Engaging in social marketing

The team could be made up of school staff representing all major programs and services, a member or members of the administration, teacher and parent representatives, and students. A resource team would complement other teams. A resource team can operate at the local school level, or district level, to facilitate integration and cohesiveness. A resource team gathers, integrates, redesigns, and communicates data, using a variety of tools to be further described in this chapter.

Culture and School Evaluation

The James Irvine Foundation established the Campus Diversity Initiative (CDI) for higher education, which includes resources for evaluation (http://www.aacu.org).

Public elementary and secondary schools can use the CDI. The CDI is committed to attending to the culture and context of prevention programs and draws on "democratic evaluation theory" (Samuels & Ryan, 2011). It uses formative and summative assessments such as internal data and assessments not created by teachers or schools to reflect on the needs and interests of the school community. New assessments can be created when they are needed. This approach is designed to examine the contextual factors around a program and provide opportunities to dialogue and work with others who disagree with them. Underrepresented stakeholders' views are included in an in-depth manner. Teams in this model are assembled to reflect the racial, ethnic, and economic community. The team attempts to understand shared and disparate values and experiences. Culture can be in the forefront of discussions as data is collected and interpreted in relation to all students in the school. In the same way that high-stakes assessment data aggregates data, school professionals will want to aggregate internal data that is collected as well and uncover hidden assumptions. Action plans need to consider all information and plan for close monitoring.

Building Capacity

Developing capacity for change is complicated because each school or school district is unique in regard its history, culture, staff, and politics (Bond, Glover, Godfrey, Butler, & Patton, 2001). Building capacity is directed toward the system rather than toward individuals. When changes are attempted in schools, teams must attend to building capacity (Zimmerman, 2008). In system terminology, capacity building involves moving people from their current state to where they need to be. Because change such as the implementation of prevention programs is stressful, change agents must be prepared to lead, understand how change occurs, and provide the support necessary for change to take place. Educational professionals need to see the change as something other than an add-on. Building capacity involves providing professional development and increasing teachers' sense of self-efficacy through shared decision-making and students' progress. Developing supportive school cultures for change and encouraging collaboration are vital. One strategy that is helpful is asking well-respected teachers to serve as role models and opinion leaders to foster acceptance of a new program.

The Early Ongoing Collaboration and Assistance (EOCA) is a Wisconsin initiative with a vision for system change to ensure quality education in the state (Sanetti, Kratochwill, Volpiansky, & Ring, 2011). Its framework involves four components:

- Building capacity by developing a shared vision and commitment with administrative leadership and support in a collaborative environment
- Adopting processes such as resource mapping and collaboration for meeting student needs
- Making informed decisions around evidence-based prevention and intervention
- Ensuring sustainability with ongoing professional support and both family and community involvement

Michigan has designed a similar initiative. The Michigan model considers building local capacity a critical lever for change (Redding, 2009). Local capacity rests on a system of support. It involves moving beyond identified student problems to causes. It rests on the local school to accept responsibility for improvement, working within systems versus promulgating fragmented services and evaluating the effectiveness of the system of support. It begins with assessing school functions and moves on to resource mapping.

Resource Mapping

The first step to remedying the fragmentation of services in schools is to clarify programs and services within schools or school districts already in place, in order to identify better ways to use the resources (Adelman & Taylor, 1999). Resource mapping, or asset mapping, is a process conducted by a prevention or resource team to identify and evaluate existing resources already in place in a school. Resource mapping may lead to rearranging or redeploying resources to improve school mental health services. It may identify gaps in services or identify redundant services. Resource mapping also helps demonstrate the process of addressing problems or the process of improving resources for all stakeholders and the local community (Center for Mental Health in Schools at UCLA, 2006). Resource mapping identifies programs, services, equipment, funding, leadership, personnel, etc. More specifically, the team might look at whether or not various mental health activities are coordinated (or integrated) with one another. The team might consider which activities need improvement or which need to be cut. They also need to consider what services may be missing. The Center for Mental Health in Schools at UCLA provides tools online for this process. The EOCA (see above) also provides a number of forms for resource mapping along with descriptions of the process. Sanetti, Kratochwill, et al. (2011) point out that resource mapping is an ongoing and stage-based process (p. 14). The four stages of resource mapping are as follows:

- A pre-mapping stage to assign roles and establish procedures for team members
- A mapping stage during which resources are identified in the school and community

- A strategic implementation stage during which resources are analyzed
- An evaluate, refresh, recycle stage for strategic planning and sustaining efforts

Lane, Colan, and Reicher (2011) have demonstrated the use of resource mapping to build capacity for implementation of Positive Behavior Interventions and Supports at the high school level.

Readiness for Change

Readiness for change must be addressed if change is to be successful. "Readiness for change" refers to school professionals' shared commitment in implementing a prevention program and incorporating preventive strategies into their daily work. Readiness for change refers to a shared belief that the work is going to be accomplished with success (Weiner, 2009). Readiness is affected by past experiences with change, the skills and knowledge in place, and willingness to engage in the proposed activities (Spiro, 2009). In addition, professionals must value the change and feel positively about the demands they will be required to make. Sufficient resources must be available. If readiness is high, people will work hard, be more persistent, and be less resistant. If readiness is low, much more structure and encouragement will be necessary before attempting school change.

Organizational readiness for change is a multilevel construct. Readiness can be addressed with individuals, departments, or at the whole-school level (Weiner, 2009). Implementing prevention programs or other school change involves collective action. It is a "team sport" that can get uncomfortable when some members of the staff feel ready and others do not. Motivation can vary among staff members. Some may value change; others may feel they have little choice and so go along with the group. Some will feel obligated; others may be against change. Change efficacy is higher when school professionals feel confident that they can implement a new program. Low confidence decreases motivation. When the school professionals want to implement a new program and feel confident that they can do so, organizational readiness will be high. Organizational readiness can involve availability of resources, but psychological readiness can either facilitate or sabotage change efforts.

Different strategies would be needed to increase readiness for change depending on whether school professionals were considered to be low (need for high structure by leaders), medium (collaborative planning with moderate structure), or high (letting the group make decisions) in readiness (Spiro, 2009). When there is significant variation in readiness, it may be best to either form smaller work groups or use strategies appropriate for the lowest "readiness" group. There are readiness tools available for use, but available readiness tools have limited reliability and validity (Weiner, 2009). Spiro provides a "Readiness Rubric" for staff members and for organizations as a whole that may be useful for resource teams. One of the strategies involves planning an "early win" to increase confidence as the innovation is implemented. Another involves techniques that minimize resistance. The National Child Welfare Workforce Institute website (http://www.ncwwi.org/) lists a number of organizational readiness for change tools, including evidence-based practice attitude scales, dimensions of organizational readiness, and organizational climate measures.

Needs Assessment

When a school team decides to address a mental health problem, it is critical to know the results that the team wants to achieve *before* determining actions to take to reach that goal (Watkins et al., 2012). The team looks at the goals and objectives they have generated to determine if subsequent actions can be justified based on the results that the various actions are designed to achieve. The end result is to improve performance of students, teams, or the school itself.

An early decision for the team is dealing with the needs assessment, which starts the process of addressing prevention concerns. A needs assessment is a proactive (to increase student resilience) or reactive (reduce bullying) systematic process for decision-making that justifies decisions before they are made. The needs assessment will guide decisions throughout the process from addressing concerns to evaluating the results of actions taken by a school. Needs assessment involves gathering data from *many* sources and the viewpoints of all stakeholders in order to make intelligent decisions and recommendations.

A needs assessment is a decision-making tool (Watkins et al., 2012). Needs are gaps (lack of skills) between current behaviors and the desired behaviors or competencies of students. A needs assessment begins with determining the decisions that the team will make once the assessment is completed. It starts with a plan for identifying needs, analyzing them, and making recommendations for action(s). The team must decide what information is required, where the information can be located, and which data collection tools will be used. They must pilot test the information gathering tools, decide which tools to use, gather the required data, and link action steps to the data that is collected.

Tools for planning, monitoring, evaluating, and communicating around mental health needs of students include a variety of needs assessment strategies. Tools may include structured interview questions, questionnaires, surveys, focus groups, logic models, fishbone diagrams, and concept mapping. Watkins et al. (2012) provide details (strengths, weaknesses, and uses) in regard to all of the various choices of tools. This resource can be accessed online. A needs assessment cannot rely on only one tool. The team must select the tools that fit the goals and outcomes desired. The needs assessment should involve all stakeholders, i.e., administration, staff, parents, students, and community representatives. Tools are selected based on a cost–benefit analysis, feasibility, acceptability, expertise of team members, and past experience. Some data will already be available to a team, such as student demographics, student achievement data, enrollment counts, dropout rates, graduation rates, and discipline records. The assessment is not completed until the team has *enough* data to make the decisions that were planned.

Needs assessment strategies and tools can be located online. The Wisconsin Department of Public Instruction (http://winss.dpi.wi.gov) provides school climate surveys, self-reflection tools for teachers and administrators, and characteristics of successful school surveys in Spanish and Lao. The NCLB website provides comprehensive needs assessment information and tools (http://portal.esc20.net). The National Association of School Psychologists (NASP) provides guidelines for a school needs assessment interview (http://www.nasponline.org). The Michigan Department of Education provides a number of tools for assessing school community needs as does the Kansas State Department of Education. The National Association of Secondary School Principals website describes how to implement a quality needs assessment (http://www.nassp.org). Helpful information about *methods* for conducting an educational needs assessment is available (http://www.cals.uidaho.edu). A completed needs assessment and recommendations for school-based mental health services and supports for Napa County (2007) provides an example of information that can be garnered from a needs assessment.

Needs Assessment to Prevent Bullying

Preventing bullying in American schools is a hot issue. Currently, bullying prevention efforts are assessed using anonymous self-report measures. Needs assessment questionnaires define bullying for students and then ask how often individual students have been bullied or have bullied others in the past couple of months (Vaillancourt et al., 2010). Students choose from a range of responses. Bullying prevention questionnaires are used for needs assessment rather than for screening total school student populations, for several reasons screening tools are time-consuming, expensive to administer and analyze, require informed consent from parents, and require assent from students. The Olweus Bully/Victim Questionnaire (BVQ; Olweus, 1996) enjoys wide acceptance and use in schools in many countries, including the United States. Ontario researchers conducted a study of two questions adapted from the Olweus Bully/Victim Questionnaire because these questions are used to determine prevalence of bullying in worldwide prevalence studies. Researchers next asked more detailed questions in a second trial (Vaillancourt et al., 2010). These critical screening items from the Olweus' scales identified noninvolved students very well and identified student experiences with overt (physical and verbal) bullying. The questions did not provide information about social or cyberbullying, and therefore the tool may underestimate bullying prevalence. Data indicated that when a student reports that he or she is a victim of bullying when responding to the Olweus questionnaire, it is most likely true.

Peer nomination is a needs assessment technique that is well validated to assess relationships among students (Lee & Cornell, 2010). This technique asks students to nominate peers they feel are victims of bullying or who bully others. School professionals conduct the assessment, determine the number of nominations a student is given, and use this to identify bully or victim status. This technique is sensitive to relational aggression. Lee and Cornell (2010) compared the peer nomination technique to the BVQ and found that although there was a modest correlation, peer nominations identified more bullies than the BVQ, but self-reported victimization was similar using both approaches. When school staff members are attempting to determine the prevalence of bullying and additionally identify students heavily involved, it may be better to use more than one technique.

Alternatives and additions to questionnaires to assess negative student behaviors might include reviews of disciplinary records in a school and school climate surveys. Tableman and Herron (2004) list several school climate surveys. The Delaware School Climate Survey-Student (DSCS-S) (Bear, Gaskins, Blank, & Chen, 2011) is new. The California School Climate Survey and the California School Parent Survey (http://chks.wested.org) are helpful tools. The National School Climate Center (NSCC) (http://www.schoolclimate.org) recommends the Comprehensive School Climate Inventory (CSCI), comprises student, parent/guardian, school personnel, and community scales. The Center for the Study and Prevention of Violence (CSPV) (http://www.colorado.edu) recommends the Safe Communities Safe Schools (SCSS) School Climate Surveys.

Focus Groups

Focus groups are qualitative approaches used for a wide variety of purposes (Table 13.1). Qualitative approaches are inductive and interactive as compared to quantitative approaches (Kress & Shoffner, 2007). The technique is not new. Focus groups have been used as far back as the 1920s. Focus groups have been described

Table 13.1 Uses for focus groups

- Gather data about opinions, perceptions, attitudes, beliefs, and insights of a select group
- As one component of a needs assessment as long as the individuals selected for the group represent the population of interest or an important subpopulation
- To assist in program development of mental health services
- As a means of determining needs
- To determine whether or not a program or its components are feasible
- To determine response to the pilot study of a new program
- As part of outcomes evaluation
- For soliciting input to make policy decisions
- To generating possible solutions when things go wrong
- As a process assessment to make programmatic changes
- To evaluate staff training
- To stay in touch with parents or community members
- To improve assessment methods
- To gather background information
- To demonstrate accountability

Sources: Heary and Hennessy (2002) and Jayanthi and Nelson (2002)

as guided discussions (Nagel & Gagnon, 2008). They are used to gather data of a select group. Focus groups are not used for solving problems, for reaching general consensus, or for determining what all members of the school community think. It is important to keep in mind that focus groups were never considered to be stand-alone tools (Kidd & Parshall, 2000).

In a focus group, 6–12 participants are asked predetermined, structured, and open-ended questions to encourage the discussion of various themes (Heary & Hennessy, 2002; Kress & Shoffner, 2007). Typically, there are several initial questions to help participants feel comfortable, followed by several additional questions on the themes of interest, and a final question. A trained and experienced moderator clarifies the purpose of the group, the expected roles, maintains focus, and encourages members to dialogue with one another. Interaction among participants is important. A recorder observes nonverbal behaviors, takes detailed notes, and summarizes the session for participants. After a focus group or several focus groups have been conducted, the records are analyzed by hand or by computer for content and themes. Ethical issues include the fact that what individuals have to say is not confidential, and the discussion could be stressful. The lack of confidentiality, what will be done with notes taken, what kind of information must be shared, and when information will be shared should be explained for participants (Heary & Hennessy, 2002).

Focus groups have the reputation of being culturally sensitive and empowering. They can be useful when working with individuals who have had limited power and influence in the past or in the particular school district (Kress & Shoffner, 2007; Morgan & Krueger, 1993). A focus group is likely to gather more infor-mation than other methods and will most likely obtain at a range of opinions or experiences. The focus group process tends to feel respectful to participants and is more stimulating than other approaches. A large amount of data can be col-lected in a short amount of time. Focus groups generate more data than an indi-vidual interview approach and are particularly useful when trying to determine how satisfied participants and teachers may be with a new program (Heary & Hennessy, 2002; Kidd & Parshall, 2000). Focus group data combines well with other approaches. Confidence in focus group data can be enhanced by conduct-ing multiple focus groups and by including other data sources. Focus groups are not useful for testing hypotheses as in an experimental study, they cannot be used for drawing inferences about a whole-school population, and there is a risk of intimidation for participants should the group be led by a less-skilled member of the school staff. Focus group leaders can reduce bias by asking questions addressing both the strengths and limitations of a prevention program (Kress & Shoffner, 2007).

Examples of Use of Focus Groups

Focus groups have been used successfully with teachers and students around a wide variety of prevention topics (Kress & Shoffner, 2007). Wang et al. (2006) used a series of focus groups with students, school professionals, parents, and grocery store owners to gain some insight into the cultural appropriateness of an obesity prevention program among low SES African American students in Chicago. The themes that came out of the focus groups helped researchers understand the social and cultural aspects of obesity and school practices, barriers and facilitators to issues around eating (preferences, food preparation, accessibility), weight management, and body images. Students suggested a number of ideas to help with the development of interventions.

The extent to which focus groups can be useful is illustrated in a series of studies. Focus groups were used with multiethnic parents as background by another set of researchers who wanted to develop an obesity prevention program (McGarvey et al., 2006). Researchers determined that beliefs and perspectives were specific to each group in the study. The groups included low-income African American, Caucasian, Hispanic, and Vietnamese parents. This data was critically important for program development. Another group of researchers compared the use of a focus group to a brainstorming technique with high school students. The goal was to recruit students who smoke into a smoking cessation group (Sussman, Burton, Dent, Stacy, & Flay, 1991). Use of the focus group worked better than the brainstorming technique.

Bean and Rolleri (2005) used focus groups with African American and Latino parents, and their adolescents, around parent–child connectedness. A study of cyberbullying was conducted with middle and high school students using focus groups (Aatston, Kowalski, & Limber, 2007). They found that students, girls in particular, felt that cyberbullying is a problem that was not talked about in schools and shared that school staff members were not helpful. Students provided some ideas for dealing with cyberbullying but did not know how to respond when they observed cruel online behaviors.

Charlesworth and Rodwell (1997) examined whether or not focus groups could be used with children as a tool in a program evaluation. They determined that the approach is quite feasible for use with children. The focus group elicited unexpected information. The advantages of using focus groups with children include the fact that there is less pressure on a child as compared to an interview. The child is considered an expert when he or she participates in a focus group. Children are spontaneous. And focus group data has high face validity. The length of the session needs to be shorter for children, with fewer participants, and at least three students who will talk readily. Focus groups have been used with children as young as kindergarten, although with very young students more active approaches such as card sorting may be used more easily. The age range of students in a focus group should not be too great. When the focus group is used for research with children, written parental consent and student assent are both needed. Children need an appropriate explanation of the goals of the session, their role in the focus group process, and how the information gathered will be used. Children need to be told that they do not have to participate and can withdraw at any time.

Logic Model

A logic model is an extremely useful preventive tool. A program logic model tells viewers how the system works. It includes both theory and basic assumptions. It links short- and long-term outcomes with activities. It creates a shared understanding of the program's goals and process (Tucker, Liao, Giles, & Liburd, 2006). The components of a logic model include resources, activities, outputs, outcomes, impacts, and any external factors that may affect the program. Logic models are visual representations designed in a variety of sizes and layouts.

The logic model helps staff understand the rationale (causal factors) or logic of a new preventive program (Renger & Titcomb, 2002). Developing a logic model is important because implementing a program successfully depends on how well the process was conceptualized by stakeholders from the very beginning. The logic model is used for planning, implementation, and later on for program evaluation. A logic model can be simple with three elements such as a problem statement involving antecedents, activities, and outcomes. These are placed in a table format with each of the components described in a column. More commonly, there would be additional columns. Components, activities, target groups, short-term outcomes, long-term outcomes, and assessments may be included. Creating the logic model helps the planning team make certain that program components are clearly identified and that there is a strong focus on them. In addition, the logic model highlights factors or variables that may be overlooked, identifies needed resources, and links activities with both causal factors and outcomes. Outcomes will be clear if indicators are specified. Specifying the indicators of various outcomes can lead to an additional column that includes the measurement tools for each step of the process. Examples of logic models for various programs can be found online. The *Olweus Bullying Prevention Program* has a logic model (http://www.episcenter.psu.edu). Another example is a logic model for reducing and preventing youth tobacco use found online (http://www.uwex.edu).

A simple reason why the logic model is a good tool is the fact that it has no cost (Hayes, Parchman, & Howard, 2011). Additionally, the team developing a logic model must focus, think critically, and work together to create the logic model. Outcome indicators can be thought of as milestones on the way to accomplishing the goal of putting a prevention program in place (Hayes et al., 2011). The logic model tells professionals what data to collect and how to move ahead. Once team members agree on the logic model, the process can begin. Keep in mind, however, that it is not unusual to make corrections in the logic model as implementation proceeds.

More advanced development of logic models might involve concept mapping. Concept mapping can be used to identify the critical components of a program (Anderson et al., 2006). Additionally, the map visually shows the relationships between the program elements. Developing a concept map is a structured process involving project planning, idea generations, and analysis. First, all stakeholders are identified, each of whom submits ideas in response to a prompt. The team members then place their ideas into categories that they generate. These are reviewed to eliminate repetitions. A team creates a matrix from the responses. Finally from this data, a logic map can be constructed showing program inputs, activities, and outcomes. The logic model is then representative of the opinions of stakeholders.

The PRECEDE–PROCEED Planning Model

PRECEDE–PROCEED is a planning model used to integrate various theories of change and put them into action for preventive work. The PRECEDE aspect of the model stands for "predisposing, reinforcing, and enabling" constructs in educational/environmental diagnosis and evaluation (Green, Kreuter, Deeds, & Partridge, 1980; in Gielen, McDonald, Gary, & Bone, 2008, p. 409). PRECEDE indicates that educational diagnosis must occur first before planning takes place. PROCEED stands for policy, regulatory, and organizational constructs in educational and environmental development. This part of the model appreciates the fact that the approach to prevention and other interventions must be ecological. Problems take place in a larger context than the individual or even the school. The model has four planning phases to include an implementation phase and three evaluation phases. Some phases can be skipped when evidence is available. The premise of the model is that change will be successful if there is active participation by stakeholders in prioritizing problems to be addressed, in formulating goals, and in determining solutions. This model is a good example that allows a review of some of the concepts already covered and places them in a framework that demonstrates the planning process.

The PRECEDE–PROCEED process begins with a social assessment that comprises various data collection including interviews and focus groups (Gielen et al., 2008). The goal of this assessment is to spell out needs and desires, determine the system's problem-solving capacity, evaluate readiness to change, and list resources. Engaging a community partnership may be important and can provide more resources. The next phase involves gathering data that is already available in the school, information about the identified problem(s), and the factors that may influence the problem(s). In the case of risky behavior, this would include at-risk students' behavior, who and what affects the behavior, and how the environment supports or hinders the behavior. Identifying environmental factors is extremely important. Next, a team might look at theories of behavior change and the constructs that make up the theories to determine how they can be used to understand the behavioral and environmental factors that contribute to the problem. Schools need to investigate school norms for behavior and know how to change organizational policy (smoking prevention) or individual behavior (use of helmets in sports activities).

At this point, antecedent and reinforcing factors need to be implemented in order to start the change process (Gielen et al., 2008). Next, resources, barriers, facilitators, and policies needed for implementation are addressed. The most effective strategies are the ones that match the program, the students' needs, and the theory that fits the concern. Building a sustainable program requires a good match between the program and the local ecology, as well as mapping the preventive interventions to the identified factors affecting the problem (Gielen et al., 2008). Plans for data collection are made including process evaluation, impact evaluation, and outcomes evaluation. Process evaluation measures how well the program is implemented. Impact evaluation determines changes in predisposing, reinforcing, and enabling factors as well as measuring behavioral and environmental factors. Outcomes evaluation measures program effects. The resource or planning team is ready to implement the program at this point. The PRECEDE–PROCEED model requires extensive data collection. School-based teams need at least one member skilled in data collection (such as a school psychologist) to train the team, teachers, or those implementing the program in data collection.

Screening

Preventive services can reach a large population of students. Since the majority of students actually receiving mental health services receive them in schools, the President's New Freedom Commission on Mental Health (2003) strongly supported school mental health services, including programs and screening for mental health difficulties (Weist, Rubin, Moore, Adelsheim, & Wrobel, 2007). Because there are many barriers to providing mental health services in schools such as weak funding, lack of training and evidence-based practices, high turnover of staff, academic priorities, and challenges involving families, the recommendation for mental health screening presents a formidable barrier and challenge.

Universal screening is a systematic process of determining the risk status of a population of children without incurring significant costs and leading to identifying a mental health or behavioral problem before there is a need for referral and diagnosis (Feeney-Kettler, Kratochwill, Kaiser, Hemmeter, & Kettler, 2010). Universal screening is proactive (Weist et al., 2007). Even though mental health-screening programs are voluntary, they require informed consent of families along with student assent; community concerns persist. Some families feel that mental health screening is a violation of family privacy. Other families worry about stigma. Both issues contribute to community resistance to screening programs.

Ethical concerns around a mental health-screening program need to be addressed as schools consider expanding services including the ability to deliver services to students needing services, the possibilities of misidentification, community acceptance, and family rights (Chafouleas, Kilgus, & Wallach, 2010). Schools may not be able to service all of the students that a screening program might identify, although this would not eliminate any responsibility to identify students in need. However, it would be wise for a school considering mental health screening to determine the ability of school staff to service students identified, and if resources were too limited, community partnerships would need to be built with community agencies before initiating screening (Weist et al., 2007). The possibility of misidentification needs to be considered. Typically when screening, a higher level of false positives may be ethically supported in that schools would not want to miss students; yet, some may disagree with this position.

Increased interest in screening for emotional and behavioral problems also raises equity issues. For example, a number of studies have indicated that teachers rate African American children more hyperactive and inattentive than Caucasian children. There is little to no data on use of screening tools for students who are not as yet fluent in English (Dowdy, Dever, DiStephano, & Chin, 2011). This suggests that identification tools themselves may be part of the problem. We do not as yet have definitive data to show how screening tools may be affected by factors such as ethnicity, language, or gender. It is important to evaluate the appropriateness, technical adequacy, and usability of screening tools with diverse student populations. One serious concern is the possibility of over-identification of students with racial and ethnic differences, which would raise questions around the fairness of mental health screening (Chafouleas et al., 2010). Still another ethical concern has to do with acceptance by the community of a mental health-screening program. Parents worried about possible stigmatization or those who do not believe that schools should be involved with behavioral or mental health screening may raise objections. Frontline school staff would need to work hard to teach the community the value of screening efforts. Connecting negative behavior and mental health difficulties to academics may help convince parents of the value of screening. Stated goals might involve preventing behavior and emotional problems so they do not interfere with school performance. Screening needs to be closely connected to supports that provide for students who are identified at risk. Careful monitoring of a screening program is necessary.

Professionals themselves have raised the issue of family rights associated with mental health screening. IDEA (2004; 34 C.F.R. 300.302 and 34 C.F.R. 300.300) indicates that screening used to determine instruction, or screening conducted as a component of the general school activity, does not require consent from parents. Individual evaluations for special education services do require parental consent (Chafouleas et al., 2010). School professionals are not as clear about mental health screening, in that negative behaviors and mental health difficulties could certainly interfere with school performance, but may not be considered to be part of expected day-to-day practices. In cases in which a school has a multitiered model of service delivery, it is more reasonable to think that the assessment of students used to design supports that would be delivered as part of regular school practices would fall under the purview of normal educational practices. In this case screening would require that parents be notified in advance, the screening process and the results of screening carefully explained, and parents would have the option to decide *for* their children to participate or not participate in screening. Still, concerns will continue until social–emotional learning and behavioral supports become solidly integrated into regular school practices. In searching for screening tools, schools must also consider the *Protection of Pupil Rights Amendment* (PPRA, 2002) (http://www2. ed.gov), which requires consent when students are surveyed using items that are considered "protected information." These include psychological problems of the student and certain behaviors. The necessity for parental permission may depend on whether the screening tool involves questions around internalizing behaviors which may require permission if they fall under PPRA (2002) guidelines.

An essential task of school mental health services is to attend to the mental health status of all students in the school or district (Dowdy, Ritchey, & Kampaus, 2010). Conducting mental health evaluations on individual students is an expensive and time-consuming proposition. Schools do not have the resources to meet every student's needs alone, as some students with very severe needs will require resources outside of the schools. One approach to identifying mental health problems in the school as a whole is to conduct anonymous screening of all students with a tool such as the Youth Risk Behavior Surveillance System (YRBSS) of the CDC. This is a biannually administered instrument for high school students. The data from this tool would show evidence of a more general problem that might exist in a particular community and could be used to measure progress in addressing identified problems in addition to screening for the presence of a particular mental health problem in the student population. Another approach would be a multiple-gating screening model where all students would be screened to determine risk factors. Those who were determined to be at risk would be given a more in-depth assessment. A few students would eventually receive a comprehensive evaluation. As critical as needs for services may be, as of 2005, less than 2 % of schools in the United States were estimated to screen their student populations for mental health difficulties.

Given significant concerns around mental health problems along with improved screening technology, universal screening is more feasible than it has been in the past (Dowdy et al., 2010). There are several advantages to universal screening. Universal screening determines both the problems and the strengths of a student population. It collects trends in student functioning over time and provides needed data to identify preventive activities. It prioritizes resources to address the most critical issues in behavior and mental health. It helps create local norms and determines the effectiveness of efforts to improve student functioning. Universal screening determines risk rather than disorders in identifying mental health problems before they have become full blown, although universal screening can also be used to identify assets and resiliency. Use of a broadband screening tool is preferred for screening. Screening for a variety of problems makes more sense than focusing on a single problem such as suicide prevention.

There are some general considerations that school teams need to consider when choosing a universal screener. The construct or domain of interest, the population (age group or developmental level), the informants (teachers, parents, caregivers, students), costs, and the complications of administering and scoring the screening tools are each important (Feeney-Kettler et al., 2010). An expert, such as a school psychologist on the planning team, needs to evaluate the psychometric properties of the tools under consideration. The sensitivity and specificity of the tools must be determined. Sensitivity refers to the proportion of children who are correctly identified by the tools. Specificity refers to children who should not be identified and indeed are not identified by the screener. These determine the accuracy of the tool and help determine cut scores and decision rules. The screening tool must fit the local population, costs must not be excessive, and the tool must be acceptable to the school community and parents. The screener must have "treatment utility," which refers to its ability to lead to preventive interventions. Screening tools need to be pilot tested to determine if they match local needs and are acceptable to the local population (Dowdy et al., 2010). The bottom line is whether or not the screener meets the needs of the school and is both time and cost-efficient.

A Few Specific Screening Tools

There are problems with screening tools for social/emotional and behavioral concerns. Some focus on only one mental problem. Some do not measure the competencies that are related to critical outcomes. Some require much too much time (teacher rankings or long questionnaires for teachers) (DiStephano & Morgan, 2010). Add to these concerns information about the use of screening tools with minority students is just beginning. Examples of screening tools addressing a single mental health problem include the *Short Mood and Feelings Questionnaires* (SMFQ). This tool can be used for students 7–8 years of age through 18 years of age. It discriminates well for students who have more severe symptoms (Sharp, Goodyer, & Croudace, 2006). There are child and parent versions of the 13-item SMFQ. When they are used together, they show high accuracy (Rhew et al., 2010). The SMFQ measures affective and cognitive symptoms rated as true, sometimes true, or not true over the past 2 weeks. The tool has good internal reliability. Although this tool has been studied in school settings, it may be more appropriate in a clinic setting.

The *Screen for Child Anxiety Related Emotional Disorders* (SCARED) is a screening tool for childhood anxiety-related issues (Boyd, Ginsberg, Lambert, Cooley, & Campbell, 2003). The tool has 41 items with good test–retest reliability. Boyd et al. explored how the screening tool would work for African American students and determined that while a five-factor structure worked well for Caucasian students, a three-factor structure emerged for African American teens. This is a good example of work being done to determine minority differences when using screening tools.

Looking at screeners that may have broader appeal for schools, there is a small group of promising tools. One of these is the *Behavioral and Emotional Screening System Teacher Rating System for Children and Adolescents* (BASC-2 BESS: Kamphaus & Reynolds, 2007). The BESS TRS-CA screener was developed from two forms of the BASC. Items were taken from four areas. Adaptive Skills, Externalizing Problems, Internalizing Problems, and School Problems dimensions are the four areas (DiStephano & Morgan, 2010). The BESS TRS-CA measures one construct and produces results that are compatible across individuals. There is a parent and a teacher version. Cross-informant agreement is "medium" (reported in Feeney-Kettler et al., 2010). Internal consistency and test–retest reliability are both high. The tool compared well to other measures although it is less sensitive when predicting internalizing problems. It is expensive, but there is software available that allows for both individual and group score reports. It can be used for monitoring large groups of children. Scoring can be adjusted and it is available in Spanish.

Given the increasing recognition of social and emotional competence in relation to academic success and the concerns around mental health screening in general, researchers are looking to develop screening tools to measure strengths, specifically, factors related to resiliency. Strengths-based assessments involve measurement of skills that improve ability to cope with stress, create a sense of accomplishment, contribute to positive relationships with peers, and promote social and academic development (LeBuffe, Shapiro, & Naglieri, 2009). Strengths-based approaches are more acceptable to stakeholders, identify replacement behaviors, and lead to prevention.

An example of a strengths-based tool and also an example of examining how screening tools differ for different populations is the work of Romer, Ravitch, Tom, and Merrell (2011) who looked at gender differences on a relatively new screening tool. The *Social Emotional Assets and Resilience Scales* (Sears: Merrell, 2011) is a cross-informant social and emotional screening tool measuring knowledge and skills associated with resilience. This is strengths-based measure that can be used as a screening tool and also as a progress-monitoring tool. The tool measures protective factors, which predict social, emotional, and behavioral outcomes possibly better than tools measuring only risk factors. More specifically, the tool measures aspects of social competence, self-regulation, and problem solving, as well as social and emotional knowledge. There are four versions of the SEARS to include a teacher report form for students K-12 (SEARS-T), a parent report for rating children in the 5- to 18-year-old age group (SEARS-P), a child self-report version for students in grades 3–6, and an adolescent self-report for students in grades 7–12 (SEARS-A). The tools have good test–retest reliability, strong internal consistency, and positive correlations with other measures. Further evaluation of the data examining gender differences determined that separate norms for boys and girls were not needed in that differences were so small.

Another strengths-based screening tool is the *Devereux Student Strengths Assessment, DESSA-mini* (Naglieri, LeBuffe, & Shapiro, 2011). The DESSA-mini is a brief 8-item tool with parallel forms used for screening and progress monitoring. It yields a total score, the Social–Emotional Total (SET). There are four forms. All four have excellent internal reliability, sensitivity, specificity, and both positive and negative predictive power. SET scores from all forms predict the total score of the full 72-item DESSA, 91–96 % of the time, and are similar to other screening tools. The DESSA-mini helps identify children at risk who would benefit from social–emotional learning prevention programs. The DESSA-mini can also be used for progress monitoring. The full DESSA can be administered for students who are identified at risk (LeBuffe et al., 2009). A special feature of this tool is that assessment planning and intervention suggestions based on the DESSA are available.

The *SSIS Performance Screening Guides* (Gresham & Elliott, 2008) are part of a comprehensive model, which includes screening guides, rating scales, a classwide intervention program, and intervention guides aimed at prevention

(Elliott & Gresham, 2008). The purpose of this tool is to screen for possible behavior problems that might interfere with peer relationships and academics. Three levels of the tool cover preschool, elementary, and secondary school levels. The areas covered include prosocial behaviors, motivation to learn, and basic skills. The focus is on "keystone" classroom behaviors and skills. Progress-monitoring options are available. The screener uses a criterion-referenced judgment system similar to proficiency levels of basic skills, rather than using norms. Initially the system is complex to use, but teachers adapt and improve with use. The fact that the system provides more in-depth assessments and an intervention program is appealing.

Many screening tools have been designed for specific child and adolescent behaviors. SAMHSA (2011) has developed a valuable guide (http://www.samhsa.gov), which contains two matrices: a matrix of mental health and combined screening tools and a matrix of substance use/abuse screening tools. The matrices compare tools on a variety of variables. For example, the matrix of mental health tools compares seven screening tools in regard to the target conditions, whether or not the scales contain high-risk items, the age range of the tools and format, administration time, reading level, and translations. Two of the scales are appropriate for use in schools. These tools would constitute second-tier screening tools in that they have too many questions for easy use to screen an entire population of students.

Once screening data is collected, the team needs to plan around the highest priority needs and examine hypothesized causal factors creating or interfering with desired outcomes. Data must be synthesized. Recommendations are summarized in a report or presentation, and the information is disseminated throughout the school district and local community (Watkins et al., 2012). Tools for analyzing needs assessment data include the nominal group technique, which is a group consensus building and ranking activity. In addition, multi-criteria and tabletop analyses, fishbone diagrams, concept mapping (a method of making a visual representation), and many others may be used.

Online Screening and Progress-Monitoring Assists

Two online companies provide universal screeners that are used by schools that have response to intervention in place. Pearson Corporation has incorporated the *Behavioral and Emotional Screening System* (BESS; Kamphaus & Reynolds, 2007) and portions of the *Social Skills Improvement System Performance Screening Guide* (SSIS; Elliott & Gresham, 2008) to create AIMSweb Behavior (http://aimsweb-qa.ratchet.com/). This allows schools to screen for both behavioral and emotional issues. There are forms for teachers and students in English and Spanish, which rate prosocial behaviors and student motivation. Importantly, there is a progress-monitoring component as well. Forms can be completed online if desired which generate reports. Individual and whole-group reporting in these areas can be combined with academic results. The system provides strategies for assisting students who are determined to be at risk.

BESST Web (https://besstweb.com) is a behavioral/emotional social skills system to identify social–emotional needs. The system is in line with the Illinois Board of Education Social–Emotional Learning Standards. Students are screened with a short Benchmark Assessment Tool (BAT), and scores are entered online to identify at-risk or "at some risk" students. The BAT is a universal screener completed by teachers (K-8), and there is a student self-report for students in grades 6 through 8. The BAT is somewhat different from other screeners in that it is considered to be a GOM (General Outcome Measure) rather than a mastery-based tool. A GOM is similar to curriculum-based measurement tools. GOMS are generic in that they were developed from social–emotional learning theory, rather than designed from a specific curriculum.

A second tool, the Performance Assessment Tool (PAT) (https://besstweb.com), indicates the proficiency with which a student can develop or improve the skills in the social–emotional domain. The items are expansions of skills identified by the BAT (samples can be located on the BESST Web site). This tool measures general progress and facilitates targeting specific behaviors that need to be addressed at the Tier 2 level. "Tracking sheets" are available for the mental health staff providing secondary prevention activities. This provides a "running record" of progress in specific skills that can demonstrate growth (or lack of growth) over a short period (8 weeks). Research continues around the BAT and PAT tools.

Process or Formative Evaluation

According to the WHO (2011), process indicators measure how well a preventive intervention is progressing in the process of change. Process indicators explain how the work is being done versus the result of the program. Process indicators must be measurable, valid, and should mean the same thing to everyone involved. Process indicators must be able to be checked and be sensitive enough to show changes being made. A core set of indicators includes the most critical aspects of implementation (Meusel et al., 2008).

Research over many years shows that process or formative assessment can have powerful effects on outcomes and on decreasing gaps among student groups (Ysseldyke & McLeod, 2006). In well-designed prevention work, process evaluations of curricula or programs will have already been described through the development of a logic model, along with the tools that will be used to make decisions about the implementation of prevention programs and the progress of indicators of outcomes. Process evaluation allows school teams to examine how well a preventive program is being received by implementers and participants. Process evaluation allows school teams to distinguish between components of intervention, see how contextual factors are influencing the intervention, see how subgroups are affected, and help with interpretation of outcomes later on (Oakley et al., 2008). The data used for process evaluation can be either quantitative, qualitative, or both. Common types of process assessments include focus groups, student observations, and interviews with teachers. The goal is to answer questions such as whether or not the program is being followed well (quality of implementation), how are students and staff responding, and are any mediators interfering with progress. When process data is examined while a program is ongoing (before outcome data is collected), there may be less bias in the interpretation and reporting of outcome data. Interpretation of eventual outcomes must be determined directly from data.

Process evaluation focuses on the inputs, activities, and outputs sections of a logic model (CDC, 2008). Input indicators have to do with resources that are invested such as funds, staff, and materials. Activity indicators have to do with events, lessons, media used, etc. Output indicators have to do with products such as the number of students involved, the number of sessions implemented, the actual components that were used, and any alterations or changes in behavior/attitudes/ beliefs. Process evaluation helps assess activities and links these to outcomes. Process evaluations tend to involve observations and opinions. Process evaluations can occur just once, or frequently, as a prevention program is implemented. Program monitoring may involve the amount and types of activities, the number of students involved, the number of training sessions for those implementing the program, and unique events that occurred during the implementation period. The data collected can be used to compare the program to a standard or expectation and help determine whether or not specific populations of students are being reached in order to fine-tune the intervention. Local fidelity of implementation can be compared to the original study, which determined the efficacy of the program, and can help school professionals determine if they are moving in the right direction. Should a program not reach the established goals, the process evaluation data may help the staff identify the specific aspects of the program that may explain the outcomes.

There has been a great deal of work done on implementing SEL programming. The Sustainable Schoolwide Social and Emotional Learning (SEL): Implementation Guide and Toolkit (Devaney, O'Brien, Resnik, Keister, & Weissberg, 2006) provides implementation worksheets and checklists as well as outcomes evaluations and surveys for SEL programming. Some of the evidence-based programs that have been extensively studied have evaluation tools available for use by schools. The PATHS program (Kusché & Greenberg, 1994a, 1994b) offers evaluation kits for preschool/kindergarten and grades 1–6 classrooms. The kits (Kusché & Greenberg, 2005) provide tools for process evaluation and student evaluation. The process evaluation tools include recording the lessons that were actually taught. Teachers, who are implementing the program, evaluate successes and report on their own satisfaction with the curriculum. The student evaluations are completed twice a year in order to monitor each student's or group of students' progress. The authors also provide information on how to interpret results. The EPI Center (http://www.episcenter.psu.edu) includes a monitoring form and observation logs for implementing the PATHS program and a wide variety of outcome tools.

School-Wide Positive Behavior Interventions and Supports is a respected model for prevention of behavior problems in schools. Research data indicates that the elements of this model can be implemented with integrity in school settings (Horner, Sugai, & Anderson, 2010). Implementation of SW-PBIS at Tier 1 results in a reduction in problem behavior, which is often measured by counting office discipline referrals and out-of-school suspensions, as well as measuring improved perceptions of school safety. SW-PBIS implementation was previously measured using the School-Wide Evaluation Tool, an observation and interview assessment, which provided information about implementation (SET; Horner et al., 2004). The weaknesses of this tool included the lengthy time involved in data collection along with an issue with scoring. A newer tool replacing the original is the School-Wide Benchmarks of Quality (BoQ; Kincaid, Childs, & George, 2010). The BoQ scale has 53 items measuring the degree of implementation fidelity of SW-PBIS. This tool is both reliable and valid for assessing universal positive behavior supports. A SW-PBIS coach first completes the BoQ using a scoring guide. Each person on the implementation team then completes a simplified version, and the coach compares the ratings to determine if there are differences. The BoQ takes less time than the original SET tool, it is easier to use, and the scoring is improved allowing for a finer analysis of factors related to successful implementation of the school-wide program. The BoQ has been revised with use (Kincaid et al., 2010). It is used for assessing and monitoring PBS team activities.

To meet challenges of data collection, the U.S. Department of Education Office of Special Education Programs (OSEP) funded the National Center on Student Progress Monitoring to provide technical assistance for progress-monitoring practices that work. When teachers or mental health staff members keep track of what they are doing during implementation of a preventive program, they can make changes and avoid failure. Involving school staff in process evaluation helps professionals involved feel more invested. This is true for giving ongoing feedback as well. In addition to fixing problems, data collection allows school professionals to get a reading on the impact of the program, make safe adaptations, and make the intervention more efficient. Unnecessary components can be dropped after consulting with program developers and making this decision will have been based on data (Simonsen & Sugai, 2007). Process evaluation is particularly important when implementing a preventive program that has not been implemented with a population that was exactly the same as the target school or when a school is implementing a program that was not originally conducted in a school.

Culturally Responsive Evaluation

Evaluations of programs can cause stress when the process is intrusive or when the evaluation points out practices that were tacitly accepted in the past. Safeguards to the rights of disadvantaged groups are critically important (English, 1997). An evaluation will be seriously compromised if representatives of populations of ethnicity and culture in the community are not included on the team (Wehipeihana, Davidson, McKegg, & Shanker, 2010). In addition, data needs to be understood and shared within each groups' cultural worldview. Program evaluations take place in context and cannot be separated from organizational and social structures (Samuels & Ryan, 2011).

The needs of marginalized groups must be taken into account and addressed. School professionals must take care that power imbalances do not affect the evaluation.

Race and low SES can influence mental health worker perceptions and can affect minority students' and families' attitudes (Collett, 2011). These variables have been associated with negative health outcomes. Schools need to provide services that are ethical, competent, and effective for all students. There is data to support the fact that prevention programs can be designed to incorporate culturally appropriate norms of minority students and families and at the same time address the risk factors that several different ethnic minority groups share (Rodney, Johnson, & Srivastava, 2005). Schools also need to learn to develop culturally oriented evaluations that involve all stakeholders as team members, designers, and implementers of the evaluation (Ryan, Chandler, & Samuels, 2007). Each school has a unique culture and students in a school have their own peer culture. Culturally responsible evaluation entails deep knowledge of the students in a school and the local community. Evaluators need to understand what matters to these populations when it comes to implementing prevention programs. Practitioners need to consider whether preventive programs are culturally relevant to students who participate in these programs. When training with teachers who are implementing programs, team-building exercises might be added to implementation training to introduce a discussion of culture and values.

U.S. Department of Health and Human Services (2008, updated 2010) developed a framework that would be integrated into plans for evaluating projects, strategies, practices, and interventions to support ethnic and minority health problems. The framework addresses the identified problems, the key factors, and available data. The framework identifies what evidence-based effort is being proposed to address the problem. The framework involves identification of expected outcomes and impacts and how will these be measured, tracked, evaluated, and reported. Considerations in this effort include increased awareness of health disparities, improved cultural and linguistic competency and diversity of practitioners, measurable racial/ethnic minority-specific objectives, and development of specific performance measures for evaluating programs. The key recommendation is the collection of racial and ethnic data to help health care providers plan, identify disparities, and better meet needs.

Outcomes or Summative Evaluation

Because evidence-based programs can fail, the outcome evaluation is particularly important:

- In environments that are different from those in the original studies (Ives, 2006)
- When used with students who are different from those in the original studies
- Because the program was not implemented with fidelity
- Because implementers or students didn't value it, or it was too much work

Table 13.2 Resources for program evaluation

- The Child Welfare Information Gateway (https://www.childwelfare.gov)
- The Office of Justice Programs (https://www.bja.gov)
- The Collaborative for Academic, Social, and Emotional Learning has resources for "Needs and Outcomes" (http://casel.org)
- The National Resource Center for Community-Based Child Abuse Prevention offers a compendium of 70 tools including a logic model builder, measurement tools by protective factor, and how to construct your own evaluation tool (http://friendsnrc.org)
- The Centers for Disease Control and Prevention (http://www.cdc.gov) has a compendium of assessment tools for measuring bullying participation, for measuring violence-related attitudes, behaviors, and influences (Dahlberg, Toal, Swahn, & Behrens, 2005)
- The Incredible Years website (http://www.incredibleyears.com) has tools for evaluating program effectiveness
- The Lions Quest website (http://www.lions-quest.org) is a rich resource for evaluation tools
- *These are a few examples. There is new material posted frequently online to assist schools and community agencies involved in prevention activities*

According to WHO (2011) output indicators can be short term (more knowledge) or long term (changed student behaviors). Although data collection is important for all programming, a new program with limited efficacy will be in critical need of an outcome evaluation (Meusel et al., 2008).

Outcome evaluation depends on what the school team is trying to demonstrate (Meusel et al., 2008). The goal may be behavior change or if this is too ambitious, influencing risk factors or strengthening protective factors may meet needs. School staff may want to design an outcome evaluation that is complex using experimental or quasi-experimental designs. Or school practitioners may have a goal that involves whether or not a well-researched, evidence-based program will work in their particular school. They may be interested in how they can improve a prevention program already in place. In these cases the outcome evaluation does not have to be so complex. A simple evaluation would comprise a posttest compared to pretest or to a baseline. It is better to collect a few different indicators using different methods for different groups (students, teachers, parents) for the several program objectives to confirm results. This process is called data triangulation. Program outcomes can be used for advocacy, fund-raising, or simply support and the views of stakeholders will be important. It is important to think about what kinds and amounts of data will best fit local goals.

More quantitative data can be more impressive and persuasive, but it is also important not to ask too many questions. A school team needs to determine what is really needed, taking into consideration time and resources (Meusel et al., 2008). Collecting data and analyzing it is a waste of time if the data isn't used, reported, and communicated. A suggestion to increase the ability of an evaluation to measure change may be to administer a survey after the intervention and ask participants to recall their opinions or behavior before the activity. This would be followed with a post-intervention tool. The ability to measure change using this technique may be improved according to the U.S. Department of Health and Human Services (2008, updated 2010, p. 212). Many government and agency websites provide resources for evaluating prevention programs (Table 13.2).

An Example of Outcomes Evaluation

Second Step is a school-based social–emotional curriculum for elementary and middle school children covering three sets of skills. The sets include anger and emotional management, empathy, and impulse control (Cooke et al., 2007). Researchers implemented the *Second Step* program at the third and fourth grades in eight elementary and two middle schools in an ethnically diverse town in Connecticut. They collected data from five of the eight elementary schools. This study serves as an example of a multicomponent evaluation. Data collection involved pre- and post-implementation self-report questionnaires developed from four other surveys. In addition, behavioral observations were collected within 2 weeks of baseline data collection and within 2 weeks post-intervention. Disciplinary records were collected. Teachers completed a year-end survey asking about whether or not they felt that the program helped students, to what degree they implemented the program, whether or not they felt supported by the administration, whether or not they used extension activities, and whether or not they could integrate the program into regular classroom activities. Teacher training satisfaction data was also collected. A subset of parents was also trained, and they in turn self-rated their own skills acquisition.

Results of the study indicated that one in four students participating in the *Second Step* curriculum reported positive changes in behavior (Cooke et al., 2007). Implementation was considered successful as reports indicated a high level of implementation fidelity, although the evaluation tool chosen could not quantify the fidelity of implementation. Observations did not show changes in negative behavior, but prosocial behaviors were observed to increase. Discipline referrals were compared to the previous year data at the same time of year, because discipline referrals typically increase as the school year progresses. The tool did not work as well as anticipated. Program participants reported only a slight decline in discipline referrals. An unintended consequence may have been an increase in the use of referrals as is found in bullying prevention studies, because of increased teacher awareness. The program was well received by students and their teachers and is an example of a multi-tool, multi-respondent outcomes evaluation that could be a model for practitioners.

Prevention in Action Challenge: Five Challenges

1. Mental health screening in schools can be a controversial topic. Explore the pros and cons of mental health screening in schools. Create a chart listing both the pros and cons. Respond to the lists, arguing each point.
2. Identify a social, emotional, or behavioral problem in a school you know well. Conduct a search to determine if there is needs assessment tool online for that particular problem behavior (drug use, suicide, dropping out, etc.). Also determine if there is a logic model available which can be located online for prevention of the behavior.
3. The ClassMaps Survey (Doll, Zucker, & Brehm, 2004) is a 55-item rating scale to be completed by students, to measure student perceptions in eight different areas including a variety of interpersonal relationships. The tool also measures classroom autonomy, classroom engagement, and academic self-efficacy (Doll, Spies, LeClair, Kurien, & Foley, 2010). Data that is collected is shared with students in the classroom. Students participate with the teacher in problem solving (Doll et al., 2013). There are 6 items on the intermediate grades tool measuring anxiety, i.e., "worries" (http://sehd.ucdenver.edu). All six items measure worry in regard to the student's perception of *other student's* behavior. Discuss whether these items would be a good screening tool for students' anxiety symptoms, and why or why not administration of tools of this type would require parental permission to administer.
4. Discuss the difference between a logic model and a theory of change.
5. Find several logic models online or create a logic model for a particular school or school district to address a problem of concern.

Chapter 14
Prevention in Action

One of the most urgent issues for schools presently is preventing youth violence and aggression. In addition to the pain and disruption these behaviors create when an incident occurs, violence and aggression additionally predict later problem behaviors (Hahn et al., 2007). While the most serious forms of violent behaviors rarely take place in schools, less serious behaviors are not uncommon. Behaviors such as fighting, bullying, threatening others, and even bringing weapons to schools can make faculty and students alike feel as if it isn't safe to be in school.

Schools certainly address the possibility of violence. Somewhat extreme reactions such as zero tolerance policies aside, Hahn and the Task Force on Community Preventive Services (2007) report that more than 90 % of schools teach skills and techniques for avoiding violence. Yet, this instruction is quite limited if you count the number of actual hours of instruction per year. Published evaluations of school-based programs that are implemented to address all students in a school vary according to the specific program that a school selects to implement. Some programs are theory-based which is critically important in prevention work. Hahn et al. (2007) offered *Second Step* as an example of a stronger theory-based program. *Second Step* uses social learning theory, which poses that changing the way students experience and think about social problems, along with built-in opportunities for practice, will improve behaviors that lead to conflict and aggression.

Hahn et al. (2007) completed a comprehensive review of universal school-based programs to prevent violence and determined that these programs are effective in general, with the caveat that some are more effective than others. A particular concern of these researchers was that effectiveness of universal programs *decreases* over time in many cases due to decreases in implementation fidelity. Another complication is that many studies of universal prevention programs were primarily conducted as research studies and disseminating these successfully is challenging. Research studies are often more effective than ongoing preventive programs implemented in schools. Hahn and colleagues' meta-analysis demonstrated a 15 % reduction in violent behavior. This was not connected to the level of schooling or to the socioeconomic status of the students (Hahn et al., 2007; Prothrow-Stith, 2007).

G.L. Macklem, *Preventive Mental Health at School: Evidence-Based Services for Students*, 277
DOI 10.1007/978-1-4614-8609-1_14, © Springer Science+Business Media New York 2014

Prothrow-Stith (2007) reminds us that school-based violence prevention programs are a component of public health prevention strategies that have been proposed and advocated for since 1985. We know that programs implemented in schools cannot eliminate aggressive and violent behaviors, and universal programs may not be able to affect the behaviors of the most aggressive children. Universal programs may not be strong enough or implemented long enough to change well-entrenched or more severe behaviors. Yet there is hope that well-implemented preventive programs in schools can mitigate aggressive behavior. Wilson and Lipsey (2007) also conducted a meta-analysis of school-based prevention programs designed to decrease aggressive/disruptive behaviors. They also determined that well-implemented universal preventive efforts are of practical significance. The programs reviewed by Wilson and Lipsey did not overlap substantially with the studies reviewed by Hahn et al. (2007); yet, the findings were more consistent than may have been anticipated. Both reviews concluded that programs that schools select for implementation can be effective and can be effective at all school levels. Wilson and Lipsey argued that violence prevention programs were most effective for elementary level children in high-risk settings. Program duration was particularly important in whether or not programs were effective. Hahn et al. (2007) concluded that universal prevention is important and the opportunity to effect change through universal programming is an opportunity that is "difficult to overestimate" (p. S127).

As important as universal programming may be, schools need to do more than provide universal programming. It is time to move toward comprehensive mental health preventive programming in schools. Some schools are already moving in this direction and can serve as models.

Attempts to Develop More Comprehensive Services in Schools

There have been a number of attempts to develop comprehensive preventive programming supporting school mental health. According to the National Center for Education Research, one approach to comprehensive programming is social and character development programming (Ruby & Doolittle, 2010). An example of this approach is the *Positive Action* program, which includes a K-12 universal curriculum of 140 lessons for each grade. The program additionally addresses school climate using a kit with a principal's manual, interventions for counselors, and both family and community involvement (Flay & Slagel, 2006; Snyder et al., 2010). Also included is a parent manual for use at home. A trial of the *Positive Action* program in Hawaii of 20 schools showed moderate to large effect sizes for reducing absenteeism, retentions, and suspensions along with positive effects on reading and math.

In one of the first published examples of integrating SEL programs, Domitrovich et al. combined the *PAX-Good Behavior Game* (GBG; Embry, Staatemeier, Richardson, Lauger, & Mitich, 2003) and the *Promoting Alternative Thinking Strategies* (*PATHS*) curriculum (Kusché & Greenberg, 1994a, 1994b) to form the *PATHS to PAX Program*. Researchers are working to determine if this combination will be more effective than programs implemented in isolation. The *GBG* is a group-based token economy system. Students are organized into teams and are reinforced for their positive behaviors. The *PAX* version involves groups working together to maintain appropriate behavior. Teaching strategies include behavioral cues, additional practice strategies, and the exchange of written compliments. A large number of studies on the *GBG* have demonstrated its power to reduce disruptive, aggressive, and inattentive behaviors. A pilot study has been completed involving six schools, which implemented the *PATHS to PAX* model with fifth grade students. Students in the study were primarily disadvantaged African American students. Teacher satisfaction and implementation were high. A randomized controlled trial in 27 urban schools is underway. The Excellence in School Mental Health Initiative (ESMHI) project in Baltimore is built on *PATHS to PAX* at the universal level (Domitrovich, Bradshaw, et al., 2010). *Coping Power* (Lochman & Wells, 2002) and the *Incredible Years* programs (Jones, Daley, Hitchings, Bywater, & Eames, 2007; Webster-Stratton, 1994) are used at the selective level (Tier 2). All of these are supported by efforts to improve the school climate and to improve relationships among staff, parents, and students.

Another effort to integrate models combines student and family preventive interventions (Connell, Dishion, Yasui, & Kavanagh, 2007). This group developed the *Adolescent Transitions Program* (ATP: Dishion, Kavanagh, Schneiger, Nelson, & Kaufman, 2002) to integrate a universal intervention, comprised of consultations with parents, and feedback regarding student behaviors using the *Family Check-Up* intervention (FCU: Dishion & Kavanagh, 2003) and family management treatment. The *Triple P–Positive Parenting Program* is a multilevel prevention system for families of children 12 years of age and younger (Prinz, Sanders, Shapiro, Whitaker, & Lutzker, 2009). This program has a universal level, a selected level, and a primary care level. It is designed to prevent antisocial behaviors, to promote competencies, and to improve parenting skills. The *FAST Track Program* is a multilevel program (CPPRG, 2011), which utilizes the *PATHS* curriculum in the elementary school, along with social skills groups, and parent training with positive outcomes.

The most recent discussions around combining programming into a comprehensive model of school mental health involve the integration of several compatible programs such as the combination of Positive Behavioral Interventions and Supports (PBIS) and Social–Emotional Learning (SEL) (http://casel.org/). The Johns Hopkins Center for Prevention and Early Intervention is conducting extensive effectiveness trials of evidence-based prevention and treatment interventions for elementary and middle schools. They are combining interventions and programs in order to develop a continuum of prevention efforts. They are working on developing an integrated prevention model that combines up to four evidence-based and promising, universal preventive interventions: *PATHS*, GBG, *PBIS*, and *Classroom Check-Up* (CCU: Reinke, Lewis-Palmer, & Merrell, 2008).

There are actually a number of possible combinations of programs that can be integrated. Bohanon and Wu (2011) describe a study of 61 schools in the upper Midwest implementing combinations of models to include *PBIS* alone, *PBIS + RtI + SEL*, *PBIS + SEL*, and *SEL* alone. To date they have determined that schools most likely to report using universal screening tools and a decision-making school team tended to be implementing multiple combinations of models. Schools combining PBIS with another three-tiered model and collecting disciplinary data reported zero expulsions. The schools combining *PBIS* and *SEL* components did better when a school-based mental health professional, such as a school psychologist, was part of monthly planning meetings for universal programming. The outcomes data that is collected when schools implemented *PBIS*, *RtI*, and *SEL* was particularly beneficial.

In an effort to demonstrate the concepts of preventive work as it applies to schools, it may be helpful to identify several efforts in which school departments of education in various areas have attempted to better meet the mental health needs of students. One way to approach this is to look first at prevention models or frameworks and then look to see how these efforts have been implemented in specific cases. One model that has been proposed is the Center for Substance Abuse Prevention (CSAP)'s Strategic Prevention Framework (http://www.samhsa.gov). This is not the only model available, but it is based on research in the public health field and also on studies of evidence-based programs. Relevant to mental health concerns and the current interest in SEL is CASEL's 10-Step Implementation Plan (CASEL, 2008). These models are briefly summarized, and an example of a school district application for each is described.

The Strategic Prevention Framework

In the 1990s, the CSAP attempted to help communities build partnerships to deal with problems at the local level. The limitation of this effort was that community coalitions tended to choose programs they "liked" for subjective reasons, rather than selecting effective, evidence-based programs and strategies (http://captus.samhsa. gov). The results were disappointing. Schools and communities easily became discouraged and decided not to attempt prevention work. CSAP needed to refocus school and community partnerships on evidence-based approaches that would fit the local communities seeking grants. The result of CSAP concerns was the development of the Strategic Prevention Framework State Incentive Grant Program. The framework developed for the grants is geared toward broad changes across related systems. Additionally, the framework demands the use of programs and practices supported by evidence.

The first step in the Strategic Prevention Framework (SPF) (see Table 14.1) involves needs assessment in order to determine the problem that the community wants to address (http://captus.samhsa.gov). The needs assessment might involve data already available, epidemiological data, or newly collected data. The data helps the community partnership determine which problem, or problems, to tackle. The data may also help determine the impact of problems on students and may help identify relevant factors and possible solutions impacting problems. This first step includes investigating risk and protective factors that relate to the identified problem.

Table 14.1 Aides for schools planning implementation of prevention programming

The Strategic Prevention Framework (SPF) (SAMHSA)	CASEL's 10-Step Implementation Plan (http://casel.org/wp-content/uploads/Leading-an-SEL-School-EDC1.pdf)
The five steps of the SPF (http://captus.samhsa.gov/access-resources/about-strategic-prevention-framework-spf)	Phase 1: Readiness
Step 1: Assess needs	Step 1: School leaders commit to school-wide SEL
Step 2: Build local capacity	Step 2: School leaders engage stakeholders and form a steering committee
Step 3: Develop a comprehensive strategic plan	Phase 2: Planning
Step 4: Implement evidence-based prevention policies, programs, and practices	Step 3: The school community develops, articulates, and effectively communicates a shared vision of student social, emotional, and academic development
Step 5: Monitor and evaluate program effectiveness	Step 4: The steering committee conducts a needs and resources assessment
The community toolbox (http://ctb.ku.edu/en/tablecontents/sub_section_main_210.aspx)	Step 5: The steering committee develops an action plan
1. Creating and maintaining coalitions and partnerships	Step 6: The school community selects an evidence-based SEL program
2. Assessing community needs and resources	Phase 3: Implementation
3. Analyzing problems and goals	Step 7: Program developers provide initial staff development for those launching the program
4. Developing a framework or model of change	Step 8: Teachers piloting the program launch SEL in select classrooms
5. Developing strategic and action plans	Step 9: All school staff engage in instruction and integrate SEL school-wide
6. Building leadership	Step 10: The school community revisits activities and adjusts for improvement
7. Developing an intervention	Sustainability factors
8. Increasing participation and membership	Ongoing professional development
9. Enhancing cultural competence	Ongoing assessment and evaluation
10. Advocating for change	Infrastructure and school-wide integration
11. Influencing policy development	Family–school community partnerships
12. Evaluating the initiative	Ongoing communication
13. Implementing a social marketing effort	
14. Writing a grant application for funding	
15. Improving organizational management and development	
16. Sustaining the work or initiative	

A school-based resource assessment and a community readiness assessment are involved. Those involved in the preventive effort must be aware of diversity needs and barriers, making sure that all stakeholders are involved in the process.

The second step in the SPF has to do with building "capacity," which must be addressed before a program is implemented. This step addresses educating those who will be affected, obtaining buy-in, identifying potential collaborators, involving partners, and preparing the implementers and the systems that will be involved. Planning is the third SPF step. Planning is related to both implementation and sustainability. A logic model is extremely helpful to build a comprehensive and data-driven plan. Programs and activities must be reviewed to make sure that they have sufficient support. Decisions must be made with full involvement of all stakeholders. Implementation is the fourth SPF step. Specific programs and preventive interventions must be selected that fit the community and be implemented with fidelity. In determining fit, CSAP recommends adding to a program rather than changing core components. Any cultural adaptations that are needed must be accomplished carefully. An action plan and staff training are critical, as administrative and stakeholder support is strengthened through education.

The final SPF step is evaluation. Evaluation that involves all stakeholders is important. Outcomes of both formative (during implementation) and summative evaluation (post-intervention) must be communicated and shared. Specific questions from the original data analysis are addressed, evaluated, and answered. Changes are made as needed. The ultimate goal is to sustain positive outcomes. CSAP strongly recommends that programs that do not work should be discarded.

Technical assistance is available (http://captus.samhsa.gov). Carnevale Associates provides an *Information Brief* with a very helpful chart of the steps, milestones, and products (http://www.drugpreventionlenawee.com).

The Strategic Prevention Framework in Practice

Eddy et al. (2012) used SPF as a model to address underage alcohol use in Eau Claire, Wisconsin. Preventing or delaying alcohol use in school-aged students is a priority at the national level. Eddy and colleagues published their project as a demonstration of use of the SPF tool, given not very much had been published to demonstrate the framework in action as of 2012. The population addressed in the project was 95 % Caucasian, with 2.7 % Asian students (Eddy et al., 2012). Survey data was collected and the results identified students' early onset drinking as the key behavior to address. Both national data and the local community data collected indicated that early use of alcohol was a "serious" problem. Alcohol was readily available to students in the local area. Local capacity was built as school districts collaborated with the Eau Claire County (ECC) Health Department, law enforcement, physicians, and youth organizations to address the problem. Fifteen organizations formed an alliance and hired a project coordinator. Training in SPF was provided to all participants.

The strategic plan included interventions at the school, family, and community levels. Evidence-based programming for students, parents, and the community were selected. The *All Stars* prevention program (Hansen, 1996) was selected for universal implementation (Eddy et al., 2012). OJJDP considers the *All Stars* program "promising." NREPP rates *ALL Stars* 2.2 out of 4.0 (last updated December 3, 2013). The program looked even stronger when "readiness for dissemination" was considered (rated by NREPP, in 2007). NREPP rates programs on a 0–4 scale using criteria. The list of criteria is available online. The program was given an overall rating of 3.4 out of 4.0.

In addition, some schools in ECC were implementing the *LifeSkills* program (Epstein, Botvin, Diaz, Baker, & Botvin, 1997). This program was given an overall rating of 3.9 out of 4.0 by NREPP in regard to quality of the research to support the program, along with a rating 4.0 in regard to dissemination (rated in 2008). However, in this case, the *All Stars* program was considered preferable perhaps because it covered a wider age range than the *LifeSkills* program. Four middle schools were selected for the project because they did not have an evidence-based program in place. Two evidence-based family strengthening programs were chosen for implementation: *Guiding Good Choices* (Spoth, Redmond, Haggerty, & Ward, 1995) and *Staying Connected with Your Teen* (Haggerty, MacKenzie, Skinner, Harachi, & Catalano, 2006; Haggerty, Skinner, MacKenzie, & Catalano, 2007). Finally *Communities Mobilizing for Change on Alcohol* was selected in order to raise community awareness of the problem (Wagenaar et al., 1999). The *All Stars* program was implemented in community settings initially, and then in the four middle schools over several years time (Eddy et al., 2012). Parent sessions were offered free of charge. A policymakers' breakfast meeting was held to take action.

The community was saturated with messages (Eddy et al., 2012). Activities included newsletters, skits, photo-documentation of advertising, information sheets, mailings, compliance checks on businesses and venders, and other actions. This effort provides an interesting example of the use of social norms theory and social marketing. Social norms theory is an effort to correct misperceptions that adolescents may have about a problem behavior (Hahn-Smith & Springer, 2005).

Social marketing is a tool to influence social behaviors. It is used to help individuals choose to adopt healthy and prosocial behavior (Weinreich, 2011). Social marketing is used to make changes at the community level when other organizations in the community are supporting the effort. The idea is to reach the target audience(s) and motivate change by prompting, asking for a commitment to change, and influencing community norms with engaging messages and images. The method of disseminating information in social marketing is broad using media such as posters and messages located where the students or their parents spend their time. The goal is to get the message out in the public by presenting accurate information about peer behaviors and group norms. Perkins, Craig, and Perkins (2011) used social norms to decrease bullying in middle schools, which serves as an example. They noted that schools are peer intensive environments and student norms in schools are rigid. Adolescents tend to overestimate permissiveness of some negative behaviors and overestimate the prevalence of negative behaviors as well. Perkins et al. were able to affect a change in bullying with a poster image campaign conveying accurate messages around peer support for and participation in bullying. They found that overall exposure made a difference.

The final step of the Eddy et al. efforts and of the SPF model in practice was evaluation. Students who received the program in middle school were surveyed when they reached tenth grade and the data was compared to data from the National Survey of Drug Use and Health. Improvement was seen in all measures of alcohol use. The average age of first use of alcohol increased from 12.3 to 13.1 years. Parental disapproval as reported by students increased, and students reported that alcohol was increasingly difficult to obtain. Study limitations included use of self-reports, not all schools participated at each data point, comparative data was not always available, and there were no control groups. However, the study demonstrated that schools could use the strategic prevention framework to implement preventive programming, schools could responsibly collect data, an entire community could be engaged in prevention, and positive results could be obtained that were important for students and families.

CASEL's 10-Step Implementation Plan

The movement to prevent mental health difficulties in students is illustrated by CASEL's efforts to integrate social–emotional programming into schools. Key variables in SEL involve explicit teaching of student skills and the creation of safe learning environments (CASEL, 2008). The 10-step CASEL model stresses the importance of school leadership as the single best predictor of success when implementing prevention programming and helping students. Engagement and active support are needed from school administrators if change is going to take place in schools in the United States.

CASEL's model (see Table 14.1) is described as a model that was developed and influenced by the SPF, along with several other models. It is designed around three phases. Phase 1 (Readiness) involves a commitment and buy-in on the part of school leaders (Step 1). It also involves the commitment of resources and formation of a steering committee made up of all stakeholders (Step 2). Phase 2 (Planning) encompasses four steps: development of a shared vision woven into the school's mission or school improvement plans, a needs and resources assessment, an action plan, and selection of an evidence-based SEL program. The evidence-based program that is selected must be a universal program for all students in all grades creating a shared framework of language and strategies. All students would be explicitly trained using a sequenced, active, and focused skills instruction approach (Durlak, Weissberg et al., 2011). The program must have evidence of effectiveness in regard to outcomes, professional development, and teaching strategies. Phase 3 (Implementation) of the model involves staff development, a pilot of the program in select classrooms, staff training for all, implementation K-12, and adaptations to the plan when determined by data to be necessary. A pilot program allows the planning team to determine if adaptations are needed, or if consultation from the program developer and technical assistance will be needed. Once the pilot has been evaluated and adapted if necessary, the full staff can be trained and the program or curriculum widely implemented. Continual assessment improves chances of success. The broader community needs to appreciate the core components of the chosen SEL curriculum. Planning for sustainability is critical. This includes ongoing professional development, continuation of family/school/community partnerships, ongoing communication, and ongoing assessment/evaluation. This 10-step model in three phases clearly articulates a pathway for schools and districts to follow.

The CASEL 10-Step Model in Practice

Massachusetts has had a long history of innovation in education. This forward-looking effort has somehow been neglected in recent years. The state which passed the first legislation to provide services for children with special needs (PL 94-142), on which IDEA was based, with a capitol city that prides itself on housing some of the greatest hospitals in the United States, by the early 2000s, was not providing for its neediest children. MGL 321 of the Acts of 2008, An Act Regarding Children's Mental Health, came about as a result of Massachusetts' abysmal services for children with severe mental health needs (http://www.nami.org/Content/ContentGroups/CAAC/st02804.pdf). One result of the 2008 legislation was formation of a Behavioral Health and Public Schools Task Force. The Task Force was comprised of multiple agencies in the state including representatives of school psychology training schools.

The Behavioral Health and Public Schools Task Force developed a framework to help schools create safe and supportive learning environments. The framework addressed leadership, professional development, access to resources and services, academic and nonacademic strategies, policies and protocols, and collaboration with families. The Task Force also designed and piloted an assessment tool to measure schools capacity to implement the framework. The tool identifies needs. The final report of the Task Force contained recommendations to implement and require the use of the framework by Massachusetts' schools. This effort resulted in the writing of An Act Relative to Safe and Supportive Schools, which has been introduced into the Massachusetts legislature (http://www.mspa-online.com). This legislation would implement the recommendations of the Task Force, published in 2011. If passed, the bill would require all schools in Massachusetts to develop action plans for creating safe and supportive school environments. It would establish a commission to assist in implementation of action plans and would provide a grant program to fund model schools as well as provide technical assistance.

Massachusetts had passed An Act Relative to Bullying in Schools, Chapter 92 of the Acts of 2010, a short time earlier (http://www.malegislature.gov).

This law defined bullying and cyberbullying, prohibited bullying and retaliation, and required school districts to provide age-appropriate bullying prevention in each grade in the form of a universal evidence-based prevention curriculum. The law also required the publication of "guidelines" for the implementation of social and emotional learning curricula in schools (Section 16). The published guidelines (last updated in August 2011, http://www.doe.mass.edu) specify implementation of a minimum of eight lessons of a prevention program, each year, along with monitoring the implementation of programs. In order to prevent fragmentation, the guidelines recommend aligning SEL programming with other initiatives. The SEL Alliance for Massachusetts (SAM) (http://www.sel4mass.org), an independent group of individuals of several hundred members, has been working hard to introduce SEL into schools in Massachusetts by influencing legislators. The group advocates use of the existing infrastructure of schools to teach students specific emotional control skills, to practice strategies that are taught, and to reduce violence and addiction through education. These pieces of legislation together may influence schools in Massachusetts in significant ways.

Boston, Massachusetts: Needs Assessment

Boston is one of the oldest cities in America. It is a city built around ten distinct neighborhoods. More than 120 schools are spread throughout the city (Amador et al., 2013). Families in Boston speak over 100 different languages. The student population served by the Boston Public Schools is 43 % Hispanic, 33.7 % African American, 12.6 % White, and 8.3 % Asian American. A significant percentage of students are from low-income families (69.5 %) and 44.8 % of students' first language is not English.

In 2000, a Boston citywide coalition known as the Full-Service Schools Roundtable was established (http://www.fssroundtable.org). The mission of the Roundtable involved using integrated school–community partnerships to support the healthy development and academic success of students in Boston schools. This made sense for Boston in that the majority of students come from low-income families and the poverty rate at many schools is 80 % or higher (Weiss & Siddall, 2012). In 2007, the Roundtable focused work on systems-level change with the goal of providing comprehensive, strategic, and intentional services to students (Weiss & Siddall, 2012, p. 7). At the end of the school year 2009–2010, the Roundtable conducted a survey of the Boston Public Schools principals to develop a "services map," which would serve as a baseline for partnership work. Data collected from 93 % of Boston Public Schools covered three main areas to include prevention, social/emotional/behavioral support/mental health, and the availability of school-based health centers.

According to survey results, a majority of Boston schools offered prevention services including emotional and mental health services (Weiss & Siddall, 2012). Partner organizations were major providers of emotional/mental health prevention and mental health services in city schools. However, between 20 and 50 % of high schools did not offer services for alcohol and substance abuse, sexually transmitted diseases, pregnancy, suicide, or tobacco use. Two-thirds of middle schools did not offer prevention services in regard to sexually transmitted diseases or pregnancy. Seventy-five percent of middle schools did not offer tobacco, alcohol, or substance abuse prevention. In regard to mental health services specifically, 98 % of schools provided individual counseling, 62 % provided small group counseling, and 61 % provided consultation to teachers (Weiss & Siddall, 2012). However only half of the schools responding offered services such as crisis intervention, classroom-based prevention work, family therapy, and/or referral.

The report clearly stated that unmet needs remained high (Weiss & Siddall, 2012). Schools could access Medicaid and health insurance to provide some of the needed services. But even when mental health services were available in some schools, the collected data indicated the mental health services were not adequate to meet the need. Boston Public Schools had made an effort to increase services for students by bringing community providers into many of the schools. However, the 17 mental health providers that had been brought into the Boston Public Schools provided inconsistent services, with only a handful of schools reporting a full complement of service providers. Some schools were hard at work patching together a team of service providers to service the most critical problems in their schools, while less critical needs went unmet.

Weiss and Siddall (2012) recommended coordination of partnerships. In order to be effective, partnerships needed "to be properly designed and vetted" and "coordinated effectively" (p. 4). Schools' priority needs had to be addressed. These needed to be aligned with the Boston School District's strategic goals. Critically important, they needed to be *equitably distributed* among all schools and student populations. Few schools in Boston were found *to include a wide spectrum* of mental health services. Survey participants rated the need for mental health services as a "high priority" at most schools.

The Mauricio Gastón Institute for the Latino Community at the University of Massachusetts at Boston (http://www.umb.edu) provided another source of baseline data. Latino students in the Boston Public Schools made up 43.0 % of the enrollment in 2012 and were thereby the largest racial/ethnic group in the school district. The Boston Public Schools enrolled the largest number of Latino students in the state. In 2009, Latino students had the highest rates of poverty, mobility, chronic absence (missing 10 % or more of the school year), and grade retention, of all students in the Boston district. Latino students also evidenced high rates of disability, suspensions, and limited English proficiency compared to other races. This report unfortunately did not include specific information about mental health status and care. However, Alegria, Vallas, and Pumariega (2010) reported national data indicating that public schools in general have serious racial and ethnic disparities in health care. While White children often receive treatment for emotional complications, minority children more often find themselves in the juvenile justice system not having received needed mental health care. There are many risk factors that minorities face compromising their mental health. Coker et al. (2009) suggested sociodemographics might be related to *use* of health care for Hispanic children.

Table 14.2 Massachusetts trainers group

The *Massachusetts Trainers Group* includes faculty from the six school psychology training
programs in the state, a representative of the state school psychology association, and several
head school psychologists:

Andria Amador, CAGS, NCSP, Assistant Director, Behavioral Health Services, Boston, MA

Bob Lichtenstein, Ph.D., NCSP, Massachusetts School of Professional Psychology

Terry Bontrager, Ph.D., and Melissa Pearrow, Ph.D., Department of Counseling & School
Psychology, UMass, Boston

John M. Hintze, Ph.D., University of Massachusetts, Amherst

Laura Rogers, Ed.D., Tufts University

Chieh Li, Psy.D., NCSP, Northeastern University

Diane Tighe Cooke, Ph.D., and Denise Foley, D.Ed., Worcester State University

David Gotthelf, Ph.D., NCSP, Coordinator for Therapeutic Services/Head School
Psychologist, Newton Public Schools

Joan Struzziero, Ph.D., School Psychologist Scituate High School and adjunct faculty at
UMass, Boston, and Northeastern University

Bob Babigian, CAGS, NCSP, School Psychologist, President of the Massachusetts School
Psychologists Association

Planning

Andria Amador, CAGS, NCSP, Acting Director of Student Services and Assistant
Director of Behavioral Health Services for the Boston Public Schools, interpreted
the mental health needs of students and the legislative efforts in the state, as an
"opportunity" to make changes and improve services (Amador et al., 2013).
Together with representatives of the 52 school psychologists and other mental health
professionals who worked in the Boston Public Schools, Amador decided to put
into action the national movement to bring comprehensive mental health services
into schools. She used the needs assessment data as the trigger to create a model that
could not only make a difference for the children of the Boston Public Schools but
would also create a model that others might use in diverse urban school districts.
The Boston situation was unique in that the recent legislation mandating improved
mental health services in the state supported Amador's vision. It should be noted
that it is *unusual for school psychologists to generate and lead comprehensive
school reform* given the pressures and complexities of their work in schools, but this
is indeed what has occurred.

Amador had already developed an impressive professional development program for the Boston school psychologists and mental health professionals. She had
also developed a close alliance with the Massachusetts School Psychologists
Association, serving on the Board of Directors and executive committee (http://
www.mspa-online.com), and had become involved with the leaders of school psychology in Massachusetts, who meet on a regular basis (Table 14.2).

When it comes to systems change, a champion or change agent is needed to provide the coordination and vision to help others see that change can be accomplished
(Gustafson et al., 2003; Stjernberg & Philips, 1993). The change agent creates the

climate for implementing change. Amador's association with the training schools, the fact that the Boston Public Schools already had established some relationships with community mental health agencies; her ardent determination to provide the best in professional development for her staff; and her remarkable political or "people" ability to bring together diverse groups allowed her to generate a working group of partners with various expertise to design a preventive effort using the most current thinking in prevention and in systems theory.

Prothrow-Stith (2007) insists that partnering with experts is critical. The University of Massachusetts at Boston had already developed such a partnership with the Boston Public Schools. Amador and her mental health/behavioral professionals within the Boston Public Schools and consulting partners from the UMass-Boston Counseling and School Psychology training program worked together to create a model of mental health services for the city. Initially, goals were established to include addressing unmet needs of students and addressing inequities in access to services. Responding to state and national initiatives and expanding the role of school psychologists for all domains of practice following the 2012 NASP Practice Model (NASP, 2010) were additional goals.

The UMass-Boston training program for school psychologists provided assistance in several ways. One important contribution was the services of a school psychology doctoral student, Erik Maki, to support Amador 1 day a week. Maki's knowledge of how mental health agencies work was very helpful as partnerships were redesigned. In Boston, as indicated by the Weiss and Siddall report (2012), community mental health services supported the work of school-based mental health staff, but the agencies tended to work independently within the schools. Beyond this, not all schools had established partnerships with community services resulting in inequities. The services also varied, depending on the school and the specific agency servicing that school. Importantly, the services were not overseen by the school district. As vital as these services may have been, progress and outcomes monitoring was nonexistent.

When school mental programs incorporate mental health professionals from the community to work together to help school-aged students, particularly when these professionals are brought into the school, there are many challenges. For example, there are differences in philosophy, confidentiality considerations, training, knowledge bases, professional backgrounds, and work contingencies such as fee-for-service billing (Ball, Anderson-Butcher, Mellin, & Green, 2010; Mellin & Weist, 2011). A study by Kelly et al. (2010) determined that a group of social workers used a clinical casework orientation and their choices in practice had not changed in the past 10 years. These differences make collaboration between schools and agencies challenging.

Mellin and Weist (2011) point out the importance of collaboration in urban communities where there are often limited resources along with extensive problems such as poverty, racism, and violence. The President's New Freedom Commission on Mental Health (2003) (http://govinfo.library.unt.edu) recommended collaboration between community services and schools in order to improve access to mental health services. However, in order to make this work, training and coaching to implement evidence-based practices would be needed. Teachers and other school staff members need to develop trusting relationships with outside-the-school service providers. School staff professionals need to be open to collaboration. There are issues for community providers around frequent staff turnover, lack of understanding of school cultures, lack of understanding of school policies, power differentials, clarity of roles, and responsibilities and procedures. Making this collaboration work was no easy task.

The Boston solution by Amador and her colleagues was to form a school-based mental health collaborative. Guidelines were created to clarify roles and expectations. Standards of practice were developed. A Memorandum of Agreement was negotiated to created equity in access for all students. Mandatory training for all 250 mental health providers involved in the Boston Public Schools was put in place.

The UMass-Boston partnership with the Boston Public Schools was considered mutually beneficial. It provided for advanced training for UMass school psychology graduate students giving them opportunities for practice in all domains of professional practice and a chance to be involved in systems change as participants or leaders. For the public schools, practicing school psychologists in the schools had opportunities to supervise school psychology students expanding their own roles and learning. Building the capacities of the Boston public school students was the ultimate goal of the project.

Logic Model

Melissa Pearrow, Ph.D. of UMass-Boston, helped Amador and the in-house Boston mental health/behavioral professionals generate a logic model. This aspect of comprehensive mental health planning did not initially make sense to some of the staff, as it is a very time consuming process. Pearrow was able to help staff see the value of the process of generating a logic model. This effort helped the committee define the mission, i.e., to ensure that all students have a safe and supportive school where they can be successful.

A logic model and theory of change are necessary for successful systems change as together they lead to evaluation and sustainability and help all stakeholders get on the same page. Jordan (2010) notes that a theory-based logic model is useful for both policy development and evaluation. The logic model sets the path for implementation. In effect the logic model mandates monitoring and sets the standards for determining whether or not the program "works." A logic model also explains the process of getting to outcomes (Harris, 2005). Logic models have been used since the 1980s to help identify essential activities of a program, to set outcomes that are appropriate, and also to explain how activities and outcomes are connected (Gugiu & Rodriguez-Campos, 2007).

Vogel (2012) points out that a logic model is evaluation-informed and gets stakeholders involved in the planning process because they are going to be affected when the model is implemented. The logic model gives stakeholders a visual map.

It focuses the eventual evaluation on the principal elements of the program that will be implemented, and it provides a common understanding of the services and goals that are involved. The logic model points the way to a monitoring system and summarizes the project for possible funding and for decision-makers. Coffman (1999) recommends using a logic model to determine if the project is working as it was intended or whether changes are going to be needed. Savaya and Waysman (2005) point out that the logic model describes the program theory. When the theory is clear, complex programs are more likely to be successful.

The logic model that was designed for the Boston schools was fairly simple and very clear (Amador et al., 2013). It described the actions of students, schools, and the district. It described the short-term outcomes that would be expected as each action was implemented along with the long-term outcomes. For students, the logic model described positive skills instruction, universal screening, and access to targeted supports and services. The short-term outcomes anticipated for students included improved academic performance and increased positive behaviors. The long-term outcomes for students were academic and social competence. For schools, the activities included integrated academic and social–emotional learning along with professional development on evidence-based interventions. The short-term outcomes for schools were expected to involve improved school climate and students' engagement, along with increased skills to address needs. The long-term expectations for schools involved safe and supportive learning environments. For the Boston School District, activities included in the logic model consisted of data management and accountability (Amador et al., 2013). In addition, partnerships with families and community agencies were considered to be critically important. The short-term outcomes expected for the district involved increased capacity to provide services and improved access to, and coordination of, services. The long-term expectations for the district were high-quality and equitable behavioral health services.

The Boston logic model includes essential components of systems change and program success, collaboration with and support for families, aligned district initiative and policies, data-based decision-making, appreciation for diversity, consultation, collaboration, school and district leadership, student-centered, and differentiated instruction.

Theory of Change

Another important aspect of the Boston logic model that was designed was the inclusion of a *theory of change*. A theory of change often starts with a goal (Vogel, 2012). It justifies the use of program components. It forces planners to identify indicators that can be used to measure outcomes. It can be used to design and evaluate a district's efforts when the initiative is very complex with many components. The theory of change is described on the Boston logic model as: "Integrating behavioral health services into schools will create safe and supportive learning environments that optimize academic outcomes for all students" (Amador et al., 2013, see Table 14.3).

Table 14.3 Boston Public Schools comprehensive behavioral health model

BPS Comprehensive Behavioral Health Model
Mission: Ensuring that all students have a safe and supportive school where they can be successful

	If we do this...	We will see this...	To achieve this...
Students	Universal screening and positive skill instruction / Access to targeted supports and services	Improved academic performance / Increased positive behaviors	Academic and social competence
Schools	Integrated academic and socio-emotional learning / Professional development on evidence-based interventions	Improved school climate and student engagement / Increased skills to address students' needs	Safe and supportive learning environments
District	Data management and accountability / Partnerships with families and community agencies	Increased capacity to provide services / Improved access to and coordination of services	High-quality, equitable behavioral health services

Essential Components

Collaboration with and support for families
Aligned district initiatives and policies
Data-based decision making
Appreciation for diversity

Consultation and collaboration
School and district leadership
Student-centered
Differentiated instruction

Guided by Massachusetts Department of Elementary and Secondary Education's Behavioral Health Framework

Theory of Change: Integrating behavioral health services into schools will create safe and supportive learning environments that optimize academic outcomes for all students.

A theory of change is a kind of visual and concrete strategic *picture* of the many interventions that are required to get the results that a school district might be working toward as part of the effort to meet the mental health needs of all students (Harris, 2005). The theory of change summarizes the effort at a strategic level. The logic model, on the other hand, illustrates the work at the program level. Creating a theory of change helps a steering committee ask the difficult questions about why they hope the interventions that they are planning will result in positive changes and positive outcomes. It helps the committee question their assumptions about how the process will unfold and helps all stakeholders to be clear about which outcomes are important to them. The theory of change explains "how" and "why" the model is expected to result in creating safe and supportive learning environments. The logic model visually or graphically describes "what" will be done.

Boston Public Schools Comprehensive Behavioral Health Model

The model that Amador and her school psychologists created is now known as the *Boston Public Schools Comprehensive Behavioral Health Model*. The school psychologists on the committee publicize the model in the image of a lighthouse. The base of the lighthouse describes the foundational practices of mental health service delivery. The lighthouse rises above the foundation in three units corresponding to service delivery at the Tier 1 (universal), Tier 2 (targeted), and Tier 3 (intensive) levels. Above this are units describing highly specialized services. All of these components sit under a dome of "Behavioral Health Services." The three tiers of services include an evidence-based Tier 1 prosocial skills curriculum implemented for all students, use of universal screening to identify students in need of additional supports at Tier 2, data collection to monitor the impact of interventions, and partnerships with community mental health agencies properly trained. In this way agency staff and in-school mental health professional would "speak the same language," collect the same data, and monitor outcomes in the same way.

Community Partnerships

The community mental health partnerships providing services to the schools comprised some 25 different mental health agencies. Many Boston schools had mental health agency partners but the others did not. Some services involved fee-for-services and other services were comprehensive in that service providers attended team meetings within the schools. Financial stability was needed for the agency partners, as was a need to make sure that best practices were being implemented. Another important partnership with the Boston Public Schools was an association with Boston Children's Hospital (http://www.childrenshospital.org). Boston Children's Hospital provided some of the mental health service providers. This vital partnership proliferated into a 7-year commitment to support the partnership. The logic model allowed all who partnered with the Boston Public Schools to quickly understand the process and activities involved. The goals and details of the project were made very clear through the logic model and were embraced by all partners.

Staff and Stakeholder Buy-in

The in-house team of school psychologists, six social workers, and behavioral specialists worked together to gain support from district administrators and all school-level staff members within the Boston Public Schools. Interviews were held with key stakeholders including parents, teachers, principals, clinicians, and judges in the community. Work began by gaining buy-in from the mental health providers in-house. Change leaders needed to be creative in supporting the staff. Staff who had been quite comfortable in their roles needed to change their thinking from reactive to proactive and needed to embrace preventive approaches. To gain administrative buy-in, change agents started hosting breakfasts with principals. The breakfasts included friendly sharing of efforts to provide mental health support for students which administrators and others found engaging. Scheduling assistance was offered to administrators. Administrators teamed with the mental health professionals. A mascot contest was held. As the work became more public, Amador was invited to speak at Boston City Council meetings, which was a *highly unusual* event. School psychologists are not typically invited to speak at city council meetings. The implementation committee created a manual for training mental health staff.

Universal Screening

Once there was sufficient buy-in, a process for piloting screening tools to be used at the universal level was designed. A series of universal screening tools were selected and tested in six demographically diverse schools. A procedure was established to rate the tools using criteria. The screening team was comprised of district level administration, school psychologists and interns, and two consultants.

Screening involves brief tools, which are used to identify behaviors that predict difficulty in the future and are part of data-based decision-making (Henderson & Strain, 2009). Although the use of brief tools might be questioned, studies indicate that abbreviated rating scales used for progress monitoring result in substantially the same data as longer tools (Volpe & Gadow, 2010). Screening students to determine needs may have the added advantage of decreasing the disproportionality that is seen in the identification of students with negative and inappropriate behaviors. Screening tools help obtaining information about risk and protective factors. When schools consider the use of screening tools in the behavioral/social/emotional areas, consultation with mental health professionals such as school psychologists is important. Although most universal screening tools are academic screeners, universal screening must extend beyond academics (Cook, Volpe, & Livanis, 2010). Screening must be linked to problem-solving efforts, moderating universal screening outcomes, accurately classifying students, and must be implemented easily. Screening tools must be technically adequate. Data collected in schools should be used as part of a problem-solving approach to improve student outcomes (Burns, Scholin, & Zaslofsky, 2011). Accountability is demanded in schools today (Woods-Groves & Hendrickson, 2012).

Screening tools need to be short, not too expensive, and structured so that data can be aggregated and analyzed. An additional consideration involves data display in that graphic representations of data are very helpful along with narrative and quantitative representations. Although there are rating scales available that measure emotional and behavioral issues, they tend to be too long to use as screening tools (Volpe & Gadow, 2010). Another important aspect to screening and monitoring tools is that they are sensitive to small or moderately sized effects of the intervention (Meier, McDougal, & Bardos, 2008). Tools that are created with change-sensitive items result in larger effect sizes (Meier, 1997). Tools created with this in mind can demonstrate change as a result of a behavioral intervention and can also examine relative change across groups. Meir (2004) points out that traditional measures, such as the commonly used commercial rating scales, may be insensitive to intervention effects. Meir proposed a process of "Intervention Item Selection Rules"

(IISRs) when developing outcome measures, which would display larger effect sizes along with a reliability estimate that would be acceptable. The Behavior Intervention Monitoring Assessment System™ (BIMAS) is the only commercially available measure that was created based on this model and contains items with demonstrated change sensitivity.

The Boston team selected the BIMAS, by McDougal, Bardos, and Meier (2011), as its universal screening and monitoring tool. The BIMAS is a behavioral progress monitoring system designed to assess changes when a behavioral intervention is implemented. It is appropriate for students aged 5–18 years. It is a multi-informant tool with versions for parents, teachers, clinicians, and a self-report for older students. The standard version has 34 items, which were developed specifically to be sensitive to change. The BIMAS can be used for screening, measuring three sub-scales (conduct, negative affect, and cognitive/attention) and two adaptive scales (social and academic functioning). Each item on the "Standard" scale can be selected for individual behavioral monitoring for each version to make up a "Flex" tool for the purpose of monitoring individual behavior. Data is reported in the form of T-scores (mean of 50, standard deviation of 10). Cutoff points have been developed and are interpreted as "no concern," "mild concern," and "concern." The reliability of the tool is considered in the "good" range. The BIMAS can discriminate between clinical and nonclinical cases. Scores show good sensitivity to change and in the expected direction. All schools in a district could schedule the BIMAS Standard universal assessment and upload the data to a web-based data management and reporting system. Students could then be followed from year to year. Demographics would be linked to students. Graphs could be generated and made available at the individual and group level for screening. Once the system is in place, progress reports can be compared for a given student or a group of students. Group averages could be compared between classes, grades, and schools.

The BIMAS technical product information, provided by MHS (http://www.mhs.com), indicates that the BIMAS can be used for universal behavioral screening, progress monitoring, outcome assessment, and program evaluation. This fits both prevention best practices and RtI models used in many schools (McDougal, Bardos, & Meier, 2007). The fact that the BIMAS system can provide change data over short periods made it very appealing to the Boston school psychologists. The fact that both positive and negative effects of a program could be obtained is important as well. The BIMAS system can evaluate the effectiveness of treatment services in large population implementation of programs makes it important when a school district is interested in future funding and in establishing partnerships with agencies in the community.

Universal Evidence-Based SEL Curriculum

Key stakeholder interviews took place through the process of generating and implementing the model. A need for student social skills and self-regulation training was identified and was given precedence. This is not to say that there were no other concerns such as family stress, trauma, bullying, depression, and acculturation (in this order) according to Amador et al. (2013). A decision to implement a universal social–emotional curriculum was made.

SEL programs in general teach, model, and practice skills in many settings so that students will develop competency. Additionally, they establish caring environments to improve students' connections and engagement in school (Lazarus & Sulkowski, 2011). When implementing SEL programming, the dosage is important; a minimum of 30 min per week in skills instruction embedded in the general curricula, as part of comprehensive mental health programming, is needed according to experts (Elias, 2012). Boston chose *Second Step*, a very popular violence prevention curriculum that is used in a large number of schools across the United States. This curriculum covers grade levels kindergarten through middle school (grade 9), in order to deter aggression and promote social competence (Frey, Hirschstein, & Guzzo, 2000). Cooke et al. (2007) pointed out the challenge of demonstrating the effectiveness of prevention programs in that over a school year, students typically increase in aggressive behaviors in school so the best that outcomes data can often show, is that the aggressive behaviors of students receiving an intervention do not increase over the school year, and/or the outcome data may show that students increase their prosocial behaviors. Students who self-rate their own behaviors after receiving a preventive intervention may report increases in negative behaviors due to increased awareness. This made the choice to utilize the BIMAS system a wise decision.

A preventive curriculum needs to be evaluated early in the process of adoption so that implementation fidelity can be improved or the curriculum can be adapted when necessary. Fortunately, tools including worksheets, surveys, and checklists for implementing the *Second Step* curriculum are available for elementary and middle school levels. Cooke et al. (2007) point out that the *Second Step* curriculum is designed to first increase prosocial behavior and later to decrease negative behaviors. The *Second Step* curriculum was re-reviewed in February of 2012 by OJJDP and is listed on its Model Programs Guide (http://www.ojjdp.gov) as an "effective" program. The Promising Practices Network on Children, Families, and Communities (http://www.promisingpractices.net) last reviewed the *Second Step* program in August 2006 and gave it a "promising" rating. NREPP updated their review of the Second Step program in June, 2012. Research support was rated 2.4 on a scale of 0.0–4.0. On a "readiness for dissemination" measure including implementation materials, training, and support resources and quality assurance procedures, the overall rating was 3.8 out of 4.0.

Implementation by Boston Public Schools

Once the best-fitting screening tool was selected and evaluated, the universal curriculum was agreed upon, and all mental health providers were trained, cohort 1 for the school year 2012–2013 was established. Ten schools were chosen to participate representing the elementary, middle, and high school levels.

The first cohort of schools was selected to represent a wide range of grade levels and areas of the city. Schools were selected that had services provided by Boston Children's Hospital. Schools were selected that were open to the project because early success was critical. Schools needed to be willing to use evidence-based interventions at all three tiers of mental health service.

Implementation monitoring is supported by professional development activities in the Boston Public Schools. School psychologists participate in biweekly Professional Learning Community (PLC) activities. School principals are involved in bimonthly meetings as well to share their successes and challenges. The BIMAS will be completed by all students three times a year and as needed for students at Tiers 2 and 3. The monitoring at Tiers 2 and 3 will be based on individual student plans created by the behavior team. The Boston schools use a variety of Tier 2 interventions including anger management, transition support programs for students entering high school, and interventions for anxiety, depression, hyperactivity and inattention. Teachers provide some Tier 2 and 3 interventions such as Check in/ Check out. Additional data collection involves attendance records, assignment completion, and behavioral health and student health referrals. One school tracks office discipline referrals (ORDs) and matches this data with BIMAS data. Families have a special section on the Boston schools website. There is a Parent Resource Center and each school is involved in parent outreach. Those involved with the project will disseminate data that is collected through published papers, posters, and presentations at various conferences.

Current State of the Project

The pilot is well underway. The in-house group with its partners is seeking funding alternatives to support financial sustainability for the community mental health providers working in and partnering with the Boston Public Schools. A "steering committee" continues to work on best practices for their service delivery model. Data is being collected. The school district is providing oversight and management of the partnerships that have been established. Working continues to maximize the use of community services. Additionally, work is ongoing to determine the data sets needed to examine outcomes specified in the logic model as well as school, district, and community agency data. The model is not as yet fully implemented and outcomes evaluation data has not as yet been collected. An additional 12 schools will implement the model in 2013–2014 and additional schools will be brought into the model over a 5- to 8-year period of time. At this point, eight of the ten steps in CASEL's 10-Step Implementation Plan have been completed. The work to date is certainly impressive and is a fine example of developing a comprehensive mental health services plan and getting started. There is no doubt that this step was enormously challenging.

Boston's Comprehensive Behavioral Health Model (CBHM) is valuable in several respects even at this early stage of the process. The wider Boston community has recognized the value and importance of the project. The model represents a bottoms-up approach in that in-house school psychologists designed the model. Amador and her team of behavioral, mental health professionals are demonstrating that practitioners within schools can address mental health concerns of students at the systems level, an effort advocated by the National Association of School Psychologists Practice Model. The CBHM also demonstrates the critical nature of collaboration with community partners. It demonstrates that urban school districts in areas of high need can take steps to address disparities and significant needs for services. It demonstrates a scientific approach to preventive efforts in schools, and it demonstrates many of the concepts of a preventive science approach to solving problems. It can serve as inspiration and as a model for smaller districts as well. Systems-level change to prevent mental health problems of students and to meet the mental health needs of students at risk can be accomplished.

Prevention in Action Challenge: Complex Case Study

This case describes a very disturbing situation of a city school system in which there are overwhelming problems. The schools are dealing with poverty, homelessness, and transiency. The student population is 78 % of Hispanic, of Puerto Rican heritage. Almost half of the school-age children in the city are "food insecure" (they don't know where their next meal is coming from). Currently, more than half of children in the city schools "need improvement" or are failing in English Language Arts, and three-quarters of students "need improvement" or are failing in mathematics. The levels of special education and ELL staffing, and the training of general education teachers, are not sufficient to address the low proficiency rates of special education and LEP students. Furthermore, only a little more than half of students graduate from high school over a 4-year period in this school system. A key goal of the superintendent is to avoid district takeover by the state.

This city has the highest teen pregnancy and the highest teenage birth rate in the state. The school administration is working hard to try to change community norms with respect to the use of alcohol, tobacco, and other drugs. The crime rate is high. The poverty rate is 31 % of families, particularly high among its population of teenaged Latina mothers and their young children. Whereas in general the population rate is declining, poor families are increasing as the state sends families to this city with its large number of homeless shelters. The school system has the second-highest dropout rate in the state. Troubling gaps exist between students of different socioeconomic backgrounds. 11.2 % of Latino students dropped out in the 2010–2011 school year, as compared to 5.1 % of White students. More than 1,000 students were suspended during the 2010–2011 school year. During the 2009–2010 school year the school system registered more than 8,000 classroom incidents in grades

(continued)

(continued)

1–12, including fights and other physical attacks, sexual harassment, thefts, and threats. This resulted in 2,678 suspensions and 8,333 classroom days lost. The high school has listed 20 grounds for suspension in its handbook and eight grounds for long-term suspension and expulsion.

What approach would you suggest to address this critical situation?

How would you determine which needs to address?

Which of the many problems would you target first?

How would you get resources into the schools?

Develop a plan using the impressive work of the two school districts described in this chapter.

References

Aatston, P. W., Kowalski, R., & Limber, S. (2007). Students' perspectives on cyberbullying. *Journal of Adolescent Health, 41*(6), S59–S60. doi:10.1016/jadohealth.2007.09.003.

Adams, P. (2005). Social work practice with African American adolescent girls: A process-person-context model. In E. P. Congress & M. L. Gonzales (Eds.), *Multicultural perspectives in working with families* (2nd ed., pp. 93–110). New York: Springer.

Adams, P. (2010). Understanding the different realities, experience, and use of self-esteem between Black and White adolescent girls. *Journal of Black Psychology, 36*(3), 255–276. doi:10.1177/0095798410361454.

Adelman, H. S. (1996). Restructuring education support services and integrating community resources: Beyond the full service school model. *School Psychology Review, 25*(4), 431–445. Retrieved from http://www.nasponline.org

Adelman, H. S., & Taylor, L. (1999). Mental health in schools and system restructuring. *Clinical Psychology Review, 19*(2), 137–163. doi:10.1016/S0272-7358(98)00071-3.

Adelman, H. S., & Taylor, L. (2003). Rethinking school psychology (commentary on public health framework series). *Journal of School Psychology, 41*(1), 83–90. doi:10.1016/S0022-4405(02)00147-4.

Adelman, H. S., & Taylor, L. (2006). Mental health in schools and public health. *Public Health Reports, 121*(3), 294–298. Retrieved from http://www.publichealthreports.org

Adelman, H. S., & Taylor, L. (2008a). Best practices in the use of resource teams to enhance learning supports. In A. Thomas & A. J. Grimes (Eds.), *Best practices in school psychology V* (Vol. 5, pp. 1689–1708). Bethesda, MD: National Association of School Psychologists.

Adelman, H. S., & Taylor, L. (2008b). School-wide approaches to addressing barriers to learning and teaching. In B. Doll & J. A. Cummings (Eds.), *Transforming school mental health services* (pp. 277–306). Thousand Oaks, CA: Corwin Press.

Agboola, A. A., & Salawu, R. O. (2011). Managing deviant behavior and resistance to change. *International Journal of Business and Management, 6*(1), 235–242. Retrieved from ww.ccsenet.org

Aina, Y., & Susman, J. L. (2006). Understanding comorbidity with depression and anxiety disorders. *The Journal of the American Osteopathic Association, 106*(6), 59–514. Retrieved from http://www.jaoa.org/

Ainley, M. (2012). Students' interest and student engagement: Conceptual, operational, and empirical clarity. In S. L. Christenson, A. L. Reschly, & C. Wylie (Eds.), *Handbook of research on student engagement* (pp. 283–302). New York: Springer.

Ajzen, I. (1991). The theory of planned behavior. *Organizational Behavior and Human Decision Processes, 50*, 179–211. doi:10.1016/0749-5978(91)90020-T.

Albertine, J., Oldehinkel, A. J., Rosmalen, J. G., Veenstra, R., Dijkstra, J. K., & Ormel, J. (2007). Being admired or being liked: Classroom social status and depressive problems in early adolescent girls and boys. *Journal of Abnormal Child Psychology, 35*(3), 417–427. doi:10.1007/s10802-007-9100-0.

Albright, M. I., Weissberg, R. P., & Dusenbury, L. A. (2011). *School-family partnership strategies to enhance children's social, emotional, and academic growth*. Newton, MA: National Center for Mental Health Promotion and Youth Violence Prevention, Education Development Center.

Alegria, M., Vallas, M., & Pumariega, A. J. (2010). Racial and ethnic disparities in pediatric mental health. *Child and Adolescent Psychiatric Clinics of North America, 19*(4), 7590–7774. doi:10.1016/j.chc.2010.07.001.

Amador, A., Roop, N., Cohen, M., Pearrow, M., Maki, E., & Codding, R. (2013). *Comprehensive behavioral health model*. Mini-skills presentation. Seattle, WA: NASP Annual Convention.

American Psychological Association Task Force on Evidence-Based Practice for Children and Adolescents. (2008). *Disseminating evidence-based practice for children and adolescents: A systems approach to enhancing care*. Washington, DC: American Psychological Association.

Anderson, A. R., Christenson, S. L., & Lehr, C. A. (2004). School completion and student engagement: Information and strategies for educators. In A. S. Canter, L. Z. Paige, M. D. Roth, I. Romero, & S. A. Carroll (Eds.), *Helping children at home and school II: Handouts for families and educators* (pp. 65–68). Bethesda, MD: National Association of School Psychologists.

Anderson, L. A., Gwaltney, M. K., Sundra, D. L., Brownson, R. C., Kane, M., Cross, A. W., et al. (2006). Using concept mapping to develop a logic model for the prevention research centers program. *Preventing Chronic Disease, 3*(1). Retrieved from http://www.cdc.gov

Anderson, E. R., & Mayes, L. C. (2010). Race/ethnicity and internalizing disorders in youth: A review. *Clinical Psychology Review, 30*(3), 338–348. doi:10.1016/j.cpr.2009.12.008.

Andrews, D., & Buettner, C. (2012 update). *Evaluating supporting evidence*. Tool #33. Columbus, OH: Center for Learning Excellence. Retrieved from http://cle.osu.edu

Anfara, V. A. (2008). What research says: Varieties of parent involvement in schooling. *Middle School Journal, 39*(3), 58–64. Retrieved from http://www.amle.org

Anglin, T., Halper-Felsher, B., Kaplan, D. W., & Newcomer, S. (2011). *The science of adolescent risk-taking: Workshop report*. Washington, DC: National Academies Press. Retrieved from http://www.ncbi.nlm.nih.gov/books/NBK53417/

Appleton, J. J., Christenson, S. L., & Furlong, M. J. (2008). Student engagement with school: Critical conceptual and methodological issues of the construct. *Psychology in the Schools, 45*(5), 369–386. doi:10.1002/pits.20303.

Archambault, I., Janosz, M., Fallu, J., & Pagani, L. S. (2009). Student engagement and its relationship with early high school dropout. *Journal of Adolescence, 32*(3), 651–670. doi:10.1016/j.adolescence.2008.06.007.

Archambault, I., Janosz, M., Morizot, J., & Pagani, L. (2009). Adolescent behavioral, affective, and cognitive engagement in school: Relationship to dropout. *Journal of School Health, 79*(9), 408–415. doi:10.1111/j.1746-1561.2009.00428.x.

Arseneault, L., Walsh, E., Trzesniewski, K., Newcombe, R., Caspi, A., & Moffitt, T. E. (2006). Bullying victimization uniquely contributes to adjustment problems in young children: A nationally representative cohort study. *Pediatrics, 118*(1), 130–138. doi:10.1542/peds.2005-2388.

Ashdown, D. M., & Bernard, M. E. (2012). Can explicit instruction in social and emotional learning skills benefit the social-emotional development, well-being, and academic achievement of young children? *Early Childhood Education Journal, 39*, 397–405. doi:10.1007/s10643-0110-0481-x.

Asnaani, A., Richey, J. A., Dimaite, R., Hinton, D., & Hofmann, S. G. (2010). A cross-ethnic comparison of lifetime prevalence rates of anxiety disorders. *Journal of Nervous and Mental Disorders, 198*(8), 551–555. doi:10.1097/NMD.0b013e3181ea169f.

Atkins, M. C., Hoagwood, K. E., & Seidman, E. (2010). Toward the integration of education and mental health in schools. *Administration and Policy in Mental Health and Mental Health Services Research, 37*(1–2), 40–47. doi:10.1007/s10488-010-0299-7.

August, G. J., Realmuto, G. M., Hektner, J. M., & Bloomquist, M. L. (2001). An integrated components preventive intervention for aggressive elementary school children: The Early Risers program. *Journal of Consulting and Clinical Psychology, 69*(4), 614–626. doi:10.1037//0022-006X.69.4.614.

Austin, M. J., & Claassen, J. (2008). Impact of organizational change on organizational culture: Implications for introducing evidence-based practice. *Journal of Evidence-Based Social Work, 5*(1–2), 321–359. doi:10.1300/J394v05n01_12.

Avey, J., Wernsing, T. S., & Luthans, F. (2008). Can positive employees help positive organizational change? Impact of psychological capital and emotions on relevant attitudes and behaviors. *The Journal of Applied Behavioral Science, 44*(1), 48–70. doi:10.1177/0021886307311470.

Aveyard, P., Markham, W. A., Lancashire, E., Bullock, A., Macarthur, C., Cheng, K. K., et al. (2004). The influence of school culture on smoking pupils. *Social Science & Medicine, 58*(9), 1767–1780. doi:10.1016/S0277-9536(03)00396-4.

Axelson, D. A., & Birmaher, B. (2001). Relation between anxiety and depressive disorders in childhood and adolescence. *Depression and Anxiety, 14*(2), 67–78. doi:10.1002/da.1048.

Project AWARE: Advancing Wellness and Resilience in Education. (2013). *Now is the time: the President's plan to protect our children and our communities by reducing gun violence.* Washington, D.C.: The White House. Retrieved from (http://www.whitehouse.gov/sites/default/files/docs/wh_now_is_the_time_full.pdf)

Baban, A. & Craciun, C. (2007). Changing health-risk behaviors: A review of theory and evidence-based interventions in health psychology. *Journal of Cognitive and Behavioral Psychotherapies, 7*(1), 45–67. Retrieved from cbp.psychotherapy.ro.

Backer, T. E. (2002). *Finding the balance: Program fidelity and adaptation in substance abuse prevention: A state-of-the-art review.* Rockville, MD: Substance Abuse and Mental Health Services Administration (SAMHSA), Center for Substance Abuse Prevention (CSAP).

Bacon, T. P. (2001). Impact on high school students' behaviors and protective factors: A pilot study of the Too Good for Drugs and Violence Prevention program. *Florida Educational Research Council, Inc. Research Bulletin, 32*(3 & 4), 1–40. Retrieved from http://www.mendezfoundation.org

Baker, T. (2002). *Finding the balance: Program fidelity and adaptation in substance abuse prevention. A state-of-the-art review and executive summary.* Atlanta, GA: U.S. Department of Health and Human Services.

Baker, J. A., Kamphaus, R. W., Horne, A. M., & Winsor, A. P. (2006). Evidence for population-based perspective on children's behavioral adjustment and needs for service delivery in schools. *School Psychology Review, 35*(1), 31–46. Retrieved from http://www.nasponline.org

Baker, C. N., Kupersmidt, J. B., Voegler-Lee, M. E., Arnold, D. H., & Willoughby, M. T. (2010). Predicting teacher participation in a classroom-based, integrated preventive intervention for preschoolers. *Early Child Research Quarterly, 25*(3), 270–283. doi:10.1016/j.ecresq.2009.09.005.

Ball, A., Anderson-Butcher, D., Mellin, E. A., & Green, J. H. (2010). A cross-walk of professional competencies involved in expanded school mental health: An exploratory study. *School Mental Health, 2,* 114–115. doi:10.1007/s12310-010-9039-0.

Bandura, A. (1977). *Social learning theory.* Englewood Cliffs, NJ: Prentice-Hall.

Bandura, A. (1986). *Social foundations of thought and action: A social cognitive theory.* Englewood Cliffs, NJ: Prentice-Hall.

Bandura, A. (1988). Organizational application of social cognitive theory. *Australian Journal of Management, 13*(2), 275–302. Retrieved from http://www.asb.unsw.edu.au

Bandy, T., & Moore, K. A. (2011). What works for Latino/Hispanic children and adolescents: Lessons from experimental evaluations of programs and interventions. *ChildTrends Fact Sheet.* Retrieved from http://www.childtrends.org

Barnes, G. E., Mitic, W., Leadbeater, B., & Dhami, M. K. (2009). Risk and protective factors for adolescent substance use and mental health symptoms. *Canadian Journal of Community Mental Health, 28*(1), 1–15. Retrieved from http://www.cjcmh.com/

Barnett, W. S. (2008). *Preschool education and its lasting effects: Research and policy implications.* New Brunswick, NJ: National Institute for Early Education Research.

Barnett, W. S. (2010). Universal and targeted approaches to preschool education in the United States. *International Journal of Child Care and Education Policy, 4*(1), 1–12. Retrieved from http://childcarecanada.org

Barnett, W. S., & Frede, E. (2010). The promise of preschool: Why we need early education for all. *American Educator, 34*(1), 21–40. Retrieved from http://www.aft.org

Barnett, W. S., Jung, K., Yarosz, D. J., Thomas, J., Hornbeck, A., Stechuk, R., et al. (2008). Educational effects of the Tools of the Mind curriculum: A randomized trial. *Early Childhood Research Quarterly, 23*(3), 299–313. doi:10.1016/j.ecresq.2008.03.001.

Barrera, M., & Castro, F. G. (2006). A heuristic framework for the cultural adaptation of interventions. *Clinical Psychology: Science and Practice, 13*(4), 311–316. doi:10.1111/j.1468-2850.2006.00043.x.

Barrett, S. B., Bradshaw, C. P., & Lewis-Palmer, T. (2008). Maryland statewide PBIS initiative: Systems, evaluation, and next steps. *Journal of Positive Behavior Interventions, 10*(2), 105–114. doi:10.1177/1098300707312541.

Barrett, P. M., Lock, S., & Farrell, L. (2005). Developmental differences in universal preventive intervention for child anxiety. *Clinical Child Psychology and Psychiatry, 10*(4), 539–555. doi:10.1177/1359104505056317.

Barrett, P. M., Lowry-Webster, H., & Holmes, J. (1999). *Friends for children group leader manual* (2nd ed.). Brisbane, QLD: Australian Academic Press.

Barrett, P. M., & Pahl, K. M. (2006). School-based intervention: Examining a *universal approach to anxiety management. Australian Journal of Guidance and Counselling, 16*(1), 55–75. doi:10.1375/ajgc.16.1.55.

Bartolo, P. A. (2010). Why school psychology for diversity? *School Psychology International, 31*(6), 567–580. doi:10.1177/0143034310386532.

Bartolo, P. A., Borg, M., Cefai, C., & Martinelli, V. (2010). School psychology for diversity: Editorial. *School Psychology International, 3*, 563–566. doi:10.1177/0143034310386531.

Battistich, V., Schaps, E., Watson, M., Solomon, D., & Lewis, C. (2000). Effects of the child development project on students' drug use and other problem behaviors. *The Journal of Primary Prevention, 21*(1), 75–99. doi:10.1023/A:1007057414994.

Bauman, S. (2008). The association between gender, age, and acculturation, and depression and overt and relational victimization among Mexican American elementary students. *The Journal of Early Adolescence, 28*(4), 528–554. doi:10.1177/0272431608317609.

Bauman, S., Toomey, R. B., & Walker, J. L. (2013). Associations among bullying, cyberbullying, and suicide in high school students. *Journal of Adolescence, 36*(2), 341–350. doi:10.1016/j.adolescence.2012.12.001.

Baydala, L. T., Sewlal, B., Rasmussen, C., Alexis, K., Fletcher, F., Letendre, L., et al. (2009). A culturally adapted drug and alcohol abuse prevention program for aboriginal children and youth. *Progress in Community Health Partnerships, 3*(1), 37–46. doi:10.1353/cpr.0.0054.

Bayer, J. K., Hiscock, H., Morton-Allen, E., Ukoumunne, O. C., & Wake, M. (2007). Prevention of mental health problems: Rationale for a universal approach. *Archives of Disease in Childhood, 92*(1), 34–38. doi:10.1136/adc.2006.100776.

Bean, S., & Rolleri, L. A. (2005). *Parent–child connectedness: Voices of African-American and Latino parents and teens.* Santa Cruz, CA: ETR Associates. Retrieved from http://recapp.etr.org

Bear, G. G., Gaskins, C., Blank, J., & Chen, F. F. (2011). Delaware school climate survey-student: Its factor structure, concurrent validity, and reliability. *Journal of School Psychology, 49*(2), 157–174. doi:10.1016/j.jsp.2011.01.001.

Beauchaine, T. P., Webster-Stratton, C., & Reid, M. J. (2005). Mediators, moderators, and predictors of 1-year outcomes among children treated for early-onset conduct problems: A latent growth curve analysis. *Journal of Consulting and Clinical Psychology, 73*(3), 371–388. doi:10.1037/0022-006X.73.3.371.

Beckman, H., Hawley, S., & Bishop, T. (2006). Application of theory-based health behavior change techniques to the prevention of obesity in children. *Journal of Pediatric Nursing, 21*(4), 266–275. doi:10.1016/j.pedn.2006.02.012.

Beesdo, K., Fehm, L., Low, N. C., Gloster, A. T., & Wittchen, H. U. (2008). The role of parental psychopathology and family environment for social phobia in the first three decades of life. *Depression and Anxiety, 26*(2), 363–370. doi:10.1002/da. 20527.

Beets, M. W., Flay, B. R., Vuchinich, S., Acock, A. C., Li, K., & Allred, C. (2008). School climate and teachers' beliefs and attitudes associated with implementation of the Positive Action Program: A diffusion of innovations model. *Prevention Science, 9*(4), 264–275. doi:10.1007/s11121-008-0100-2.

Behnke, A. O., Plunkett, S. W., Sands, T., & Bámaca-Colbert, M. Y. (2011). The relationship between Latino adolescents' perceptions of discrimination, neighborhood risk, and parenting on self-esteem and depressive symptoms. *Journal of Cross-Cultural Psychology, 42*(7), 1179–1197. doi:10.1177/0022022110383424.

Behrens, D., Learn, J. G., & Price, O. A. (2013). *Improving access to children's mental health care: Lessons from a study of eleven states.* Washington, DC: Center for Health and Health Care in Schools.

Beidas, R. S., Benjamin, C. L., Puleo, C. M., Edmunds, J. M., & Kendall, P. C. (2010). Flexible applications of the Coping Cat program for anxious youth. *Cognitive and Behavioral Practice, 17*(2), 142–153. doi:10.1016/j.cbpra.2009.11.002.

Belgrave, F. Z. (2002). Relational theory and cultural enhancement interventions for African American adolescent girls. *Public Health Reports, 117*(Suppl. 1), S76–S80. Retrieved from http://www.publichealthreports.org

Belgrave, F. Z., Clark, T., & Nasim, A. (2009). Drug use among African American youth. In H. Neville, B. Tynes, & S. O. Utsey (Eds.), *Handbook of African American psychology* (pp. 469–481). Thousand Oaks, CA: Sage.

Belgrave, F. Z., Reed, M. C., Plybon, L. E., Butler, D. S., Allison, K. W., & Davis, T. (2004). An evaluation of the Sisters of Nia: A cultural program for African American girls. *Journal of Black Psychology, 30*(3), 329–343. doi:10.1177/0095798404266063.

Bell, D., Anderson, M., & Grills, C. (2011). Culture-based prevention programming for African American youth: Winners and the community prevention program of Avalon Carver Community Center. *Psych Discourse, 45*(2). Retrieved from http://pd-online.abpsi.org

Benish, S. G., Quintana, S., & Wampold, B. E. (2011). Culturally adapted psychotherapy and the legitimacy of myth: A direct-comparison meta-analysis. *Journal of Counseling Psychology, 58*(3), 279–289. doi:10.1037/a0023626.

Berkout, O. V., Young, J. N., & Gross, A. M. (2011). Mean girls and bad boys: Recent research on gender differences in conduct disorder. *Aggression and Violent Behavior, 16*(6), 503–511. doi:10.1016/j.avb.2011.06.001.

Bernal, G. (2004). *Beyond one size fits all: Adapting evidence-based interventions for ethnic minorities.* PPT. Retrieved from http://www.hogg.utexas.edu/

Bernal, G. (2009). *Cultural adaptation of psychotherapy.* Paper presented at the 13th Annual Conference on Race, Ethnicity, and Mental Health: Treatment Innovations and Cultural Adaptations of Evidence-Based Interventions, Miami, FL.

Bernal, G., Bonilla, J., & Bellido, C. (1995). Ecological validity and cultural sensitivity for outcome research: Issues for cultural adaptation and development of psychosocial treatments with Hispanics. *Journal of Abnormal Child Psychology, 23*(1), 67–82. doi:10.1007/BF01447045.

Bernal, G., Jiménez-Chafey, M. I., Domenech, R., & Melanie, M. (2009). Cultural adaptation of treatments: A resource for considering culture in evidence-based practice. *Professional Psychology: Research and Practice, 40*(4), 361–368. doi:10.1037/a0016401.

Bernal, G., & Sáez-Santiago, E. (2006). Culturally centered psychosocial interventions. *Journal of Community Psychology, 34*(2), 121–132. doi:10.1002/jcop.20096.

Bernal, G., & Scharrón-del-Río, M. R. (2001). Are empirically supported treatments valid for ethnic minorities? Toward an alternative approach for treatment research. *Cultural Diversity and Ethnic Minority Psychology, 7*(4), 328–342. doi:10.1037/1099-9809.7.4.328.

Bernstein, G. A., Layne, A. E., Egan, E. A., & Tennison, D. M. (2005). School-based interventions for anxious children. *Journal of the American Academy of Child and Adolescent Psychiatry, 44*, 1118–1127. doi:10.1097/01.chi.0000177323.40005.a1.

Bero, L., Grilli, R., Grimshaw, J., Harvey, E., Oxman, A., & Thomson, M. (1998). Closing the gap between research and practice: An overview of systematic reviews of interventions to promote the implementation of research findings. *British Medical Journal, 317*(7156), 465–468. doi:10.1136/bmj.317.7156.465.

Bershad, C., & Blaber, C. (2011). *Realizing the promise of the whole-school approach to children's mental health: A practical guide for schools.* Waltham, MA: Education Development Center.

Bert, S. C., Farris, J. R., & Borkowski, J. G. (2008). Parent training implementation strategies for *Adventures in Parenting. Journal of Primary Prevention, 29,* 243–261. doi:10.1007/s10935-008-0135-y.

Berwick, D. M. (2003). Disseminating innovations in health care. *Journal of the American Medical Association, 289*(15), 1969–1975. doi:10.1001/jama.289.15.1969.

Bienvenu, O. J., & Ginsburg, G. S. (2007). Prevention of anxiety disorders. *International Review of Psychiatry, 19*(6), 647–654. doi:10.1080/09540260701797837.

Bierman, K. L., Coie, J. D., Dodge, K. A., Greenberg, M. T., Lochman, J. E., & McMahon, R. J. (2010). The effects of a multiyear universal social–emotional learning program: The role of student and school characteristics. *Journal of Consulting and Clinical Psychology, 78*(2), 156–168. doi:10.1037/a0018607.

Bierman, K. L., Coie, J. D., Dodge, K. A., Greenberg, M. T., Lochman, J. E., McMahon, R. J., et al. (1999). Initial impact of the Fast Track prevention trial for conduct problems: I. The high-risk sample. *Journal of Consulting and Clinical Psychology, 67*(5), 631–647. doi:10.1037/0022-006X.67.5.631.

Biglan, A. (2009). *Advancing the prevention of mental, emotional, and behavioral disorders.* Paper presented at the Virginia Family Impact Seminar, Virginia Commonwealth University, Richmond, VA.

Billings, J. A. (1996). A chief state school officer's view of what's needed for comprehensive education reform. *School Psychology Review, 25*(4), 485–488. Retrieved from http://www.nasponline.org

Bingham, G. E., & Okagaki, L. (2012). Ethnicity and student engagement. In S. L. Christenson, A. L. Reschly, & C. Wylie (Eds.), *Handbook of research on student engagement* (pp. 65–95). New York: Springer.

Bird, H. R., Davies, M., Duarte, C. S., Shen, S., Loeber, R., & Canino, G. J. (2006). A study of disruptive behavior disorders in Puerto Rican youth: II. Baseline prevalence, comorbidity, and correlates in two sites. *Journal of the American Academy of Child and Adolescent Psychiatry, 45*(9), 1042–1053. doi:10.1097/01.chi.0000227878.58027.3d.

Blaber, C., & Bershad, C. (2011). *Realizing the promise of the whole-school approach to children's mental health: A practical guide for schools.* SAMHSA, Education Development Center. Retrieved from http://www.promoteprevent.org

Black, S., Washington, E., Trent, V., Harner, P., & Pollock, E. (2010). Translating the Olweus Bullying Prevention Program into real-world practice. *Health Promotion Practice, 11*(5), 733–740. doi:10.1177/1524839908321562.

Blasé, K., Ficsen, D., & Porter, F. (2012). *Core intervention components: Identifying and operationalizing "what works."* Paper presented at the OAH and ACYF Teenage Pregnancy Prevention Grantee Conference, Baltimore.

Blonigen, B. A., Harbaugh, W. T., Singell, L. D., Horner, R. H., Irvin, K. L., & Smolkowski, K. S. (2008). Application of economic analysis to School-Wide Positive Behavior Support (SWPBS) programs. *Journal of Positive Behavior Interventions, 10*(1), 5–19. doi:10.1177/1098300707311366.

Blumberg, E. J., Chadwick, M. W., Fogarty, L. A., Speth, T. W., & Chadwick, D. L. (1991). The touch discrimination component of sexual abuse training unanticipated positive consequences. *Journal of Interpersonal Violence, 6*(1), 12–28. doi:10.1177/088626091006001002.

Bodrova, E., & Leong, D. J. (1995). Scaffolding the writing process: The Vygotskian approach. *Colorado Reading Council Journal, 6,* 27–29. Retrieved from http://www.maryjofaithmorgan.com

Bodrova, E., & Leong, D. J. (1996). *Tools of the mind: The Vygotskian approach to early childhood education.* Upper Saddle River, NJ: Prentice-Hall.

Bögels, S., Stevens, J., & Majdandžić, M. (2011). Parenting and social anxiety: Fathers' versus mothers' influence on their children's anxiety in ambiguous social situations. *Journal of Child Psychology and Psychiatry, 51*(4), 599–606. doi:10.1111/j.1469-7610.2010.02345.x.

Bohanon, H., & Wu, M. (2011). Can prevention programs work together? An example of school-based mental health with prevention initiatives. *Advances in School Mental Health Promotion, 4*(4), 35–46. doi:10.1080/1754730X.2011.9715641.

Bohnert, A. M., Crnic, K. A., & Lim, K. G. (2003). Emotional competence and aggressive behavior in school-age children. *Journal of Abnormal Child Psychology, 31*(1), 79–91. doi:10.1023/A:1021725400321.

Bond, L., Butler, H., Thomas, L., Carlin, J., Glover, S., Bowes, G., et al. (2007). Social and school connectedness in early secondary school as predictors of late teenage substance use, mental health, and academic outcomes. *Journal of Adolescent Health, 40*(4), e9–e18. Retrieved from http://www.jahonline.org

Bond, L., Glover, S., Godfrey, C., Butler, H., & Patton, G. C. (2001). Building capacity for system-level change in schools, lessons from the Gatehouse project. *Health Education & Behavior, 28*, 368–383. doi:10.1177/109019810102800310.

Borbely, C. (2005). *Finding the right fit: Program fidelity and adaptation for prevention programs.* The Center for Applied Research Solutions for the California Governor's Program: Safe and Drug-Free Schools and Communities (SDFSC). *Technical Assistance Project: Prevention Brief, 1*(2), 1–18. Retrieved from http://www.ca-sdfsc.org

Borntrager, C. f., Chorpita, B. F., Higa-McMillan, C. K., Weiz, J. R., & the Network on Youth Mental Health (2009). Provider attitudes toward evidence-based practices: Are the concerns with the evidence or with the manuals? *Psychiatric Services, 60*(5), 677–681. doi:10.1176/appi.ps.60.5.677.

Botvin, G. J. (1996). Substance abuse prevention through life skills training. In R. D. Peters & R. J. McMahon (Eds.), *Preventing childhood disorders, substance abuse, and delinquency* (pp. 215–240). Thousand Oaks, CA: Sage.

Botvin, G. J. (2000). *LifeSkills training teacher's manual 2.* White Plains, NY: Princeton Health Press.

Botvin, G. J. (2004). Advancing prevention science and practice: Challenges, critical issues, and future directions. *Journal of Prevention Science, 5*(1), 69–72. doi:10.1023/B:PREV.0000013984.83251.8b.

Botvin, G. J., Baker, E., Botvin, E. M., Filazzola, A. D., & Millman, R. B. (1984). Prevention of alcohol misuse through the development of personal and social competence: A pilot study. *Journal of Studies of Alcohol, 45*(6), 550–552. Retrieved from http://www.collegedrinkingprevention.gov

Botvin, G. J., Baker, E., Dusenbury, L., Botvin, E. M., & Diaz, T. (1995). Long-term follow-up results of a randomized drug abuse prevention trial in a white middle-class population. *Journal of theAmericanMedicalAssociation,273*(14),1106–1112.doi:10.1001/jama.1995.03520380042033.

Botvin, G. J., & Griffin, K. W. (2003). Drug abuse prevention curricula in schools. In Z. Sloboda & W. J. Bukoski (Eds.), *Handbook of drug abuse prevention: Theory, science, and practice* (pp. 45–74). New York: Kluwer Academic/Plenum.

Botvin, G. J., & Griffin, K. W. (2004). Life skills training: Empirical findings and future directions. *Journal of Primary Prevention, 25*(2), 211–232. doi:10.1023/B:JOPP.0000042391.58573.5b.

Botvin, G. J., Griffin, K. W., & Nichols, T. D. (2006). Preventing youth violence and delinquency through a universal school-based prevention approach. *Prevention Science, 7*(4), 403–408. doi:10.1007s/11121-006-0057-y.

Bouckenooghe, D. (2010). Positioning change recipients' attitudes toward change in the organizational change literature. *The Journal of Applied Behavioral Science, 46*(4), 500–531. doi:10.1177/0021886310367944.

Bovey, W. H., & Hede, A. (2001). Resistance to organizational change: The role of cognitive and affective processes. *Leadership & Organization Development Journal, 22*(7–8), 372–382. doi:10.1108/01437730110410099.

Boyd, K., Ashcraft, A., & Belgrave, F. Z. (2006). The impact of mother-daughter and father-daughter relationships on drug refusal self-efficacy among African American adolescent girls in urban communities. *Journal of Black Psychology, 32*(1), 20–42. doi:10.1177/0095798405280387.

Boyd, R. C., Ginsberg, G. S., Lambert, S. F., Cooley, M. R., & Campbell, K. D. (2003). Screen for child anxiety related emotional disorders (SCARED): Psychometric properties in an African American parochial high school sample. *Journal of the American Academy of Child and Adolescent Psychiatry, 42*(10), 1188–1196. doi:10.1097/00004583-200310000-00009.

Boyle, D., & Hassett-Walker, C. (2008). Reducing overt and relational aggression among young children: The results from a two-year outcome study. *Journal of School Violence, 7*(1), 27–42. doi:10.1300/J202v07n01_03.

Brackett, M. A., Reyes, M. R., Rivers, S. E., & Elbertson, N. (2009). *Belief in SEL: Teacher scale.* New Haven, CT: Health, Emotion and Behavior Laboratory.

Brackett, M. A., Reyes, M. A., Rivers, S. E., Elbertson, N. A., & Salovey, P. (2012). Assessing teachers' beliefs about social and emotional learning. *Journal of Psychoeducational Assessment, 30*(3), 219–236. doi:10.1177/0734282911424879.

Bradshaw, C. P., Koth, C. W., Bevans, K. B., Ialongo, N., & Leaf, P. J. (2008). The impact of School-Wide Positive Behavioral Interventions and Supports (PBIS) on the organizational health of elementary schools. *School Psychology Quarterly, 23*(4), 462–473. doi:10.1037/a0012883.

Bradshaw, C. P., Mitchell, M. M., & Leaf, P. J. (2009). Examining the effects of Schoolwide Positive Behavioral Interventions and Supports on student outcomes: Results from a randomized controlled effectiveness trial in elementary schools. *Journal of Positive Behavior Interventions, 12*(3), 133–148. doi:10.1177/1098300709334798.

Bradshaw, C. P., Reinke, W. M., Brown, L. D., Bevans, K. B., & Leaf, P. J. (2008). Implementation of School-Wide Positive Behavioral Interventions and Supports (PBIS) in elementary schools: Observations from a randomized trial. *Education and Treatment of Children, 31*(1), 1–26. doi:10.1353/etc.0.0025.

Braverman, M. T., & Arnold, M. E. (2008). An evaluator's balancing act: Making decisions about methodological rigor. *New Directions for Evaluation, 120,* 71–86. doi:10.1002/ev.277.

Breslau, J., Aguilara-Gaxiola, S., Kendler, K. S., Maxwell, S., Williams, D., & Kessler, R. C. (2006). Specifying race-ethnic differences in risk for psychiatric disorder in a US national sample. *Psychological Medicine, 36*(1), 57–68. doi:10.1017/S0033291705006161.

Brewer, N. T., & Rimer, B. K. (2008). Perspectives on health behavior theories that focus on individuals. In K. Glanz, B. K. Rimer, & R. K. Viswanath (Eds.), *Health behavior and health education: Theory, research, and practice* (4th ed., pp. 149–166). San Francisco: Jossey-Bass.

Brink, S. G., Basen-Engquist, K., O'Hara-Tompkins, N. M., Parcel, G. S., Gottlieb, N. H., & Lovato, C. Y. (1995). Diffusion of an effective tobacco prevention program: Part I—Evaluation of the dissemination phase. *Health Education Research: Theory and Practice, 10*(3), 283–296. doi:10.1093/her/10.3.283.

Broderick, C. J., & Carroll, M. J. (2008). *Evaluation of the Incredible Years: September 2007–August 2008.* Denver, CO: Omni Institute. Retrieved from http://www.omni.org/

Bronfenbrenner, U. (1979). *The ecology of human development.* Cambridge, MA: Harvard University Press.

Brotman, L. M., Calzada, E., Huang, K., Kingston, S., Dawson-McClure, S., Kamboukose, D., et al. (2011). Promoting effective parenting practices and preventing child behavior problems in school among ethnically diverse families from underserved, urban communities. *Child Development, 82*(1), 258–276. doi:10.1111/j.1467-8624.2010.01554x.

Brown, E. R. C., Catalano, F., Fleming, C. B., Haggerty, K. P., & Abbott, R. D. (2005). Adolescent substance use outcomes in the Raising Healthy Children Project: A two-part latent growth curve analysis. *Journal of Consulting and Clinical Psychology, 73,* 699–710. doi:10.1037/0022-006X.73.4.699.

Brown, C. H., Guo, J., Singer, L. T., Downes, K., & Brinales, J. M. (2007). Examining the effects of school-based drug prevention programs on drug use in rural settings: Methodology and initial findings. *Journal of Rural Health, 23,* 29–36. Retrieved from http://www.ruralhealthweb.org

Brown, C. M., & Ling, W. (2012). Ethnic-racial socialization has an indirect effect on self-esteem for Asian American emerging adults. *Scientific Research, 3*, 1. doi:10.4236/psych.2012.31013.

Brownson, R. C., Colditz, G. A., & Proctor, E. K. (2012). *Dissemination and implementation research in health: Translating science to practice.* Oxford: Oxford University Press. doi:10.1093/acprof:oso/9780199751877.001.0001.

Brunwasser, S. M., Gillham, J. E., & Kim, E. S. (2009). A meta-analytic review of the Penn Resiliency Program's effect on depressive symptoms. *Journal of Consulting and Clinical Psychology, 77*(6), 1042–1054. doi:10.1037/a0017671.

Burke, L. M., & Muhlhausen, D. B. (2013). *Head Start impact evaluation report finally released.* Issue Brief (No. 382). Washington, DC: The Heritage Foundation.

Burns, M. K. (2011). School psychology research: Combining ecological theory and prevention science. *School Psychology Review, 40*(1), 132–139. Retrieved from http://www.nasponline.org

Burns, M. K., Jacob, S., & Wagner, A. R. (2008). Ethical and legal issues associated with using response-to-intervention to access learning disabilities. *Journal of School Psychology, 46*(3), 263–279. doi:10.1016/j.jsp.2007.06.001.

Burns, M. K., Scholin, S. E., & Zaslofsky, A. (2011). Advances in assessment through research: What have we learned in the past three years? *Assessment for Effective Intervention, 36*(2), 107–112. doi:10.1177/1534508410395557.

Butterfoss, F. D., Kegler, M. C., & Franciso, V. T. (2008). Mobilizing organizations for health promotion: Theories of organizational change. In K. Glanz, B. K. Rimer, & K. Viswanath (Eds.), *Health behavior and health education: Theory, research, and practice* (4th ed., pp. 335–361). San Francisco: Jossey-Bass.

Bywater, T., Hutchings, J., Daley, D., Whitaker, C., Yeo, S. T., Jones, K., et al. (2009). Long-term effectiveness of a parenting intervention for children at risk of developing conduct disorder. *The British Journal of Psychiatry, 195*, 318–324. doi:10.1192/bjp.bp.108.056531.

Caldwell, M. B., Brotman, L. M., Coard, S. I., Wallace, S. A., Stellabotte, D. J., & Calzada, E. J. (2005). Community involvement in adapting and testing a prevention program for preschoolers living in urban communities: ParentCorps. *Journal of Child and Family Studies, 14*(3), 373–386. doi:10.1007/s10826-005-6850-6.

California Postsecondary Education Commission. (2008). *Educational experiments: A field guide for conducting scientifically based research* (version 1.0). Retrieved from http://www.cpec.ca.gov/

Calvete, E., Camara, M., Estevez, A., & Villardón, L. (2011). The role of coping with social stressors in the development of depressive symptoms: Gender differences. *Anxiety, Stress, and Coping, 24*(4), 387–406. doi:10.1080/10615806.2010.515982.

Calvete, E., & Cardenoso, O. (2005). Gender differences in cognitive vulnerability to depression and behavior problems in adolescents. *Journal of Abnormal Child Psychology, 33*(2), 179–192. doi:10.1007/s10802-005-1826-y.

Camilli, G., Vargas, S., Ryan, S., & Barnett, W. S. (2010). Meta-analysis of the effects of early education interventions on cognitive and social development. *Teachers College Record, 112*(3), 579–620. Retrieved from http://spot.colorado.edu

Campbell, C. (2011). *Adapting an evidence-based intervention to improve social and behavioral competence in Head Start children: Evaluating the effectiveness of teacher-child interaction training.* Retrieved from http://digitalcommons.unl.edu/psychdiss/37

Campo, J. V. (2012). Annual research review: Functional somatic symptoms and associated anxiety and depression—Developmental psychopathology in pediatric practice. *Journal of Child Psychology and Psychiatry, 53*(5), 575–592. doi:10.1111/j.1469-7610.2012.02535.x.

Cane, J., O'Connor, D., & Michie, S. (2012). Validation of the theoretical domains framework for use in behavior change and implementation research. *Implementation Science, 7*, 37. doi:10.1186/1748-5908-7-37.

Canino, G., & Alegria, M. (2008). Psychiatric diagnosis—Is it universal or relative to culture. *Journal of Child Psychology and Psychiatry, 49*(3), 237–250. doi:10.1111/j.1469-7610.2007.01854.x.

Canino, G., Polanczyk, G., Bauermeister, J. J., Rohde, L. A., & Frick, P. J. (2010). Does the prevalence of CD and ODD vary across cultures? *Social Psychiatry and Psychiatric Epidemiology, 245*(7), 695–704. doi:10.1007/s00127-010-0242-y.

Caplan, G. (1964). *Principles of preventive psychiatry.* New York: Basic Books.

Cardemil, E. V. (2008). Commentary: Culturally sensitive treatments: Need for an organizing framework. *Cultural Psychology, 14*(3), 357–367. doi:10.1177/1354067X08092638.

Cardemil, E. V. (2010). Cultural adaptations to empirically supported treatments: A researcher agenda. *The Scientific Review of Mental Health Practice, 7*(2), 8–21. Retrieved from http://www.srmhp.org/

Cardemil, E. V., Reivich, K. J., Beevers, C. G., Seligman, M. E. P., & James, J. (2007). The prevention of depressive symptoms in inner-city middle school students: 2-year follow-up. *Behaviour Research and Therapy, 45*, 313–327. doi:10.1016/j.brat.2006.03.010.

Carpenter, C. J. (2010). A meta-analysis of the effectiveness of health belief model variables in predicting behavior. *Health Communication, 25*(8), 661–669. doi:10.1080/10410236.2010.521906.

Carrasco, M. (n.d.). *Evidence-based practices: Implications for multicultural communities.* Powerpoint presentation. Washington, DC: The National Alliance of Multi-Ethnic Behavioral Health.

Carroll, C., Patterson, M., Wood, S., Booth, A., Rick, J., & Balain, S. (2007). A conceptual framework for implementation fidelity. *Implementation Science, 2*, 40. doi:10.1186/1748-5908-2-40.

Carter, A. S., Wagmiller, S., Gray, A. O., McCarthy, K. J., Horwitz, S. M., & Briggs-Gowan, M. J. (2010). Prevalence of DSM-IV disorder in a representative, healthy birth cohort at school entry: Sociodemographic risks and social adaptation. *Journal of the American Academy of Child and Adolescent Psychiatry, 49*(7), 686–698. doi:10.1016/j.jaac.2010.03.018.

Castro, F. G., & Alarcón, E. H. (2002). Integrating cultural variables into drug abuse prevention and treatment with racial/ethnic minorities. *Journal of Drug Issues, 32*(3), 783–810. Retrieved from http://www2.criminology.fsu.edu/

Castro, F. G., Barrera, M., & Holleran Steiker, L. K. (2010). Issues and challenges in the design of culturally adapted evidence-based interventions. *Annual Review of Clinical Psychology, 6*, 231–239. doi:10.1146/annurev-clinpsy-033109-132032.

Castro, F. G., Barrera, M., & Martinez, C. R. (2004). The cultural adaptation of prevention interventions: Resolving tensions between fidelity and fit. *Prevention Science, 5*(1), 41–45. doi:10.1023/B:PREV.0000013980.12412.cd.

Castro-Olivo, S. M., & Merrell, K. W. (2012). Validating cultural adaptations of a school-based social-emotional learning programme for use with Latino immigrant adolescents. *Advances in School Mental Health Promotion, 5*(2), 78–92. doi:10.1080/1754730X.2012.689193.

Catalano, R. F., Mazza, J. J., Harachi, T. W., Abbott, R. D., Haggerty, K. P., & Fleming, C. B. (2003). Raising healthy children through enhancing social development in elementary school: Results after 1.5 years. *Journal of School Psychology, 41*, 143–164. doi:10.1016/S0022-4405(03)00031-1.

Catrambone, R., & Yuasa, M. (2006). Acquisition of procedures: The effects of example elaborations and active learning exercises. *Learning and Instruction, 16*, 139–153. doi:10.1016/j.learninstruc.2006.02.002.

Cauce, A. M., Coronado, N., & Watson, J. (1998). Conceptual, methodological, and statistical issues in culturally competent research. In M. Hernandez & M. Isaacs (Eds.), *Promising cultural competence in children's mental health services* (pp. 305–329). Baltimore: Paul H. Brookes.

Center for Mental Health in Schools. (2003). *Youngsters' mental health and psychosocial problems: What are the data?* Los Angeles: University of California at Los Angeles.

Center for Mental Health in Schools at UCLA. (2006). *A technical aid packet on resource mapping and management to address barriers to learning: An intervention for systemic change.* Los Angeles: Author.

Center for Mental Health in Schools at UCLA. (2012a). *Unit I: Motivation: Time to move beyond behavior modification. Engaging and re-engaging students and families: Four units for con-*

tinuing education. Los Angeles: School Mental Health Project. Retrieved from http://smhp. psych.ucla.edu

Center for Mental Health in Schools at UCLA. (2012b). *Unit II: Strategic approaches to enhancing student engagement and re-engagement. Engaging and re-engaging students and families: Four units for continuing education.* Los Angeles: School Mental Health Project. Retrieved from http://smhp.psych.ucla.edu

Center for Mental Health in Schools at UCLA. (2012c). *Unit III: Enhancing family engagement and re-engagement. Engaging and re-engaging students and families: Four units for continuing education.* Los Angeles: School Mental Health Project. Retrieved from http://smhp.psych.ucla.edu

Center for Substance Abuse Prevention. (2009). *Identifying and selecting evidence-based interventions revised guidance document for the strategic prevention framework state incentive grant program* (HHS Publication No. (SMA) 09-4205). Rockville, MD: Center for Substance Abuse Prevention, Substance Abuse and Mental Health Services Administration.

Center on the Developing Child at Harvard University. (2007). *A science-based framework for early childhood policy: Using evidence to improve outcomes in learning, behavior, and health for vulnerable children.* Retrieved from http://www.developingchild.harvard.edu

Centers for Disease Control and Prevention (CDC). (2008). *Introduction to process evaluation in tobacco use prevention and control.* Atlanta, GA: U.S. Department of Health and Human Services, Centers for Disease Control and Prevention, National Center for Chronic Disease Prevention and Health Promotion, Office on Smoking and Health. Retrieved from http://www. cdc.gov/

Centers for Disease Control and Prevention (CDC). (2009). *Parent training programs: Insight for practitioners.* Atlanta, GA: Centers for Disease Control, U.S. Department of Health and Human Services. Retrieved from http://www.cdc.gov

Centers for Disease Control and Prevention (CDC). (2012a). *Parent engagement: Strategies for involving parents in school health.* Atlanta, GA: U.S. Department of Health and Human Services.

Centers for Disease Control and Prevention (CDC). (2012b). Youth risk behavior surveillance-United States, 2011. *Morbidity and Mortality Weekly Report, 61*(4). Retrieved from http:// www.cdc.gov

Century, J., Rudnick, M., & Freeman, C. (2010). A framework for measuring fidelity of implementation: A foundation for shared language and accumulation of knowledge. *American Journal of Evaluation, 3*(2), 199–218. doi:10.1177/109821410366173.

Chafouleas, S. M., Kilgus, S. P., & Wallach, N. (2010). Ethical dilemmas in school-based behavioral screening. *Assessment for Effective Intervention, 35*(4), 245–252. doi:10.1177/1534508410379002.

Chandler, E., A'Vant, E. R., & Graves, S. L. (2008). Effective communication with Black families and students. *Communiqué, 37*(4). Retrieved from http://www.nasponline.org/

Chang, J. (2009). *Children's attentional and behavioral persistence and the development of externalizing behavior problems: A process oriented perspective spanning early childhood through the school-age years.* Unpublished doctoral dissertation, University of Michigan, Ann Arbor, MI.

Chaplin T. M., Gillham, J. E., Reivich, K., Elkon, A. G., Samuels, B., Freres, D. R., Seligman, M. E. (2006). Depression prevention for early adolescent girls: A pilot study of all girls versus co-ed groups. *Journal of Clinical Psychology, 62*(1), 110–126. doi:10.1177/0272431605282655.

Chaplin, T. M., Gillham, J. E., & Seligman, M. E. (2009). Gender, anxiety, and depressive symptoms: A longitudinal study of early adolescents. *The Journal of Early Adolescence, 29*(2), 307–327. doi:10.1177/0272431608320125.

Chapman, L. K., Petrie, J., Vines, L., & Durrett, E. (2012). The co-occurrence of anxiety disorders in African American parents and their children. *Journal of Anxiety Disorders, 26*, 65–70. doi:10.1016/j.janxdis.2011.08.014.

Charlesworth, L. W., & Rodwell, M. K. (1997). Focus groups with children: A resource for sexual abuse prevention program evaluation. *Child Abuse & Neglect, 21*(12), 1205–1216. doi:10.1016/ S0145-2134(97)00095-1.

Cheney, D., Lynass, L., Flower, A., Waugh, M., Iwaszuk, W., Mielenz, C., et al. (2010). The Check, Connect, and Expect program: A targeted, tier 2 intervention in the schoolwide positive behavior support model. *Preventing School Failure, 54*(3), 152–158. doi:10.1080/10459880903492742.

Chiu, M. M., Pong, S. L., Mori, I., & Chow, B. W. Y. (2012). Immigrant students' cognitive and emotional engagement at school: A multilevel analysis of students in 41 countries. *Journal of Youth and Adolescence, 41*, 1409–1425. doi:10.1007/s10964-012-9763-x.

Choi, Y., Harachi, T. W., Gillmore, M. R., & Catalano, R. F. (2006). Are multiracial adolescents at greater risk? Comparisons of rates, patterns, and correlates of substance use and violence between monoracial and multiracial adolescents. *The American Journal of Orthopsychiatry, 76*(1), 86–97. doi:10.1037/0002-9432.76.1.86.

Chorpita, B. F., & Daleiden, D. L. (2009a). *CAMHD biennial report: Effective psychosocial interventions for youth with behavioral and emotional needs.* Honolulu, HI: Hawaii Department of Health, Child and Adolescent Mental Health Division.

Chorpita, B. F., & Daleiden, E. L. (2009b). Mapping evidence-based treatments for children and adolescents: Application of the distillation and matching model to 615 treatments from 322 randomized trials. *Journal of Consulting and Clinical Psychology, 77*(3), 566–579. doi:10.1037/a0014565.

Chou, C. P., Montgomery, S., Pentz, M. A., Rohrbach, L. A., Johnson, C. A., Flay, B. R., et al. (1998). Effects of a community-based prevention program on decreasing drug use in high-risk adolescents. *American Journal of Public Health, 88*(6), 944–948. doi:10.2105/AJPH.88.6.944.

Christenson, S. L. (2002). *Families educators and the family-school partnership: Issues or opportunities for promoting children's learning competence?* Paper prepared for the 2002 Invitational Conference, The Future of School Psychology, Indianapolis, IN.

Christenson, S. L. (2004). The family-school partnership: An opportunity to promote the learning competence of all students. *School Psychology Review, 33*(1), 83–104. Retrieved from http://www.nasponline.org

Christenson, S., Palan, R., & Scullin, S. (2009). Family-school partnerships: An essential component of student achievement. *Principal Leadership, 9*(9), 10–14, 16. Retrieved from http://www.nassp.org/

Christenson, S. L., & Sheridan, S. M. (2001). *School and families: Creating essential connections for learning.* New York: Guilford Press.

Christenson, S. L., Stout, K., & Pohl, A. (2012). *Check & connect: A comprehensive student engagement intervention.* Minneapolis, MN: University of Minnesota.

Christenson, S. L., & Thurlow, M. L. (2004). School dropouts: Prevention considerations interventions, and challenges. *Current Directions in Psychological Science, 13*(1), 36–39. doi:10.1111/j.0963-7214.2004.01301010.x.

Christenson, S. L., Whitehouse, E. L., & VanGetson, G. R. (2007). Partnering with families to enhance students' mental health. In B. Doll & J. A. Cummings (Eds.), *Transforming school mental health services: Population-based approaches to promoting the competency and wellness of students services* (pp. 69–101). Thousand Oaks, CA: Corwin Press.

Chu, J. P., & Sue, S. (2011). Asian American mental health: What we know and what we don't know (Unit 3 Indigenous Approach, Article 4). *Online Readings in Psychology and Culture: International Association for Cross-Cultural Psychology.* Retrieved from http://scholarworks.gvsu.edu/

Cladwell, M. B., Brotman, L. M., Coard, S. I., Wallave, S. A., Stellabotte, D. J., & Calzada, E. J. (2005). Community involvement in adapting and testing a prevention program for preschoolers living in urban communities: ParentCorps. *Journal of Child and Family Studies, 14*(3), 373–386. doi:10.1007/s10826-6850-6.

Clark, T. T., Belgrave, F. Z., & Abell, M. (2012). The mediating and moderating effects of parent and peer influences upon drug use among African American adolescents. *Journal of Black Psychology, 38*(1), 52–80. doi:10.1177/0095798411403617.

Clarke, G. N., Hornbrook, M., Lynch, F., Polen, M., Gale, J., Beardslee, W., et al. (2001). A randomized trial of a group cognitive intervention for preventing depression in adolescent offspring of depressed parents. *Archives of General Psychiatry, 58*(12), 1127–1134. doi:10.1001/archpsyc.58.12.1127.

Coard, S. I., Wallace, S. A., Stevenson, H. C., & Brotman, L. M. (2004). Towards culturally relevant preventive interventions: The consideration of racial socialization in parent training with African American families. *Journal of Child and Family Studies, 13*(3), 277–293. doi:10.1080/15332980802032409.

Cobb, B., Sample, P., Alwell, M., & Johns, N. (2005). *The effects of cognitive-behavioral interventions on dropout for youth with disabilities. Effective interventions in dropout prevention: A research synthesis.* Clemson, SC: National Dropout Prevention Center for Students with Disabilities.

Coffee, G., & Ray-Subramanian, C. E. (2009). Goal attainment scaling: A progress—Monitoring tool for behavioral interventions. *School Psychology Forum: Research in Practice, 3*(1), 1–12. Retrieved from http://www.nasponline.org

Coffman, J. (1999). *Learning form logic models: An example of a family/school partnership program.* Brief. Boston: Harvard Family Research Project. Retrieved from http://www.hfrp.org

Cogburn, C. D., Chavous, T. M., & Griffin, T. M. (2011). School-based racial and gender discrimination among African American adolescents: Exploring gender variation in frequency and implication for adjustment. *Race Social Problems, 3*, 25–37. doi:10.1007/s12552-011-9040-8.

Cohen, J. A., Beliner, L., & Mannarino, A. (2010). Trauma focused CBT for children with co-occurring trauma and behavior problems. *Child Abuse & Neglect, 34*, 215–224. doi:10.1016/j.chiabu.2009.12.003.

Cohen, R., Kincaid, D., & Childs, K. E. (2007). Measuring school-wide positive behavior support implementation: Development and validation of the benchmarks of quality. *Journal of Positive Behavior Interventions, 9*(4), 203–213. doi:10.1177/10983007070090040301.

Coie, J. K., & Dodge, K. A. (1998). Aggression and antisocial behavior. In W. Damon & N. Eisenberg (Eds.), *Handbook of child psychology: Social, emotional, and personality development* (5th ed., Vol. 3, pp. 779–862). New York: Wiley.

Coker, T. R., Elliott, M. N., Kataoka, S., Schwebel, D. C., Mrug, S., Grunbaum, J. A., et al. (2009). Racial/ethnic disparities in the mental health care utilization of fifth grade children. *Academic Pediatrics, 9*(2), 89–96. doi:10.1016/j.acap.2008.11.007.

Colder, C., Lochman, J. E., & Wells, K. C. (1997). The moderating effects of children's fear and activity level on relations between parenting practices and childhood symptomatology. *Journal of Abnormal Child Psychology, 25*, 251–263. doi:10.1023/A:1025704217619.

Cole, P. M., Dennis, T. A., Smith-Simon, K. E., & Cohen, L. H. (2009). Preschoolers' emotion regulation strategy understanding: Relations with emotion socialization and child self-regulation. *Social Development, 18*(2), 324–352. doi:10.1111/j.1467-9507.2008.00503.x.

Collaborative for Academic, Social, and Emotional Learning (CASEL). (2008). *Leading an "SEL" school.* Newton, MA: National Center for Mental Health Promotion and Youth Violence Prevention, Educational Development Center.

Collaborative for Academic, Social, and Emotional Learning (CASEL). (2012). *2013 CASEL guide: Effective social and emotional learning programs.* Retrieved from http://casel.org

Collett, D. (2011). *An attempt to operationalize culture within healthcare: An analytical literature review.* Paper presented at the MWERA Annual Meeting, St Louis, MO.

Collie, R. J., Shapka, J. D., & Perry, N. E. (2011). Predicting teacher commitment: The impact of school climate and social-emotional learning. *Psychology in the Schools, 48*(10), 1034–1048. doi:10.1002/pits.20611.

Collie, R. J., Shapka, J. D., & Perry, N. E. (2012). School climate and social–emotional learning: Predicting teacher stress, job satisfaction, and teaching efficacy. *Journal of Educational Psychology, 104*, 1189–1204. doi:10.1037/a0029356.

Colombo, M. W. (2006). Building school partnerships with culturally and linguistically diverse families. *Phi Delta Kappan, 88*(4), 314–318. Retrieved from http://www.pdkintl.org/

Comer, J. S., Chow, C., Chan, P. T., Cooper-Vince, C., & Wilson, L. A. S. (2013). Psychosocial treatment efficacy for disruptive behavior problems in very young children: A meta-analytic examination. *Journal of the American Academy of Child and Adolescent Psychiatry, 52*(1), 26–36. doi:10.1016/j.jaac.2012.10.001.

Committee for Children. (1992). *Second Step: A violence prevention curriculum.* Seattle, WA: Author.

Committee for Children. (2001). *Steps to respect: A bullying prevention program.* Seattle, WA: Author.

Committee for Children. (2010). *Getting started information.* Seattle, WA: Second Step Early Learning Program.

Committee on the Prevention of Mental Disorders and Substance Abuse Among Children, Youth, and Young Adults: Research Advances and Promising Interventions. (2009). Implementation and dissemination of prevention programs. In M. E. O'Connell, T. Boat, & K. E. Warner (Eds.), *Preventing mental, emotional, and behavioral disorders among young people: Progress and possibilities* (pp. 297–336). Washington, DC: The National Academies Press.

Compian, L. L., Gowen, L. K., & Hayward, C. (2009). The interactive effects of puberty and peer victimization on weight concerns and depression symptoms among early adolescent girls. *The Journal of Early Adolescence, 29*(3), 357–375. doi:10.1177/0272431608323656.

Compton, M. T. (2011, June 10). *Highlights from the 2011 annual meeting of the American Psychiatric Association in sunny Honolulu, Hawaii.* From Medscape Psychiatry Treating Pediatric Anxiety: What Works?

Compton, S. N., Walkup, J. T., Albano, A. M., Piacentini, J. C., Birmaher, B., Sherrill, J. T., et al. (2010). Child/Adolescent Anxiety Multimodal Study (CAMS): Rationale, design, and methods. *Child and Adolescent Psychiatry and Mental Health, 4*(1), 1. doi:10.1186/1753-2000-4-1.

Conduct Problems Prevention Research Group (CPPRG). (2011). The effects of the fast track preventive intervention on the development of conduct disorder across childhood. *Child Development, 82*(1), 331–345. doi:10.1111/j.1467-8624.2010.01558.x.

Connell, A. M., Dishion, T. D., Yasui, M., & Kavanagh, K. (2007). An adaptive approach to family intervention: Linking engagement in family-centered intervention to reductions in adolescent problem behavior. *Journal of Consulting and Clinical Psychology, 75*(4), 568–579. doi:10.1037/0022-006X.75.4.568.

Cook, B. G., & Cook, L. (2008). Nonexperimental quantitative research and its role in guiding instruction. *Intervention in School and Clinic, 44*(2), 98–104. doi:10.1177/1053451208321565.

Cook, C. R., Volpe, R. J., & Livanis, A. (2010). Constructing a roadmap for future universal screening research beyond academics. *Assessment for Effective Intervention, 35*(4), 197–205. doi:10.1177/1534508410379842.

Cooke, M. B., Ford, J., Levine, J., Bourke, C., Newell, L., & Lapidus, G. (2007). The effects of city-wide implementation of "Second Step" on elementary school students' prosocial and aggressive behaviors. *The Journal of Primary Prevention, 28*(2), 93–115. doi:10.1007/s10935-007-0080-1.

Cooley, M. R., Boyd, R., & Grados, J. J. (2004). Feasibility of an anxiety preventive intervention for community violence exposed African-American children. *The Journal of Primary Prevention, 25*(1), 105–123. doi:10.1023/B:JOPP.0000039941.85452.ea.

Cooley-Strickland, M. R., Griffin, R. S., Darney, D., Otte, K., & Ko, J. (2011). Urban African American youth exposed to community violence: A school-based anxiety preventive intervention efficacy study. *Journal of Prevention & Intervention in the Community, 39*(2), 149–166. doi:10.1080/10852352.2011.556573.

Cooper, J. L., Masi, R., & Vick, R. (2009). *Social-emotional development in early childhood: What every policymaker should know.* New York: National Center for Children in Poverty.

Cooper, S. M., & McLoyd, V. C. (2011). Racial barrier socialization and the well-being of African American adolescents: The moderating role of mother–adolescent relationship quality. *Journal of Research on Adolescence, 21*(4), 895–903. doi:10.1111/j.1532-7795.2011.00749.x.

Corneille, M. A., Ashcraft, A. M., & Belgrave, F. Z. (2005). What's culture got to do with it? Prevention programs for African American adolescent girls. *Journal of Health Care for the Poor and Underserved, 16*(4), 38–47. doi:10.1353/hpu.2005.0109.

Corrieri, S., Heider, D., Conrad, I., Blume, A., König, H., & Riedel-Heller, S. G. (2013). School-based prevention programs for depression and anxiety in adolescence: A systematic review. *Health Promotion International*. doi: 10.1093/heapro/dat00.

Cortes, R. C., Fleming, C. B., Catalano, R. F., & Brown, E. C. (2006). Gender differences in the association between maternal depressed mood and child depressive phenomena from Grade 3 through Grade 10. *Journal of Youth and Adolescence, 35*(5), 815–826. doi:10.1007/s10964-006-9083-0.

Cosgrove, V. E., Rhee, S. H., Gelhorn, H. L., Boeldt, D., Corley, R. C., Ehringer, M. A., et al. (2011). Structure and etiology of co-occurring internalizing and externalizing disorders in adolescence. *Journal of Abnormal Child Psychology, 39*(1), 109–123. doi:10.1007/s10802-010-9444-8.

Costa, M. L., van Rensburg, L., & Rushton, N. (2007). Does teaching style matter: A randomized trial of group discussion versus lectures in orthopeadic undergraduate teaching. *Medical Education, 41*(2), 214–217. doi:10.1111/j.1365-2929.2006.02677.x.

Costantino, G., Malgady, R. G., & Rogler, L. H. (1986). Cuento therapy: A culturally sensitive modality for Puerto Rican children. *Journal of Consulting and Clinical Psychology, 54*(5), 639–645. doi:10.1037/0022-006X.54.5.639.

Costello, E. J., Mustillo, S., Erkanli, A., Keeler, G., & Anbgold, A. (2003). Prevalence and development of psychiatric disorders in childhood and adolescence. *Archives of General Psychiatry, 60*(8), 837–844. doi:10.1001/archpsyc.60.8.837.

Craig, C. (2007). *The potential dangers of a systematic, explicit approach to teaching social and emotional skills (SEAL): An overview and summary of the arguments*. Glasgow, Scotland: Center for Confidence and Well-Being.

Crone, D. A., Horner, R. H., & Hawken, L. S. (2004). *Responding to problem behavior in schools: The behavior education program*. New York: The Guildford Press.

Crosby, D. A., & Dunbar, A. S. (2012). *Patterns and predictor of school readiness and early childhood success among young children in Black immigrant families*. Washington, DC: The Migration Policy Institute.

Crosby, R. A., Salazar, L. F., & DiClemente, R. J. (2013). Ecological approaches in the new public health. In R. J. DiClemente, L. F. Salazar, & R. A. Crosby (Eds.), *Health behavior theory for public health: Principles, foundations, and applications* (pp. 231–249). Burlington, MA: Jones & Bartlett Learning.

Crosse, S., Williams, B., Hagen, S. A., Harmon, M., Ristow, L., DiGaetano, R., et al. (2011). *Prevalence and implementation fidelity of research-based prevention programs in public schools*. Rockville, MD: U.S. Department of Education.

Cuijpers, P. (2002). Effective ingredients of school-based drug prevention programs: A systematic review. *Addictive Behaviors, 27*(6), 1009–1023. doi:10.1016/S0306-4603(02)00295-2.

Cuijpers, P. (2003). Three decades of drug prevention research. *Drugs: Education, Prevention and Policy, 10*(1), 7–20. doi:10.1080/0968763021000018900.

Cuijpers, P., van Straten, A., Smit, F., Mihalopoulos, C., & Beekman, A. (2008). Preventing the onset of depressive disorders: A meta-analytic review of psychological interventions. *The American Journal of Psychiatry, 165*(10), 1272–1280. doi:10.1176/appi.ajp.2008.07091422.

Currie, J., & Thomas, D. (1999). Does head start help Hispanic children? *Journal of Public Economics, 74*(2), 235–262. doi:10.1016/S0047-2727(99)00027-4.

Curtis, S., & Norgate, R. (2007). An evaluation of the Promoting Alternative Thinking Strategies curriculum at key stage 1. *Educational Psychology in Practice: Theory, Research, and Practice in Educational Psychology, 23*(1), 33–44. doi:10.1080/02667360601154717.

Curtis, M. J., & Stollar, S. A. (1996). Applying principles and practices of organizational change to school reform. *School Psychology Review, 25*(4), 409–417. Retrieved from http://www.nasponline.org

Cusimano, M. D., & Sameem, M. (2010). The effectiveness of middle and high school-based suicide prevention programmes for adolescents: A systematic review. *Injury Prevention, 17*, 43–49. doi:10.1136/ip.2009.025502.

Cuthbert, B. (2010). Early prevention in childhood anxiety disorders. *The American Journal of Psychiatry, 167*(12), 1428–1430. doi:10.1176/appi.ajp.2010.10091316.

Cyranowski, J. M., Frank, E., Young, E., & Shear, M. K. (2000). Adolescent onset of the gender difference in lifetime rates of major depression: A theoretical model. *Archives of General Psychiatry, 57*(1), 21–27. doi:10.1001/archpsyc.57.1.21.

Dahlberg, L. L., Toal, S. B., Swahn, M. H., & Behrens, C. B. (2005). *Measuring violence-related attitudes, behaviors and influences among youths: A compendium of assessment tools* (2nd ed.). Retrieved from http://www.cdc.gov

Darnton, A. (2008). *Reference report: An overview of behavior change models and their uses.* London, UK: Centre for Sustainable Development.

Das-Munshi, J., Goldberg, D., Bebbington, P. E., Bhugra, D. K., Brugha, T. S., Dewey, M. E., et al. (2008). Public health significance of mixed anxiety and depression: Beyond current classification. *The British Journal of Psychiatry, 192*, 171–177. doi:10.1192/bjp.bp.107.036707.

Dauphinais, P., Charely, E., Robinson-Zañartu, C., Melrose, O., & Bassa, S. (2009). Home-school-community communication with indigenous American families. *Communiqué, 37*(5). Retrieved from http://www.nasponline.org/

David, H. J., von Cleve, E., & Catalano, R. F. (1991). Reducing early childhood aggression: Results of a primary prevention program. *Journal of the American Academy of Child and Adolescent Psychiatry, 30*(2), 208–217. doi:10.1097/00004583-199103000-00008.

Davis, M. K., & Gidycz, C. A. (2000). Child sexual abuse prevention programs: A meta-analysis. *Journal of Clinical Child Psychology, 29*(2), 257–265. doi:10.1207/S15374424jccp2902_11.

Davis, M. H., & McPartland, J. M. (2012). High school reform and student engagement. In S. L. Christenson, A. L. Reschly, & C. Wylie (Eds.), *Handbook of research on student engagement* (pp. 515–539). New York: Springer.

Davis, K. C., Nonnemaker, J. M., Asfaw, H. A., & Vallone, D. M. (2010). Racial/ethnic differences in perceived smoking prevalence: Evidence from a national survey of teens. *International Journal of Environmental Research and Public Health, 7*, 4152–4168. doi:10.3390/ijerph7124152.

De Arellano, M. A., Waldrop, A. E., Deblinger, E., Cohen, J. A., Danielson, C. K., & Mannarino, A. R. (2005). Community outreach program for child victims of traumatic events: A community-based project for underserved populations. *Behavior Modification, 29*(1), 130–155. doi:10.1177/0145445504270878.

De Bolle, M., De Clercq, B., Decuyper, M., & De Fruyt, F. (2011). Affective determinants of anxiety and depression development in children and adolescents: An individual growth curve analysis. *Child Psychiatry and Human Development, 42*(6), 694–711. doi:10.1007/s10578-011-0241-6.

DeAngelis, T. (2010). Social awareness + emotional skills=successful kids: New funding and congressional support are poised to being the best social and emotional learning research into more classrooms nationwide. *APA Monitor, 41*(4), 46. Retrieved from http://www.apa.org

Degnan, K. A., Almas, A. N., & Fox, N. A. (2010). Temperament and the environment in the etiology of childhood anxiety. *Journal of Child Psychology and Psychiatry, 51*(4), 497–517. doi:10.1111/j.1469-7610.2010.02228.x.

DeJong, W. (1994). *Building the peace: The Resolving Conflict Creatively Program (RCCP).* Washington, D.C.: National Institute of Justice, U.S. Department of Justice.

del Rosario, M., & Webster, J. (2007). *Family involvement information and training kit: A presentation kit for educators and parents.* Delaware, MD: Mid-Atlantic Equity Center/Delaware Department of Education.

Demetrovics, Z. (2012). Adolescent behavior and health in cross-cultural context. *Journal of Early Adolescence, 32*(1), 14–19. doi:10.1177/0272431611432713.

Denham, S. A., & Burton, R. (1996). Social-emotional interventions for at-risk preschoolers. *Journal of School Psychology, 34*, 225–245. doi:10.1016/0022-4405(96)00013-1.

Denham, S. A., & Burton, R. (2003). *Social and emotional prevention and intervention programming for preschoolers.* New York: Kluwer Academic/Plenum Press.

Denham, S. A., & Weissberg, R. P. (2004). Social-emotional learning in early childhood: What we know and where to go from here. In E. Chesebrough, P. King, T. P. Gullotta, & M. Bloom

(Eds.), *A blueprint for the promotion of prosocial behavior in early childhood* (pp. 13–50). New York: Kluwer Academic/Plenum Press.

Dent, C. W., Sussman, S., Hennesy, M., Galaif, E. R., Stacy, A. W., Moss, M., et al. (1998). Implementation and process evaluation of a school-based drug abuse prevention program: Project toward no drug abuse. *Journal of Drug Education, 28*(4), 361–375. Retrieved from http://www.baywood.com

Dent, C. W., Sussman, S., Stacy, A. W., Craig, S., Burton, D., & Flay, B. R. (1995). Two-year behavior outcomes of the Project Towards No Tobacco Use. *Journal of Consulting and Clinical Psychology, 63*(4), 676–677. doi:10.1037/0022-006X.63.4.676.

Deslauriers, L., Schelew, E., & Wieman, C. (2011). Improved learning in a large-enrollment physics class. *Science, 332*(6031), 862–864. doi:10.1126/science.1201783.

Deutsch, A. R., Crockett, L. J., Wolff, J. M., & Russell, S. T. (2012). Parent and peer pathways to adolescent delinquency: Variations by ethnicity and neighborhood context. *Journal of Youth and Adolescence, 41*(8), 1078–1094. doi:10.1007/s10964-012-9754-y.

Devaney, E., O'Brien, M. U., Resnik, H., Keister, S., & Weissberg, P. (2006). *Sustainable schoolwide social and emotional learning (SEL): Implementation guide and toolkit.* Chicago: Collaborative for Academic, Social, and Emotional Learning.

Dianda, M. R. (2008). *Preventing future high school dropouts: An advocacy and action guide for NEA state and local affiliates.* Washington, DC: Human and Civil Rights. Retrieved from http://www.nea.org/

Dilworth, J. E., Mokrue, K., & Elias, M. J. (2002). The efficacy of a video-based teamwork-building series with urban elementary school students: A pilot investigation. *Journal of School Psychology, 40*(4), 329–346. doi:10.1016/S0022-4405(02)00102-4.

Dino, G. A., Horn, K. A., Goldcamp, J., Maniar, S. D., Fernandez, A., & Massey, C. J. (2001). Statewide demonstration of Not On Tobacco: A gender-sensitive teen smoking cessation program. *The Journal of School Nursing, 17*(2), 90–97. doi:10.1177/105984050101700206.

Dishion, T. J., & Kavanagh, K. (2003). *Intervening in adolescent problem behavior: A family-centered approach.* New York: Guilford Press.

Dishion, T. J., Kavanagh, K., Schneiger, A., Nelson, S., & Kaufman, N. K. (2002). Preventing early adolescent substance use: A family-centered strategy for the public middle-school. *Prevention Science, 3*(3), 191–201. doi:10.1023/A:1019994500301.

Dishion, T. J., & Van Ryzin, M. (2011). Peer contagion dynamics in the development of problem behavior and violence: Implications for intervention and policy. *International Society for the Study of Behavioural Development, 2*(6), 6–11. Retrieved from http://www.issbd.org/

DiStephano, C., & Morgan, G. B. (2010). Evaluation of the BESS TRS-CA using the Rasch rating scale model. *School Psychology Quarterly, 25*(4), 202–212. doi:10.1037/a0021509.

Dix, K. L., Slee, P. T., Lawson, M. J., & Keeves, J. P. (2012). Implementation quality of whole-school mental health promotion and students' academic performance. *Child and Adolescent Mental Health, 17*(1), 45–51. doi:10.1111/j.1475-3588.2011.00608.x.

Dobson, K. S., Hopkins, J. A., Fata, L., Scherrer, M., & Allan, L. C. (2010). The prevention of depression and anxiety in a sample of high-risk adolescents: A randomized controlled trial. *Canadian Journal of School Psychology, 25*(4), 291–310. doi:10.1177/0829573510386449.

Doll, B., Chapla, B., Chadwell, M., Sikorski, J., Spies, R., & Franta, E. (2013). *ClassMaps consultation: Making schools places where students succeed.* Miniskills presentation. Seattle, WA: National Association of School Psychologists Annual Convention.

Doll, B., Spies, R., & Champion, A. (2012). Contributions of ecological school mental health services to students' academic success. *Journal of Educational and Psychological Consultation, 22*, 44–61. doi:10.1080/10474412.2011.649642.

Doll, B., Spies, R., Champion, A., Guerrero, C., Dooley, K., & Turner, A. (2010). The ClassMaps survey: A measure of students' perceptions of classroom resilience. *Journal of Psychoeducational Assessment, 28*, 338–348. doi:10.1177/0734282910366839.

Doll, B., Spies, R. A., LeClair, C., Kurien, S., & Foley, B. P. (2010). Student perceptions of classroom learning environments: Development of the ClassMaps survey. *School Psychology Review, 39*, 203–218. Retrieved from http://www.nasponline.org

Doll, B., Zucker, S., & Brehm, K. (2004). *Resilient classrooms: Creating healthy environments for learning*. New York: Guilford Press.

Domenech-Rodríguez, M., & Weiling, E. (2004). Developing culturally appropriate, evidence-based treatments for interventions with ethnic minority populations. In M. Rastogin & E. Weiling (Eds.), *Voices of color: First person accounts of ethnic minority therapists* (pp. 313–333). Thousand Oaks, CA: Sage.

Domitrovich, C. E., Bradshaw, C. P., Greenberg, M. T., Embry, D., Poduska, J. M., & Ialongo, N. S. (2010). Integrated models of school-based prevention: Logic and theory. *Psychology in the Schools, 47*(1), 71–88. doi:10.1002/pits.20452.

Domitrovich, C. E., Cortes, R., & Greenberg, M. T. (2001). *Head Start Competence Scale technical report*. Unpublished manuscript, Pennsylvania State University, University Park, PA.

Domitrovich, C. E., Cortes, R., & Greenberg, M. T. (2007). Improving young children's social and emotional competence: A randomized trial of the Preschool PATHS Program. *Journal of Primary Prevention, 28*(2), 67–91. doi:10.1007/s10935-007-0081-0.

Domitrovich, C., Durlak, J., Goren, P., & Weissberg, R. (2013). *Effective social and emotional learning programs: Preschool and elementary school edition*. 2013 CASEL guide. Retrieved from http://casel.org

Domitrovich, C. E., Gest, S. D., Jones, D., Gill, S., & DeRousie, R. M. S. (2010). Implementation quality: Lessons learned in the context of the Head Start REDI trial. *Early Childhood Research Quarterly, 25*(3), 284–298. doi:10.1016/j.ecresq.2010.04.001.

Dotterer, A. M., & Lowe, K. (2011). Classroom context, school engagement, and academic achievement in early adolescence. *Journal of Youth and Adolescence, 40*(12), 1649–1660. doi:10.1007/s10964-011-9647-5.

Dounay, J. (2008). *Beyond the GED: State strategies to help former dropouts earn a high school diploma*. Policy Brief. Denver, CO: Education Commission of the States. Retrieved from http://www.ecs.org/

Dowdy, E., Dever, B. V., DiStephano, C., & Chin, J. K. (2011). Screening for emotional and behavioral risk among students with limited English proficiency. *School Psychology Quarterly, 26*(1), 14–26. doi:10.1037/a0022072.

Dowdy, E., Ritchey, K., & Kampaus, R. W. (2010). School-based screening: A population-based approach to inform and monitor children's mental health needs. *School Mental Health, 2*, 166–176. doi:10.1007/s12310-010-9036-3.

Drabick, D. A., Gadow, K. D., & Sprafkin, J. (2006). Co-occurrence of conduct disorder and depression in a clinic-based sample of boys with ADHD. *Journal of Child Psychology and Psychiatry, 47*(8), 766–774. doi:10.1111/j.1469-7610.2006.01625.x.

Dretzke, J., Davenport, C., Frew, E., Barlow, J., Bayliss, S., Taylor, R. S., et al. (2009). The clinical effectiveness of different parenting programmes for children with conduct problems: A systematic review of randomised controlled trials. *Child and Adolescent Psychiatry and Mental Health, 3*(1), 7. doi:10.1186/1753-2000-3-7.

Driskell, M. M., Dyment, S. J., Mauriello, L. M., Castle, P. H., & Sherman, J. M. (2008). Relationships among multiple behaviors for childhood and adolescent obesity prevention. *Preventive Medicine, 46*, 209–215. doi:10.1016/j.ypmed.2007.07.028.

Duarte, C. S., Bird, H. R., Shrout, P. E., Wu, P., Lewis-Fernandez, R., Shen, S., et al. (2008). Culture and psychiatric symptoms in Puerto Rican children: Longitudinal results from one ethnic group on two contexts. *Journal of Child Psychology and Psychiatry, 49*(5), 563–572. doi:10.1111/j.1469-7610.2007.01863.x.

Dubas, J. S., Lynch, K. B., Galano, J., Geller, S., & Hunt, D. (1998). Preliminary evaluation of a resiliency-based preschool substance abuse and violence prevention project. *Journal of Drug Education, 28*(3), 235–255. Retrieved from http://www.baywood.com

DuBois, D. L., Holloway, B. E., Valentine, J. C., & Cooper, H. (2002). Effectiveness of mentoring programs for youth: A meta-analytic review. *American Journal of Community Psychology, 30*(2), 157–197. doi:10.1023/A:1014628810714.

Duchnowski, A. J., Kutash, K., & Friendman, R. M. (2002). Community-based interventions in a system of care and outcomes framework. In B. J. Burns & K. Hoagwood (Eds.), *Community treatment for youth: Evidence-based interventions for severe emotional and behavioral disorders* (pp. 16–37). New York: Oxford University Press.

Duncan, G. J., Dowsett, C. J., Claessens, A., Magnuson, K., Huston, A. C., Klebanov, P., et al. (2007). School readiness and later achievement. *Developmental Psychology, 43*(6), 1428–1446. doi:10.1037/0012-1649.43.6.1428.

Dunlap, G., Strain, P. S., Fox, L., Carta, J. J., Conroy, M., Smith, B. J., et al. (2006). Prevention and intervention with young children's challenging behavior: Perspectives regarding current knowledge. *Behavioral Disorders, 32*(1), 29–45. Retrieved from http://www.ccbd.net

DuPaul, G. J. (2003). Commentary: Bridging the gap between research and practice. *School Psychology Review, 32*(2), 169–173. Retrieved from http://www.nasponline.org/

Durlak, J. A., Weissberg, R. P., Dymnicki, A. B., Taylor, R. D., & Schellinger, K. B. (2011). The impact of enhancing students' social and emotional learning: A meta-analysis of school-based universal interventions. *Child Development, 82*, 405–432. doi:10.1111/j.1467-8624.2010.01564.x.

Durlak, J. A. (1997). *Successful prevention programs for children and adolescents.* New York: Plenum Press.

Durlak, J. A. (2003). The long-term impact of preschool prevention programs: A commentary. *Prevention & Treatment, 6*(1), Article 32. doi:10.1037/1522-3736.6.1.632c

Durlak, J. A., & Dupre, E. P. (2008). Implementation matters: A review of research on the influence of implementation on program outcomes and the factors affecting implementation. *American Journal of Community Psychology, 41*(3–4), 327–350. doi:10.1007/s10464-008-9165-0.

Durlak, J. A., Dymnicki, A. B., Taylor, R. D., Weissberg, R. P., & Schellinger, K. B. (2011). The impact of enhancing students' social and emotional learning: A meta-analysis of school-based universal interventions. *Child Development, 82*(1), 405–432. doi:10.1111/j.1467-8624.2010.01564.x.

Durlak, J. A., Weissberg, R. P., & Pachan, M. (2010). A meta-analysis of after-school programs that seek to promote personal and social skills in children and adolescents. *American Journal of Community Psychology, 45*, 294–309. doi:10.1007/s10464-010-9300-6.

Durlak, J. A., & Wells, A. M. (1997). Primary prevention mental health programs for children and adolescents: A meta-analytic review. *American Journal of Community Psychology, 25*, 115–152. doi:10.1023/A:1024654026646.

Dusenbury, L., Brannigan, R., Falco, M., & Hansen, W. B. (2003). A review of research on fidelity of implementation: Implications for drug abuse prevention in school settings. *Health Education Research, 18*(2), 237–256. doi:10.1093/her/18.2.237.

Dusenbury, L., & Hansen, W. B. (2004). Pursuing the course from research to practice. *Prevention Science, 5*(1), 55–59. doi:10.1023/B:PREV.0000013982.20860.19.

Dusenbury, L., Zadrazil, J., Mart, A., & Weissberg, R. (2011). *State learning standards to advance social and emotional learning: The CASEL state scan of social and emotional learning standards, preschool through high school.* Chicago: CASEL. Retrieved from http://casel.org/

Dynarski, M., Clarke, L., Cobb, B., Finn, J., Rumberger, R., & Smink, J. (2008). *Dropout prevention: A practice guide* (NCEE 2008-4025). Washington, DC: National Center for the Education Evaluation and Regional Assistance, U.S. Institute of Education Sciences.

Early Childhood Outcomes Center. (2010). *Outcomes for children served through IDEA's early childhood programs: 2010–11.* Washington, DC: Office of Special Education Programs, U.S. Department of Education.

Eastwood, J. D., Frischen, A., Fenske, M. J., & Smilek, D. (2012). The unengaged mind: Defining boredom in terms of attention. *Perspectives on Psychological Science, 7*(5), 482–495. doi:10.1177/1745691612456044.

Eddy, J. J., Gideonsen, M. D., McClafin, R. R., O'Halloran, P., Peardon, F. A., Radcliff, P. L., et al. (2012). Reducing alcohol use in youth aged 12–17 years using the strategic prevention framework. *Journal of Community Psychology, 40*(5), 607–620. doi:10.1002/jcop.21485.

Eddy, M. J., Reid, J. R., & Fetrow, R. A. (2000). An elementary school-based prevention program targeting modifiable antecedents of youth delinquency and violence: Linking the Interests of Families and Teachers (LIFT). *Journal of Emotional and Behavioral Disorders, 8*(3), 165–176. doi:10.1177/106342660000800304.

Eddy, M. J., Reid, J. R., Stoolmiller, M., & Fetrow, R. A. (2003). Outcomes during middle school for an elementary school-based preventive intervention for conduct problems: Follow-up results from a randomized trial. *Behavior Therapy, 34*(4), 535–552. doi:10.1016/S0005-7894(03)80034-5.

Edgar, M., & Call, L. (2010). *Adapting evidence-based programs to meet local needs.* Powerpoint presentation. Illinois Public Health Institute. Retrieved from http://www.iphionline.org/

Edwards, D., Hunt, M. H., Meyers, J., Grogg, K. R., & Jarrett, O. (2005). Acceptability and student outcomes of a violence prevention curriculum. *The Journal of Primary Prevention, 26,* 401–418. doi:10.1007/s10935-005-0002-z.

Egger, J., & Angold, A. (2006). Common emotional and behavioral disorders in preschool children: Presentation, nosology, and epidemiology. *Journal of Child Psychology and Psychiatry, 47*(3/4), 313–337. doi:10.1111/j.1469-7610.2006.01618.x.

Ehrenreich, J. T., Goldstein, C. M., Wright, L. R., & Barlow, D. H. (2009). Development of a unified protocol for the treatment of emotional disorders in youth. *Child and Family Behavior Therapy, 31*(1), 20–37. doi:10.1080/07317100802701228.

Eisenberg, N., Valiente, C., Spinrad, T. L., Cumberland, A., Liew, L., Reisner, M., et al. (2009). Longitudinal relations of children's effortful control, impulsivity, and negative emotionality to their externalizing, internalizing, and co-occurring behavior problems. *Developmental Psychology, 45*(4), 988–1008. doi:10.1037/a0016213.

Elbertson, N. A., Brackett, M. A., & Weissberg, R. P. (2010). School-based social and emotional learning (SEL) programming: Current perspectives. In A. Hargreaves, A. Lieberman, M. Fullan, & D. Hopkins (Eds.), *Second international handbook of educational change* (pp. 1017–1032). New York: Springer. doi:10.1007/978-90-481-2660-6_57.

Elbourne, D., Egger, M., & Altman, D. G. (2010). CONSORT 2010 explanation and elaboration: Updated guidelines for reporting parallel group randomised trials. *British Medical Journal, 340,* c869. doi:10.1136/bmj.c869.

Elder, J. P., Ayala, G. X., & Harris, S. (1999). Theories and intervention approaches to health-behavior change in primary care. *American Journal of Preventive Medicine, 17*(4), 275–284. doi:10.1016/S0749-3797(99)00094-X.

Elder, J. P., Woodruff, S. I., Sallis, J. F., de Moor, C., Edwards, C., & Wildey, M. B. (1994). Effects of health facilitator performance and attendance at training sessions on the acquisition of tobacco refusal skills among multi-ethnic, high-risk adolescents. *Health Education Research, 9*(2), 225–233. doi:10.1093/her/9.2.225.

Elias, M. J. (2011, May 12). *Why should the ESEA systematically include social–emotional and character development as essential for student's academic and life success?* Power point presentation. Presentation at a Congressional Briefing, Senate Office Building, Washington, DC. Retrieved from http://www.nasponline.org/

Elias, M. J. (2012). *Promoting social-emotional and character development is essential for students' academic and life success rationale and best practices.* Invited presentation at the 2012 Annual Conference of the Massachusetts School Psychology Association, Framingham, MA.

Elias, M. J., & Bruene-Butler, L. (2005a). *Social decision making/social problem solving: A curriculum for academic, social, and emotional learning, grades 2–3.* Champaign, IL: Research Press.

Elias, M. J., & Bruene-Butler, L. (2005b). *Social decision making/social problem solving: A curriculum for academic, social, and emotional learning, grades 4–5.* Champaign, IL: Research Press.

Elias, M. J., & Bruene-Butler, L. (2005c). *Social decision making/social problem solving for middle school students: Skills and activities for academic, social, and emotional success.* Champaign, IL: Research Press.

Elias, M. J., Bruene-Butler, L., Blum, L., & Schuyler, T. (1997). How to launch a social and emotional learning program. *Educational Leadership, 54*(8), 15–19. Retrieved from http://www.ascd.org

Elias, M. J., O'Brien, M. U., & Weissberg, R. P. (2006). *Transformative leadership for social-emotional learning.* Washington, DC: National Association of School Psychologists, Students Services. Retrieved from http://www.nasponline.org

Elias, M. J., & Weissberg, R. P. (2000). Primary prevention: Educational approaches to enhancing social and emotional learning. *Journal of School Health, 70*(5), 186–190. doi:10.1111/j.1746-1561.2000.tb06470.x.

Elias, M. J., Zins, J. E., Graczyk, P. A., & Weissberg, P. P. (2003). Implementation sustainability, and scaling up of social emotional and academic innovations in public schools. *School Psychology Review, 32*(3), 303–319. Retrieved from http://www.nasponline.org/

Ellickson, P. L., Bell, R. M., Thomas, M. A., Robyn, A. E., & Zellman, G. L. (1988). *Designing and implementing project ALERT.* Santa Monica, CA: The RAND Corporation.

Elliott, S. N., & Gresham, F. M. (2008). *The SSIS multi-level classwide social skills program, screening, intervention, and evaluation.* Paper presented at the National Association of School Psychologists Annual Convention, New Orleans, LA.

Elliott, S. N., Kratochwill, T. R., & Roach, A. T. (2003). Commentary: Implementing social-emotional and academic innovations: Reflections, reactions, and research. *School Psychology Review, 32*(3), 320–326. Retrieved from http://www.nasponline.org/

Elliott, D. S., & Mihalic, S. (2004). Issues in disseminating and replicating effective prevention programs. *Prevention Science, 5*(1), 47–53. doi:10.1023/B:PREV.0000013981.28071.52.

Ellis, B. J., Bates, J. E., Dodge, K. A., Fergusson, D. M., Horwood, L. J., Pettit, G. S., et al. (2003). Does father absence place daughters at special risk for early sexual activity and teenage pregnancy. *Child Development, 74*(3), 801–821. doi:10.1111/1467-8624.00569.

Ellis, D. A., Zucker, R. A., & Fitzgerald, H. E. (1997). The role of family influences in development and risk. *Alcohol Health and Research World, 21*(3), 218–226. Retrieved from http://www.niaaa.nih.gov

Embry, D. D., Staatemeier, G., Richardson, C., Lauger, K., & Mitich, J. (2003). *The Good Behavior Game* (1st ed.). Center City, MH: Hazelden.

English, B. (1997). Conducting ethical evaluations with disadvantaged and minority target groups. *Evaluation Practice, 18*, 49–54. doi:10.1016/S0886-1633(97)90007-6.

Ennett, S. T., Haws, S., Ringwalt, C. L., Vincus, A. A., Hanley, S., Bowling, J. M., et al. (2011). Evidence-based practice in school substance use prevention: Fidelity of implementation under real-world conditions. *Health Education Research, 26*(2), 361–371. doi:10.1093/her/cyr013.

Ennett, S. T., Ringwalt, C. L., Thorne, J., Rohrbach, L. A., Vincus, A., Simons-Rudolph, A., et al. (2003). A comparison of current practice in school-based substance use prevention programs with meta-analysis findings. *Prevention Science, 4*(1), 1–14. doi:10.1023/A:1021777109369.

Epstein, J. A., Botvin, G. J., Diaz, T., Baker, E., & Botvin, E. M. (1997). Reliability of social and personal competence measures for adolescents. *Psychological Reports, 81*(2), 449–450. doi:10.2466/pr0.1997.81.2.449.

Epstein, J. L., & Van Voorhis, F. L. (2001). More than minutes: Teachers' roles in designing homework. *Educational Psychologist, 36*(3), 181–193. doi:10.1207/S15326985EP3603_4.

Ernst, H., & Colthorpe, K. (2007). The efficacy of interactive lecturing for students with diverse science backgrounds. *Advances in Physiology Education, 31*(1), 41–44. doi:10.1152/advan.00107.2006.

Essau, C. A., Conradt, J., Sasagawa, S., & Ollendick, T. M. (2012). Prevention of anxiety symptoms in children: A universal school-based trial. *Behavior Therapy, 43*(2), 450–464. doi:10.1016/j.beth.2011.08.003.

Estell, D. B., & Perdue, N. H. (2013). Social support and behavioral and affective school engagement: The effect of peers parents, and teachers. *Psychology in the School, 50*(4), 325–339. doi:10.1002/pits.21681.

Evans, D. (2003). Hierarchy of evidence: A framework for ranking evidence evaluating healthcare interventions. *Journal of Clinical Nursing, 12*(1), 77–84. doi:10.1046/j.1365-2702.2003.00662.x.

Evers, K. E., Paiva, A. L., Johnson, J. L., Cummins, C. O., Prochaska, J. O., Prochaska, J. M., et al. (2012). Results of a transtheoretical model-based alcohol, tobacco, and other drug intervention in middle schools. *Addictive Behaviors, 37*, 1009–1018. doi:10.1016/j.addbeh.2012.04.008.

Evers, K. R., Prochaska, J. O., Van Marter, D. F., Johnson, J. L., & Prochaska, J. M. (2007). Transtheoretical-based bullying prevention effectiveness trail in middle and high schools. *Educational Research, 49*(4), 397–414. doi:10.1080/00131880701717271.

Fagan, A. A., & Eisenberg, N. (2012). Latest developments in the prevention of crime and anti-social behaviour: An American perspective. *Journal of Children's Services, 7*(1), 64–72. doi:10.1108/17466661211213689.

Falo-Stewart, W., & Klostermann, K. (2008). Substance use disorders. In J. E. Maddux & B. A. Winstead (Eds.), *Psychology: Foundations for a contemporary understanding* (2nd ed., pp. 327–348). New York: Routledge.

Faris, R., & Felmlee, D. (2011). Status struggles: Network centrality and gender segregation in same- and cross-gender aggression. *American Sociological Review, 76*(1), 48–73. doi:10.1177/0003122410396196.

Farrell, L., & Barrett, P. (2007). Prevention of childhood emotional disorders: Reducing the burden of suffering associated with anxiety and depression. *Journal of Child & Adolescent Mental Health, 12*(2), 58–65. doi:10.1111/j.1475-3588.2006.00430.x.

Farrington, D. P., & Ttofi, M. M. (2009). *School-based programs to reduce bullying and victimization* (updated 2010). Oslo, Norway: Campbell Systematic Reviews. doi:10.4073/csr.2009.6.

Feeney-Kettler, K. A., Kratochwill, T. R., Kaiser, A. P., Hemmeter, M. L., & Kettler, R. J. (2010). Screening young children's risk for mental health problems: A review of four measures. *Assessment for Effective Intervention, 35*(4), 218–230. doi:10.1177/1534508410380557.

Feis, C. L., & Simons, C. (1985). Training preschool children in interpersonal cognitive problem-solving skills: A replication. *Prevention in Human Services, 3*(4), 59–70. doi:10.1300/J293v03n04_07.

Felix, E., & Furlong, M. (2008). Best practices in bullying prevention. In A. Thomas & A. J. Grimes (Eds.), *Best practices in school psychology V* (Vol. 4, pp. 1279–1289). Bethesda, MD: National Association of School Psychologists.

Feng, X., Keenan, K., Hipwell, A. E., Henneberger, A. K., Rischall, M. S., Butch, J., et al. (2009). Longitudinal associations between emotion regulation and depression in preadolescent girls: Moderation by the caregiving environment. *Developmental Psychology, 45*(3), 798–808. doi:10.1037/a0014617.

Ferguson, C. J. (2009). An effect size primer: A guide for clinicians and researchers. *Professional Psychology: Research and Practice, 40*(5), 532–538. doi:10.1037/a0015808.

Ferguson, C. J., Miguel, C. S., Kilburn, J. C., & Sanchez, P. (2007). The effectiveness of school-based anti-bullying programs: A meta-analytic review. *Criminal Justice Review, 32*(4), 401–414. doi:10.1177/0734016807311712.

Finn, J. D., & Zimmer, K. S. (2012). Student engagement: What is it? Why does it matter? In S. L. Christenson, A. L. Reschly, & C. Wylie (Eds.), *Handbook of research on student engagement* (pp. 97–131). New York: Springer.

Finnigan, K., Daly, A., & Che, J. (2012). *The acquisition and use of evidence district-wide.* Paper presented at the Annual Meeting of the American Educational Research Association, Vancouver, Canada.

Firgens, E., & Matthews, H. (2012). *State child care policies for limited English proficient families.* Washington, DC: CLASP. Retrieved from http://www.clasp.org

Firpo-Triplett, R. (2010). *General adaptation guidelines.* ACT for Youth Center of Excellence. CDC-funded Adaptation Guidance Project. Retrieved from http://www.actforyouth.net/

Fisak, B. J., Richard, D., & Mann, A. (2011). The prevention of child and adolescent anxiety: A meta-analytic review. *Prevention Science, 12*(3), 255–268. doi:10.1007/s11121-011-0210-0.

Fishbein, M., & Ajzen, I. (1975). *Belief, attitude, intention, and behavior: An introduction to theory and research.* Reading, MA: Addison-Wesley.

Flannery, K. B., Sugai, G., & Anderson, C. M. (2009). School-Wide Positive Behavior Support in high school: Early lessons learned. *Journal of Positive Behavior Interventions, 11*(3), 177–185. doi:10.1177/1098300708316257.

Flannery-Schroeder, E., Choudhury, M., & Kendall, P. C. (2005). Group and individual cognitive-behavioral treatments for youth with anxiety disorders: One-year follow-up. *Cognitive Therapy and Research, 29*, 253–259. doi:10.1007/s10608-005-3168-z.

Flay, B. R. (2007, October 31). *Levels of evidence in prevention research*. Prepared for IOM/NRC Committee on Prevention of Mental Disorders, Washington, DC. Retrieved from https://www7.nationalacademies.org

Flay, B. R. (2009). The promise of long-term effectiveness of school-based smoking prevention programs: A critical review of reviews. *Tobacco Induced Diseases, 5*(1), 7. doi:10.1186/1617-9625-5-7.

Flay, B. R., Biglan, A., Boruch, R. F., Castro, F. G., Gottfredson, D., Kellam, S., et al. (2005). Standards of evidence: Criteria for efficacy, effectiveness and dissemination. *Prevention Science, 6*(3), 151–175. doi:10.1007/s11121-005-5553-y.

Flay, B. R., Graumlisch, S., Segawa, E., Burns, J. L., Holliday, M. Y., & The Aban Aya Investigators. (2004). Effects of 2 prevention programs on high-risk behaviors among African American youth: A randomized trial. *Archives of Pediatrics & Adolescent Medicine, 158*(4), 377–384. doi:10.1001/archpedi.158.4.377.

Flay, B., & Slagel, M. (2006). *The Positive Action family program: A pilot randomized trial*. Unpublished manuscript. Retrieved from http://www.positiveaction.net

Flores, N., & Sugai, G. (2011). *SWPBS & cultural relevance*. Paper presented at the 2011 National Implementer's Forum, Rosemont, IL.

Fonagy, P., Twemlow, S. W., Verbberg, E. M., Nelson, J. M., Dill, E. D., Little, T. D., et al. (2009). A cluster randomized controlled trial of child-focused psychiatric consultation and a school systems-focused intervention to reduce aggression. *Journal of Child Psychology and Psychiatry, 50*(5), 607–616. doi:10.1111/j.1469-7610.2008.02025.x.

Ford, J. D., & Ford, L. W. (2010). Stop blaming resistance to change and start using it. *Organizational Dynamics, 39*(1), 24–36. doi:10.1016/j.orgdyn.2009.10.002.

Ford, J. D., Ford, L. W., & D'Amelio, A. (2008). Resistance to change: The rest of the story. *Academy of Management Review, 33*(2), 362–377. Retrieved from http://aom.org

Forman, S. G., Olin, S. S., Hoagwood, K. E., Crowe, M., & Saka, N. (2009). Evidence-based interventions in schools: Developer's views of implementation barriers and facilitators. *School Mental Health, 1*(1), 26–36. doi:10.1007/s12310-008-9002-5.

Forness, S. R. (2003). Barriers to evidence-based treatment: Developmental psychopathology ad the interdisciplinary disconnect in school mental health practice. *Journal of School Psychology, 41*(1), 61–67. doi:10.1016/S0022-4405(02)00144-9.

Fox, L., Dunlap, G., Hemmetter, M. L., Hoseph, G., & Strain, P. (2003). The teaching pyramid: A model for supporting social competence and preventing challenging behavior in young children. *Infants and Children, 58*(4), 48–52. doi:10.1002/cbl.20134.

Fox, L., & Hemmeter, M. L. (2009). A program-wide model for supporting social emotional development and addressing challenging behavior in early childhood settings. In W. Sailor, G. Dunlap, G. Sugai, & R. Horner (Eds.), *Handbook of positive behavior support* (pp. 177–202). New York: Springer.

Fox, L., Jack, S., & Broyles, L. (2005). *Program-wide positive behavior support: Supporting young children's social-emotional development and addressing challenging behavior*. Tampa, FL: University of South Florida de la Parte, Florida Mental Health Institute.

Fram, M. S., & Kim, J. (2008). Race/ethnicity and the start of child care: A multi-level analysis of factors influencing first child care experiences. *Early Childhood Research Quarterly, 23*(4), 575–590. doi:10.1016/j.ecresq.2008.04.002.

Franklin, C. G., Kim, J. S., Ryan, T. N., Kelly, M. S., & Mongomery, K. L. (2012). Teacher involvement in school mental health interventions: A systematic review. *Children and Youth Services Review, 34*, 973–982. doi:10.1016/j.childyouth/2012.01.027.

Frazier, A. M., & Chester, P. A. (2009). Culturally and linguistically diverse populations: Serving GLBT families in our schools. *Perspectives on communication disorders and sciences in culturally and linguistically diverse populations*. doi:10.1044/cds16.1.11. Retrieved from http://div14perspectives.asha.org

Fredricks, J. A., Blumenfeld, P. C., & Paris, A. H. (2004). School engagement: Potential of the concept, state of evidence. *Review of Educational Research, 74*(1), 59–109. doi:10.3102/00346543074001059.

Fredricks, J., & McColskey, W. (2011). *Measuring student engagement in upper elementary through high school: A description of 21 instruments* (Issues & Answers Report, REL 2011-No. 098). Washington, DC: U.S. Department of Education, Institute of Educational Sciences, National Center for Education Evaluation and Regional Assistance, Regional Educational Laboratory Southeast. Retrieved from http//ies.ed.gov/ncee/edlabs

French, S. D., Green, S. E., O'Connor, D. A., McKenzie, J. E., Francis, J. J., Michie, S., et al. (2012). Developing theory informed behavior change interventions to implement evidence into practice: A systematic approach using the theoretical domains framework. *Implementation Science, 7*, 38. doi:10.1186/1748-5908-7-38.

Frey, K. S., Hirschstein, M. K., & Guzzo, B. A. (2000). Second Step: Preventing aggression by promoting social competence. *Journal of Emotional and Behavioral Disorders, 8*(2), 102–112. doi:10.1177/106342660000800206.

Frey, K. S., Nolen, S. B., Van Schoiack, E. L., & Hirschstein, M. K. (2005). Effects of a school-based social-emotional competence program: Linking children's goals, attributions and behavior. *Journal of Applied Developmental Psychology, 26*(2), 171–200. doi:10.1016/j.appdev.2004.12.002.

Frey, A. J., Park, K. L., Browne-Ferrigno, T., & Korfhage, T. L. (2010). The social validity of program-wide Positive Behavior Support. *Journal of Positive Behavior Interventions, 12*(4), 222–235. doi:10.1177/1098300709343723.

Froelich, J., Doepfner, M., & Lehmkuhl, G. (2002). Effects of combined cognitive behavioural treatment with parent management training in ADHD. *Behavioural and Cognitive Psychotherapy, 30*, 111–115. doi:10.1017/S1352465802001108.

Fullan, M. (1996). Professional culture and educational change. *School Psychology Review, 25*(4), 496–500. Retrieved from http://www.nasponline.org

Fullan, M. (2006). *Change theory: A force for school improvement*. Jolimont, VIC: CSE Centre for Strategic Education.

Fuller, B., & Coll, C. G. (2010). Learning from Latinos: Contexts, families, and child development in motion. *Developmental Psychology, 46*(3), 559–565. doi:10.1037/a0019412.

Furman, R., Negi, N. J., Iwamoto, D. K., Rowan, D., Shukraft, A., & Gragg, J. (2010). Social work practice with Latinos: Key issues for school workers. *Social Work, 54*(2), 167–174. doi:10.1093/sw/54.2.167.

Furr-Holden, C. D., Milam, A. J., Reynolds, E. K., MacPherso, L., & Lejuez, C. W. (2012). Disordered neighborhood environments and risk-taking propensity in late childhood through adolescence. *Journal of Adolescent Health, 50*, 100–102. doi:10.1016/j.jadohealth.2011,04.008.

Galambos, N. L., Leadbeater, B. J., & Barker, E. T. (2004). Gender differences in and risk factors for depression in adolescence: A 4-year longitudinal study. *International Journal of Behavioral Development, 28*(1), 16–25. doi:10.1080/01650250344000235.

Gallerani, C. M., Garber, J., & Martin, N. C. (2010). The temporal relation between depression and comorbid psychopathology in adolescents at varied risk for depression. *Journal of Child Psychology and Psychiatry, 51*(3), 242–249. doi:10.1111/j.1469-7610.2009.02155.x.

Gangwisch, J. E., Babiss, L. A., Malaspina, D., Turner, J. B., Zammit, G. K., & Posner, K. (2010). Earlier parental set bedtimes as a protective factor against depression and suicidal ideation. *Sleep, 33*(1). Retrieved from http://www.journalsleep.org

Garber, J. (2006). Depression in children and adolescents: Linking risk research and prevention. *American Journal of Preventive Medicine, 31*, S104–S125. doi:10.1016/j.amepre.2006.07.007.

Garber, J., Clarke, G. N., Weersing, V. R., Beardslee, W. R., Brent, D. A., Gladstone, T. R., et al. (2009). Prevention of depression in at-risk adolescents: A randomized controlled trial. *Journal of the American Medical Association, 301*(21), 2215–2224. doi:10.1001/jama.2009.788.

Garcia-Dominic, O., Wray, L. A., Treviño, R. P., Hernandez, A. E., Yin, Z., & Ulbrecht, J. S. (2010). Identifying barriers that hinder onsite parental involvement in a school-based health promotion program. *Health Promotion Practice, 11*(5), 703–713. doi:10.1177/1524839909331909.

Garg, A. X., Hackam, D., & Tonelli, M. (2008). Systematic review and meta-analysis: When one study is just not enough. *Clinical Journal of the American Society of Nephrology, 3*(1), 253–260. doi:10.2215/CJN.01430307.

Garrison, C., Jeung, B., & Inclan-Rodriguez, R. (Eds.). (2009). Making graduation a priority. *Trends: Issues in Urban Education, 26*, 1–5. Washington, DC: National Education Association.

Gavin, A. R., Chae, D. H., Alegria, M., Jackson, J. S., & Takeuchi, D. (2010). The associations between socio-economic status and major depressive disorder among Blacks, Latinos, Asians, and non-Hispanic Whites: Findings from the Collaborative Psychiatric Epidemiology Studies. *Psychological Medicine, 40*(1), 51–61. doi:10.1017/S0033291709006023.

Gee, G. C., Ro, A., Shariff-Marco, S., & Chae, D. (2009). Racial discrimination and health among Asian Americans: Evidence, assessment, and directions for future research. *Epidemiologic Reviews, 31*(1), 130–151. doi:10.1093/epirev/mxp009.

Geller, S. (1999). *Al's pals: Kids making healthy choices*. Richmond, VA: Wingspan, LLC.

George, H. P., & Kincaid, D. K. (2008). Building district-level capacity for Positive Behavior Support. *Journal of Positive Behavior Interventions, 10*(1), 20–32. doi:10.1177/1098300707311367.

Gielen, A. C., McDonald, E. M., Gary, T. L., & Bone, L. R. (2008). Using the precede-proceed model to apply health behavior theories. In K. Glanz, B. K. Rimer, & K. Viswanath (Eds.), *Health behavior and health education: Theory, research, and practice* (4th ed., pp. 407–433). San Francisco: Jossey-Bass.

Gillen-O'Neel, C., Ruble, D. N., & Fuligni, A. J. (2011). Ethnic stigma, academic anxiety, and intrinsic motivation in middle childhood. *Child Development, 82*(5), 1470–1485. doi:10.1111/j.1467-8624.2011.01621.x.

Gillham, J. E. (1994). Preventing depressive symptoms in school children. *Dissertation Abstracts International: Section B. Sciences and Engineering, 55*.

Gillham, J., & Reivich, K. (2004). Cultivating optimism in childhood and adolescence. *The Annals of the American Academy of Political and Social Science, 591*(1), 146–163. doi:10.1177/0002716203260095.

Gillham, J. E., Reivich, K. J., Freres, D. R., Chaplin, T. M., Shatté, A. J., Samuels, B., et al. (2007). School-based prevention of depressive symptoms: A randomized controlled study of the effectiveness and specificity of the Penn Resiliency Program. *Journal of Consulting and Clinical Psychology, 75*(1), 9–19. doi:10.1037/0022-006X.75.1.9.

Gilliam, W. S. (2008). *Implementing policies to reduce the likelihood of preschool expulsion*. FCD Policy Brief No. Seven. Foundation for Child Development. Retrieved from http://medicine.yale.edu

Gini, G., & Pozzoli, T. (2009). Association between bullying and psychosomatic problems: A meta-analysis. *Pediatrics, 123*(3), 1059–1065. doi:10.1542/peds.2008-1215.

Gini, G., Pozzoli, T., & Hauser, M. (2011). Bullies have enhanced moral competence to judge relative to victims, but lack moral compassion. *Personality and Individual Differences, 50*(5), 603–608. doi:10.1016/j.paid.2010.12.002.

Ginsburg, G. S., Becker, K. D., Kingery, J. N., & Nichols, T. (2008). Transporting CBT for childhood anxiety disorders into inner-city school-based mental health clinics. *Cognitive and Behavioral Practice, 15*(2), 148–158. doi:10.1016/j.cbpra.2007.07.001.

Ginsburg, G. S., & Drake, K. L. (2002). School-based treatment for anxious African-American adolescents: A controlled pilot study. *Journal of the American Academy of Child and Adolescent Psychiatry, 41*(7), 768–775. doi:10.1097/00004583-200207000-00007.

Ginsburg, G. S., Kimberly, D., Becker, K. D., Drazdowski, T. K., & Tein, J. (2012). Treating anxiety disorders in inner city schools: Results from a pilot randomized controlled trial comparing CBT and usual care. *Child and Youth Care Forum, 42*(1), 1–19. doi:10.1007/s10566-011-9156-4.

Glanville, J. M., Lefebvre, C., Miles, J. N., & Camosso-Stefinovic, J. (2006). How to identify randomized controlled trials in MEDLINE: Ten years on. *Journal of the Medical Library Association, 94*(2), 130–136. Retrieved from http://www.mlanet.org

Glanz, K., & Rimer, B. K. (2008). Perspectives on using theory: Past, present, and future. In K. Glanz, B. K. Rimer, & K. Viswanath (Eds.), *Health behavior and health education: Theory, research, and practice* (4th ed., pp. 509–518). San Francisco: Jossey-Bass.

Glanz, K., Rimer, B. K., & Viswanath, K. (2008). Theory, research, and practice in health behavior and health education. In K. Glanz, B. K. Rimer, & K. Viswanath (Eds.), *Health behavior and health education: Theory, research, and practice* (4th ed., pp. 23–38). San Francisco: Jossey-Bass.

Glor, E. D. (2007). Identifying organizations fit for change. *The Innovation Journal: The Public Sector Innovation Journal, 12*(1), Article 5. Retrieved from http://www.innovation.cc

Glover, A., & Dent, E. B. (2005). *Conceptualizing ethnicity, justice, and resistance during organizational change.* Lecture notes. Retrieved from http://www.learningace.com

Golden, S. D., & Earp, J. A. (2012). Social ecological approaches to individuals and their contexts: Twenty years of health education & behavior health promotion interventions. *Health Education & Behavior, 39*(3), 364–372. doi:10.1177/1090198111418634.

Goldratt, E. M. (1990). *What is this thing called Theory of Constraints?* Croton-on-Hudson, NY: North River Press.

Goldstein, M. J., & Noguera, P. A. (2006). Designing for diversity: Incorporating cultural competence in prevention programs for urban youth. *New Directions for Youth Development, 111*, 29–40. doi:10.1002/yd.180.

Goodkind, J. R., Lanoue, M. D., & Milford, J. (2010). Adaptation and implementation of cognitive behavioral intervention for trauma in schools with American Indian youth. *Journal of Clinical Child and Adolescent Psychology, 39*(6), 858–872. doi:10.1080/15374416.2010.517166.

Gordon, R. (1987). An operational classification of disease prevention. In J. A. Steinberg & M. M. Silverman (Eds.), *Preventing mental disorders.* Rockville, MD: U.S. Department of Health and Human Services.

Gordon, R., Ji, P., Mulhall, P., Shaw, B., & Weissberg, R. P. (2011). *Social and emotional learning for Illinois students: Policy, practice and progress. The Illinois report 2011* (pp. 69–83). Urbana, IL: The Institute of Government and Public Affairs.

Gore, F. M., Bloem, P. J., Patton, G. C., Ferguson, J., Joseph, V., Coffey, C., et al. (2011). The global burden of disease in young people aged 10–24 years: A systematic analysis. *The Lancet, 377*(9783), 2093–2102. doi:10.1016/S0140-6736(11)60512-6.

Gorman, J. M. (1996). Comorbid depression and anxiety spectrum disorders. *Depression and Anxiety, 4*(4), 160–168. doi:10.1002/(SICI)1520-6394(1996)4:4<160::AID-DA2>3.0.CO;2-J.

Gortmaker, S. L., Peterson, K., Wiecha, J., Sobol, A. M., Dixit, S., Fox, M. K., et al. (2011). Reducing obesity via a school-based interdisciplinary intervention among youth. *Archives of Pediatrics & Adolescent Medicine, 153*(4), 409–418. doi:10.1001/archpedi.153.4.409.

Gottfredson, D. C., Cross, A., Wilson, D., Rorie, M., & Connell, N. (2010). An experimental evaluation of the All Stars prevention curriculum in a community after school setting. *Prevention Science, 11*(2), 142–154. doi:10.1007/s11121-009-0156-7.

Grabe, S., Hyde, J. S., & Lindberg, S. M. (2007). Body objectification and depression in adolescents: The role of gender, shame, and rumination. *Psychology of Women Quarterly, 31*(2), 164–175. doi:10.1111/j.1471-6402.2007.00350.x.

GRADE Working Group. (2004). Grading quality of evidence and strength of recommendations. *British Medical Journal, 328*(7454), 1490. doi:10.1136/bmj.328.7454.1490.

Graham, J. (1999). *It's up to us: Giraffe Heroes Program for high school.* Langley, WA: Giraffe Project.

Granberg, E. M., Simons, R. L., Gibbons, F. J., & Melby, J. N. (2008). The relationship between body size and depressed mood: Findings from a sample of African American middle school girls. *Youth Society, 39*(3), 294–315. doi:10.1177/0044118X07301952.

Gray, M. (1996). *Evidence-based healthcare.* London: Churchill Livingstone.

Green, L. W., Kreuter, M. W., Deeds, S. G., & Partridge, K. B. (1980). *Health education planning: A diagnostic approach.* Mountain View, CA: Mayfield.

Greenberg, M. T., Domitrovich, C., & Bumbarger, B. (2000). *Preventing mental disorder in school-aged children: A review of the effectiveness of prevention programs.* Washington, DC: U.S. Department of Health and Human Services.

Greenberg, M. T., Domitrovich, C. E., & Bumbarger, B. (2001). The prevention of mental disorders in school-aged children: Current state of the field. *Prevention & Treatment, 4*(1), 1–59. doi:10.1037/1522-3736.4.1.41a.

Greenberg, M. T., & Kusche, C. A. (1998). *Promoting Alternative Thinking Strategies.* Boulder, CO: Institute of Behavioral Sciences, University of Colorado.

Greenberg, M. T., Weissberg, R. P., O'Brien, M. U., Zins, J. E., Fredericks, L., Resnik, H., et al. (2003). Enhancing school-based prevention and youth development through coordinated social, emotional, and academic learning. *American Psychologist, 58*(6/7), 466–474. doi:10.1037/0003-066X.58.6-7.466.

Greenwood, C. R. (2009). Treatment integrity: Revisiting some big ideas. *School Psychology Review, 38*(4), 547–553. Retrieved from http://www.nasponline.org/

Greenwood, C. R., & Kim, J. M. (2012). Response to intervention (RTI) services: An ecobehavioral perspective. *Journal of Educational and Psychological Consultation, 22*, 79–105. doi:10.1080/10474412.2011.649648.

Greenwood, P. W., Welsh, B. C., & Rocque, M. (2012). *Implementing proven programs for juvenile offenders: Assessing state progress*. Association for the Advancement of Evidence-Based Practice.

Gregory, A., Skiba, R. J., & Noguera, P. A. (2010). The achievement gap and the discipline gap: Two sides of the same coin? *Educational Researcher, 39*(1), 59–68. doi:10.3102/0013189X09357621.

Gresham, F. M. (2009). Evolution of the treatment integrity concept: Current status and future directions. *School Psychology Review, 38*(4), 533–540. Retrieved from http://www.nasponline.org/

Gresham, F. M., & Elliott, S. N. (2008). *Social skills rating scales*. Minneapolis, MN: NCD Pearson.

Griffiths, A., Lilles, E., Furlong, M. J., & Sidhwa, J. (2012). In S. L. Christenson, A. L. Reschly, & C. Wylie (Eds.), *Handbook of research on student engagement* (pp. 563–584). New York: Springer.

Grimes, J., & Tilly, W. D., III. (1996). Policy and process: Means to lasting educational change. *School Psychology Review, 25*(4), 465–476. Retrieved from http://www.nasponline.org

Griner, D., & Smith, T. B. (2006). Culturally adapted mental health intervention: A meta-analytic review. *Psychotherapy: Theory, Research, Practice, Training, 43*(4), 531–548. doi:10.1037/0033-3204.43.4.531.

Grossman, D. C., Neckerman, H. J., Koepsell, T. D., Liu, P. Y., Asher, K. N., Beland, K., et al. (1997). Effectiveness of a violence prevention curriculum among children in elementary school: A randomized controlled trial. *Journal of the American Medical Association, 277*(20), 1605–1611. doi:10.1001/jama.1997.03540440039030.

Grover, R. L., Ginsburg, G. S., & Ialongo, N. (2006). Psychosocial outcomes of anxious first graders: A seven-year follow-up. *Depression and Anxiety, 24*(6), 410–420. doi:10.1002/da.20241.

Guarnaccia, P. J., Martinez, I., Ramirez, R., & Canino, G. (2005). Are ataques de nervious in Puerto Rican children associate with psychiatric disorder? *Journal of the American Academy of Child and Adolescent Psychiatry, 44*(11), 1184–1192. doi:10.1097/01.chi.0000177059.34031.5d.

Guerra, N. G., & Williams, K. R. (2010). Implementing bullying prevention in diverse settings: Geographic, economic, and cultural influences. In E. M. Vernberg & B. K. Biggs (Eds.), *Preventing and treating bullying and victimization* (pp. 319–336). New York: Oxford University Press.

Guerra, N. G., Williams, K. R., & Sadek, S. (2011). Understanding bullying and victimization during childhood and adolescence: A mixed methods study. *Child Development, 82*(1), 295–310. doi:10.1111/j.1467-8624.2010.01556.x.

Guerrero, C., & Leung, B. (2008). Communicating effectively with culturally and linguistically diverse families. *Communiqué, 36*(8), 19. Retrieved from http://www.nasponline.org/

Gugiu, P. C., & Rodriguez-Campos, L. (2007). Semi-structured interview protocol for constructing logic models. *Evaluation and Program Planning, 30*, 339–350. doi:10.1016/j.evalprogplan.2007.08.004.

Gunter, L., Caldarella, P., Korth, B. B., & Young, K. R. (2012). Promoting social and emotional learning in preschool students: Study of *Strong Start Pre-K*. *Early Childhood Education Journal, 40*, 151–159. doi:10.1007/s10643-012-0507-z.

Gustafson, D. H., Sainfort, F., Eichler, M., Adams, L., Bisognano, M., & Steudel, H. (2003). Developing and testing a model to predict outcomes of organizational change. *Health Services Research, 38*(2), 751–776. doi:10.1111/1475-6773.00143.

Gutkin, T. B. (2012). Ecological psychology: Replacing the medical model paradigm for school-based psychological and psychoeducational services. *Journal of Educational and Psychological Consultation, 22*, 1–20. doi:10.1080/10474412.2011.649652.

Guttmannova, K., Szanyi, J. M., & Cali, P. W. (2007). Internalizing and externalizing behavior problem scores: Cross-ethnic and longitudinal measurement invariance of the Behavior Problem Index. *Educational and Psychological Measurement, 68*(4), 676–694. doi:10.1177/0013164407310127.

Hadorn, D. C., Baker, D., Hodges, J. S., & Hicks, N. (1996). Rating the quality of evidence for clinical practice guidelines. *Journal of Clinical Epidemiology, 49*(7), 749–754. doi:10.1016/0895-4356(96)00019-4.

Hage, S. M., & Romano, J. L. (2010). History of prevention and prevention groups: Legacy for the 21st century. *Group Dynamics: Theory, Research and Practice, 14*(3), 199–210. doi:10.1037/a0020736.

Haggerty, K. P., MacKenzie, E. P., Skinner, M. L., Harachi, T. W., & Catalano, R. F. (2006). Participation in 'Parents Who Care': Predicting program initiation and exposure in two different program formats. *Journal of Primary Prevention, 27*(1), 47–65. doi:10.1007/s10935-005-0019-3.

Haggerty, K. P., Skinner, M. L., MacKenzie, E. P., & Catalano, R. F. (2007). A randomized trial of Parents Who Care: Outcomes at 24-month follow-up. *Prevention Science, 8*(4), 249–260. doi:10.1007/s11121-007-0077-2.

Hahn, R., Fuqua-Whitley, D., Wethington, H., Lowy, J., Crosby, A., Fullilove, M., et al. (2007). Effectiveness of universal school-based programs to prevent violent and aggressive behavior: A systematic review. *American Journal of Preventive Medicine, 33*(2S), S114–S129. doi:10.1016/j.amepre.2007.04.012.

Hahn, E. J., Noland, M. P., Rayens, M. K., & Christie, D. M. (2002). Efficacy of training and fidelity of implementation of the Life Skills Training Program. *Journal of School Health, 72*(7), 282–287. doi:10.1111/j.1746-1561.2002.tb01333.x.

Hahn-Smith, S., & Springer, F. (2005). Social norms theory. *Prevention Tactics, 8*(9), 1–6. Retrieved from http://www.cars-rp.org

Hale, W., Raaijmakers, Q., Muris, P., van Hoof, A., & Meeus, W. (2008). Developmental trajectories of adolescent anxiety disorder symptoms: A 5-year prospective community study. *Journal of the American Academy of Child & Adolescent Psychiatry, 47*(5), 556–564. doi: 10.1097/CHI.0b013e3181676583.

Hale, W. W., Raaijmakers, Q., Muris, P., van Hoof, A., & Meeus, W. (2009). One factor or two parallel processes? Comorbidity and development of adolescent anxiety and depressive disorder symptoms. *Journal of Child Psychology and Psychiatry, 50*(10), 1218–1226. doi:10.1111/j.1469-7610.2009.02115.x.

Halifors, D., & Godette, D. (2002). Will the 'principles of effectiveness' improve prevention practice? Early findings from a diffusion study. *Health Education Research, 17*(4), 461–470. doi:10.1093/her/17.4.461.

Hall, D. M., Cassidy, E. F., & Stevenson, H. C. (2008). Acting "tough" in a "tough" world: An examination of fear among urban African American adolescents. *Journal of Black Psychology, 34*(3), 381–398. doi:10.1177/0095798408314140.

Hammen, C. (2009). Adolescent depression: Stressful interpersonal contexts and risk for recurrence. *Current Directions in Psychological Science, 18*(4), 200–204. doi:10.1111/j.1467-8721.2009.01636.x.

Hammond, C. (2007). *Dropout risk factors and exemplary programs: A technical report.* Clemson, SC: National Dropout Prevention Center. Retrieved from http://www.doe.virginia.gov/support/prevention/dropout_truancy/resourc es/dropout_risk_factors.pdf

Han, S. S., & Weiss, B. (2005). Sustainability of teacher implementation of school-based mental health programs. *Journal of Abnormal Child Psychology, 33*(6), 665–679. doi:10.1007/s10802-005-7646-2.

Hankin, B. L., & Abramson, L. Y. (2001). Development of gender differences in depression: An elaborated cognitive vulnerability-transactional stress theory. *Psychological Bulletin, 127*(6), 773–796. doi:10.1037/0033-2909.127.6.773.

Hanley, S., Ringwalt, C., Ennett, S. T., Vincus, A. A., Bowling, J. M., Haws, S. W., et al. (2010). The prevalence of evidence-based substance use prevention curricula in the nation's elementary schools. *Journal of Drug Education, 40*(1), 51–60. Retrieved from http://www.baywood.com

Hansen, W. B. (1996). Pilot test results comparing the All Stars program with seventh grade D.A.R.E.: Program integrity and mediating variable analysis. *Substance Use and Misuse, 31*(10), 1359–1377. Retrieved from http://informahealthcare.com

Harachi, T. W., Catalano, R. F., Kim, S., & Choim, Y. (2001). Etiology and prevention of substance use among Asian American youth. *Prevention Science, 2*(1), 57–65. doi:10.1023/A:1010039012978.

Harden, B. J., Sandstrom, H., & Chazan-Cohen, R. (2012). Early Head Start and African American families: Impacts and mechanisms of child outcomes. *Early Childhood Research Quarterly, 27*(4), 572–581. doi:10.1016/j.ecresq.2012.07. 006.

Hargreaves, M. B. (2010). *Evaluating system change: A planning guide.* Princeton, NJ: Mathematica Policy Research.

Harlacher, J. E. (2008). *Social and emotional learning as a universal level of support: Evaluating the follow-up effects of Strong Kids on social and emotional outcomes.* Unpublished doctoral dissertation, University of Oregon, Eugene, OR.

Harris, E. (2005). An introduction to theory of change. *The Evaluation Exchange, 11*(2). Retrieved from http://www.hfrp.org

Harris, A. D., McGregor, J. C., Perencevich, E. N., Furuno, J. P., Zhu, J., Peterson, D. E., et al. (2006). The use and interpretation of quasi-experimental studies in medical informatics. *Journal of the American Medical Informatics Association, 13*(1), 16–23. doi:10.1197/jamia. M1749.

Harrist, A. W., & Bradley, K. D. (2003). "You can't say you can't play": Intervening in the process of social exclusion in the kindergarten classroom. *Early Childhood Research Quarterly, 19*, 185–205. doi:10.1016/so885-2006(03)00024-3.

Harthun, M. L., Dustman, P. A., Reeves, L. J., Hecht, M. L., & Marsiglia, F. F. (2008). Culture in the classroom: Developing teacher proficiency in delivering a culturally-grounded prevention curriculum. *Journal of Primary Prevention, 29*(5), 435–454. doi:10.1007/s10935-008-0150-z.

Hawkins, J. D., Catalano, R. F., Morrison, D. M., O'Donnell, J., Abbott, R. D., & Day, L. E. (1992). The Seattle Social Development Project: Effects of the first four years on protective factors and problem behaviors. In J. McCord & R. E. Tremblay (Eds.), *Preventing antisocial behavior: Interventions from birth through adolescence* (pp. 139–161). New York: Guilford Press.

Hawkins, J. D., Kosterman, R., Catalano, R. F., Hill, K. G., & Abbott, R. D. (2005). Promoting positive adult functioning through social development intervention in childhood: Long-term effects from the Seattle Social Development Project. *Archives of Pediatrics & Adolescent Medicine, 159*(1), 25–31. doi:10.1001/archpedi.159.1.25.

Hawkins, J. D., Kosterman, R., Catalano, R. F., Hill, K. G., & Abbott, R. D. (2008). Effects of social development intervention in childhood 15 years later. *Archives of Pediatrics & Adolescent Medicine, 162*(12), 1133–1141. doi:10.1001/archpedi.162.12.1133.

Hawkins, J. D., Oesterle, S., Brown, E. C., Arthur, M. W., Abbott, R. D., Fagan, A. A., et al. (2009). Results of a type w translations research trial to prevent adolescent drug use and delinquency: A test of communities that care. *Archives of Pediatrics & Adolescent Medicine, 163*(9), 789–798. doi:10.1001/archpediatrics.2009.141.

Hawkins, J. D., Von Cleve, E., & Catalano, R. F., Jr. (1991). Reducing early childhood aggression: Results of a primary prevention program. *Journal of the American Academy of Child and Adolescent Psychiatry, 30*(2), 208–217. doi:10.1097/00004583-199103000-00008.

Hayes, H., Parchman, M. L., & Howard, R. (2011). A logic model for evaluation and planning in a primary care practice-based research network (PBRN). *Journal of the American Board of Family Medicine, 24*(5), 576–582. doi:10.3122/jabfm.2011.05.110043.

Heary, C. M., & Hennessy, E. (2002). The use of focus group interviews in pediatric health care research. *Journal of Pediatric Psychology, 27*(1), 47–57. doi:10.1093/jpepsy/27.1.47.

Hecht, M. L., Marsiglia, F. F., Elek, E., Wagstaff, D. A., Kulis, S., Dustman, P., et al. (2003). Culturally-grounded substance use prevention: An evaluation of the keepin' it R.E.A.L. curriculum. *Prevention Science, 4*, 233–248. doi:10.1080/00909882.2010.490848.

Heckman, J. J., Moon, S. H., Pinto, R., Savelyev, P. A., & Yavitz, A. Q. (2010). The rate of return to the HIghScope Perry Preschool Program. *Journal of Public Economics, 94*(1–2), 114–128. doi:10.1016/j.jpubeco.2009.11.001.

Heckman, J. J., Moon, S. H., Pinto, R., Savelyev, P. A., & Yavitz, A. Q. (2011). *Inference with imperfect randomization: The case of the Perry Preschool Program*. Cambridge, MA: National Bureau of Economic Research. Retrieved from http://jenni.uchicago.edu

Hemmeter, M. L., Fox, L., Jack, S., Broyles, L., & Doubet, S. (2007). A program-wide model of positive behavior support in early childhood settings. *Journal of Early Intervention, 29*, 337–355. doi:10.1177/105381510702900405.

Henderson, M., Ecob, R., Wight, D., & Abraham, C. (2008). What explains between-school differences in rates of smoking? *BMC Public Health, 8*, 218. doi:10.1186/1471-2458-8-218.

Henderson, A. T., & Mapp, K. L. (2002). *A new wave of evidence: The impact of school, family, and community connections on student achievement*. Austin, TX: Southwest Educational Development Laboratory.

Henderson, J., & Strain, P. (2009). *Screening for social emotional concerns: Considerations in the selection of instruments*. Tampa, FL: Technical Assistance Center on Social Emotional Intervention for Young Children, University of South Florida.

Hendricks, C. O. (2005). The multicultural triangle of the child, the family, and the school: Culturally competent approaches. In E. P. Congress & M. J. Gonzalz (Eds.), *Multicultural perspectives in working with families* (2nd ed., pp. 71–92). New York: Springer.

Hendy, J., & Barlow, J. (2012). The role of the organizational champion in achieving health system change. *Social Science & Medicine, 74*(3), 348–355. doi:10.1016/j.socscimed2011.02.009.

Herman, K. C., Borden, L. A., Reinke, W. M., & Webster-Stratton, C. (2011). The impact of the Incredible Years parent, child, and teacher training programs on children's co-occurring internalizing symptoms. *School Psychology Quarterly, 26*(3), 189–201. doi:10.1037/a0025228.

Hernandez, D., Denton, N. A., & Blanchard, V. L. (2011). Children in the United States of America: A statistical portrait by race-ethnicity, immigrant origins, and language. *The Annals of the American Academy of Political and Social Science, 633*(1), 102–127. doi:10.1177/0002716210383205.

Hesseler, D., & Katz, L. F. (2010). Brief report: Associations between emotional competence and adolescent risky behavior. *Journal of Adolescence, 33*(1), 241–246. doi:10.1016/j.adolescence.2009.04.007.

Hill, A. L., Degnan, K. A., Calkins, S. D., & Keane, S. P. (2006). Profiles of externalizing behavior problems for boys and girls across preschool: The roles of emotion regulation and inattention. *Developmental Psychology, 42*(5), 913–928. doi:10.1037/0012-1649.42.5.913.

Hilt-Panahon, A., Kern, L., Divatia, A., & Gresham, F. (2007). School-based interventions for students with or at risk for depression: A review of the literature. *Advances in School Mental Health Promotion, 1*, 32–41. doi:10.1080/1754730X.2008.9715743.

Hinde, E. R. (2004). School culture and change: An examination of the effects of school culture on the process of change. *Essays in Education, 12*. Retrieved from http://www.usca.edu

Hipwell, A. E., Stepp, S., Feng, X., Burke, J., Battista, D. R., Loeber, R., et al. (2011). Impact of oppositional defiant disorder dimensions on the temporal ordering of conduct problems and depression across childhood and adolescence in girls. *Journal of Child Psychology and Psychiatry, 52*(10), 1099–1108. doi:10.1111/j.1469-7610.2011.02448.x.

Hirshfeld-Becker, D. R., Micco, J., Henin, A., Bloomfield, A., Biederman, J., & Rosenbaum, J. (2008). Behavioral inhibition. *Depression and Anxiety, 25*(4), 357–367. doi:10.1002/da.20490.

Ho, J. K., McCabe, K. M., Yeh, M., & Lau, A. S. (2010). Evidence-based treatments for conduct problems among ethnic minorities. In R. C. Murrihy, A. D. Kidman, & T. H. Ollendick (Eds.),

Clinical handbook of assessing and treating conduct problems in youth (pp. 455–489). New York: Springer. doi:10.1007/978-1-4419-6297-3_18.

Ho, P. M., Peterson, P. N., & Masoudi, F. A. (2008). Evaluating the evidence: Is there a rigid hierarchy? *Circulation, 118*, 1675–1684. doi:10.1161/CIRCULATIONAHA.107.721357.

Hoagwood, K., Burns, B. J., Kiser, L., Ringeisen, H., & Schoenwald, S. K. (2001). Evidence-based practice in child and adolescent mental health services. *Psychiatric Services, 52*, 1179–1189. doi:10.1176/appi.ps.52.9.1179.

Hoagwood, K., & Johnson, J. (2003). School psychology: A public health framework: From evidence-based practices to evidence-based policies. *Journal of School Psychology, 41*(1), 2–21. doi:10.1016/S0022-4405(02)00141-3.

Hoffman, D. M. (2009). Reflecting on social emotional learning: A critical perspective on trends in the United States. *Review of Educational Research, 79*(2), 533–556. doi:10.3102/0034654308325184.

Holleran, L. K., Taylor-Seehafer, M. A., Pomeroy, E. C., & Neff, J. A. (2005). Substance abuse prevention for high risk youth: Exploring culture and alcohol and drug use. *Alcoholism Treatment Quarterly, 23*(2/3), 164–184. doi:10.1300/J020v23n02_10.

Honberg, R., Diehl, S., Kimball, A., Gruttadaro, D., & Fitzpatrick, M. (2011). *State mental health cuts: A national crisis.* A report by the National Alliance on Mental Illness. NAMI. Retrieved from http://www.nami.org

Hoop, J. G., DiPasquale, T., Hernandez, J. M., & Roberts, L. W. (2008). Ethics and cultures in mental health care. *Ethics & Behavior, 18*(4), 353–372. doi:10.1080/10508420701713048.

Hooshman, S., Willoughby, T., & Good, M. (2012). Does the direction of effects in the association between depressive symptoms and health-risk behaviors differ by behavior? A longitudinal study across the high school years. *Journal of Adolescent Health, 50*(2), 140–147. doi:10.1016/j.jadohealth.2011.05.016.

Hoover-Dempsey, K. V., & Sandler, H. M. (1997). Why do parents become involve in their children's education? *Review of Educational Research, 67*(1), 3–42. doi:10.3102/00346543067001003.

Hopson, L. M., & Steiker, L. K. (2008). Methodology of adapted versions of an evidence-based prevention program in reducing alcohol use among alternative school students. *Children and Schools, 30*(2), 116–127. doi:10.1093/cs/30.2.116.

Hopson, L. M., & Steiker, L. K. (2010). Effectiveness of adapted versions of an evidence-based prevention program in reducing alcohol use among alternative school students. *Children and Schools, 32*(2), 81–92. doi:10.1093/cs/cds039|hwp:master-id:cs;cds039.

Hornby, G., & Lafaele, R. (2011). Barriers to parental involvement in education: An explanatory model. *Educational Review, 63*(1), 37–52. doi:10.1080/00131911.2010.488049.

Horner, R. H., Sugai, G., & Anderson, C. M. (2010). Examining the evidence base for School-Wide Positive Behavior Support. *Focus on Exceptional Children, 42*(6), 1–16. Retrieved from http://www.lovepublishing.com

Horner, R. H., Sugai, G., Smolkowski, K., Eber, L., Nakasato, J., Todd, A. W., et al. (2009). A randomized, wait-list controlled effectiveness trial assessing School-Wide Positive Behavior Support in elementary schools. *Journal of Positive Behavior Interventions, 11*(3), 133–144. doi:10.1177/1098300709332067.

Horner, R. H., Todd, A., Lewis-Palmer, T., Irvin, L., Sugai, G., & Boland, J. (2004). The school-wide evaluation tool (SET): A research instrument for assessing School-Wide Positive Behavior Support. *Journal of Positive Behavior Interventions, 6*(1), 3–12. doi:10.1177/10983007040060010201.

Hu, M., Grielser, P., Schaffran, C., & Kandel, D. (2011). Risk and protective factors for nicotine dependence in adolescence. *Journal of Child Psychology and Psychiatry, 52*(10), 1063–1072. doi:10.1111/j.1469-7610.2010.02362.x.

Huang, L. N., Hepburn, K. S., & Espiritu, R. C. (2003). To be or not to be evidence-based? *Data Matters: An Evaluation Newsletter, 6*, 2–3.

Huang, C., & Huang, I. (2009). Resistance to change: The effects of organizational intervention and characteristic. *Review of Business Research, 9*(1), 110–114. Retrieved from http://www.iabe.org

Huberty, T. J. (2004). *Depression: Helping students in the classroom*. Bethesda, MD: National Association of School Psychologists. Retrieved from http://www.nasponline.org

Huey, S. J., & Polo, A. J. (2008). Evidence-based psychosocial treatments for ethnic minority youth. *Journal of Clinical Child and Adolescent Psychology, 37*(1), 262–301. doi:10.1080/15374410701820174.

Huey, S., & Polo, A. (2010). Assessing the effects of evidence-based psychotherapies with ethnic minority youths. In J. R. Weisz & A. E. Kazdin (Eds.), *Evidence-based psychotherapies for children and adolescents* (2nd ed., pp. 451–465). New York: Guilford Press.

Hughes, J. N., & Barrois, L. K. (2010). The developmental implications of classroom social relationships and strategies for improving them. In B. Doll, W. Pfohl, & J. S. Yoon (Eds.), *Handbook of youth prevention science* (pp. 194–217). New York: Routledge.

Humensky, J., Kuwabara, S. A., Fogel, J., Wells, C., Goodwin, B., & Van Voorhees, B. W. (2010). Adolescents with depressive symptoms and their challenges with learning in school. *The Journal of School Nursing, 26*(5), 377–392. doi:10.1177/1059840510376515.

Humphries, M. L., Keenan, K., & Wakschlag, L. S. (2012). Teacher and observer ratings of young African American children's social and emotional competencies. *Psychology in the Schools, 49*(4), 311–327. doi:10.1002/pits.21604.

Hunter, L. (2003). School psychology: A public health framework III. Managing disruptive behavior in schools: The value of a public health and evidence-based perspective. *Journal of School Psychology, 41*, 39–59. doi:10.1016/S0022-4405(02)00143-7.

Huser, M., Cooney, S., Small, S., O'Connor, C., & Mather, R. (2009). *Evidence-based program registries. What works, Wisconsin research to practice series*. Madison, WI: University of Wisconsin-Madison/Extension. Retrieved from http://whatworks.uwex.edu/

Hussain, S., Anwar, S., & Majoka, M. (2011). Effect of peer group activity-based learning on students' academic achievement in physics at secondary level. *International Journal of Academic Research, 3*(1), 940–944. Retrieved from http://www.ijar.lit.az/

Hutcherson, S. T., & Epkins, C. C. (2009). Differentiating parent- and peer-related interpersonal correlates of depressive symptoms and social anxiety in preadolescent girls. *Journal of Social and Personal Relationships, 26*(6–7), 875–897. doi:10.1177/0265407509345654.

Hwang, W. (2006). The psychotherapy adaptation and modification framework: Application to Asian Americans. *American Psychologist, 61*(7), 702–715. doi:10.1037/0003-066X.61.7.702.

Hwang, W. (2009). The formative method for adapting psychotherapy (FMAP): A community-based developmental approach to culturally adapting therapy. *Professional Psychology: Research and Practice, 40*(4), 369–377. doi:10.1037/a0016240.

Hwang, W., Jyers, H., Abe-Kim, J., & Ting, J. Y. (2008). A conceptual paradigm for understanding culture's impact on mental health: The cultural influences on mental health (CIMH) model. *Clinical Psychology Review, 28*(2), 211–227. doi:10.1016/j.cpr.2007.05.001.

Hyde, P. S. (2012). *A public health approach to prevention of behavioral health conditions*. Presentation at Project LAUNCH Grantees' Spring Training Institute. Retrieved from http://store.samhsa.gov/

Ijaz, S., & Vitalis, A. (2011). Resistance to organizational change: Putting the jigsaw together. *International Review of Business Research Papers, 7*(3), 112–121.

In-Albon, T., & Schneider, S. (2007). Psychotherapy of childhood anxiety disorders: A meta-analysis. *Psychotherapy and Psychosomatics, 76*(1), 15–24. doi:10.1159/000096361.

Individuals with Disabilities Education Improvement Act of 2004 (IDEA). (2004). Pub. L. No. 108-446, 632, 118 Stat. 2647. Retrieved from http://www.copyright.gov/legislation/pl108-446.pdf

Ingram, R., & Smith, L. T. (2008). Mood disorders. In J. E. Maddux & B. A. Winstead (Eds.), *Psychopathology: Foundations for a contemporary understanding* (2nd ed., pp. 191–197). New York: Routledge.

Inman, D. D., van Bakergem, K. M., LaRosa, A. C., & Garr, D. R. (2011). Evidence-based health promotion program for schools and communities. *American Journal of Preventive Medicine, 40*(2), 207–219. doi:10.1016/j.amepre.2010.10.031.

Institute of Medicine (IOM). (1994). *Reducing risks for mental disorders: Frontiers for preventive intervention research.* Washington, DC: National Academy Press.

Interian, A., Allen, L. A., Gara, M. A., & Escobar, J. I. (2008). A pilot study of culturally adapted cognitive behavior therapy for Hispanics with major depression. *Cognitive and Behavioral Practice, 15*(1), 67–75. doi:10.1016/j.cbpra.2006.12.002.

Ives, R. (2006). *Monitoring and evaluating youth substance abuse prevention programmes.* Vienna: United Nations Office on Drugs and Crime. Retrieved from http://www.unodc.org

Izard, C. E., King, K. A., Trentacosta, C. J., Laurenceau, J. P., Morgan, J. K., Krauthamer-Ewing, E. S., et al. (2008). Accelerating the development of emotion competence in Head Start children. *Development and Psychopathology, 20*(1), 369–397. doi:10.1017/S0954579408000175.

Jacob, S. (2008). Best practices in developing ethical school psychology practice. In A. Thomas & A. J. Grimes (Eds.), *Best practices in school psychology V* (Vol. 6, pp. 1921–1932). Bethesda, MD: National Association of School Psychologists.

Jacobs, J. A., Jones, E., Gabella, B. A., Spring, B., & Brownson, R. C. (2012). Tools for implementing an evidence-based approach in public health practice. *Prevention of Chronic Disease, 9,* 110324. doi:10.5888/pcd9.110324.

James Bell Associates. (2009). *Evaluation brief: Measuring implementation fidelity.* Arlington, VA: Author.

Jansen, K. J. (2000). The emerging dynamics of change: Resistance, readiness, and momentum. *Human Resource Planning, 23*(2), 53–55. doi:10.4018/jkm.2005040104.

Janssens, K. A., Rosmalen, J. G., Ormel, J., Van Oort, F. V., & Oldehinkel, A. J. (2010). Anxiety and depression are risk factors rather than consequences of functional somatic symptoms in a general population of adolescents: The TRAILS study. *Journal of Child Psychology and Psychiatry, 51*(3), 304–312. doi:10.1111/j.1469-7610.2009.02174.x.

Jayanthi, M., & Nelson, J. S. (2002). *Savvy decision making: Administrator's guide to using focus groups in schools* (pp. 1–19). Thousand Oaks, CA: Sage.

Jaycox, L. H. (2004). *Cognitive behavioral intervention for trauma in schools.* Longmont, CO: Sopris West Educational Services.

Jaycox, L. H., Burnam, M. A., Meredith, L. S., Tanielian, T., Stein, B. D., Chandra, A., et al. (2010). *The teen depression awareness project: Building on evidence base for improving teen depression care.* Santa Monica, CA: The RAND Corporation. Retrieved from http://www.rand.org/pubs/research_briefs/2010/RAND_RB9495.pdf

Jaycox, L. H., McCaffrey, D. F., Ocampo, B. W., Shelley, G. A., Blacke, S. M., Peterson, D. J., et al. (2006). Challenges in the evaluation and implementation of school-based prevention and intervention programs on sensitive topics. *American Journal of Evaluation, 27*(3), 320–336. doi:10.1177/1098214006291010.

Jaycox, L. H., Reivich, K. J., Gillham, J., & Seligman, M. E. P. (1994). Preventing depressive symptoms in school children. *Behavior Research and Therapy, 32*(8), 801–816. doi:10.1016/0005-7967(94)90160-0.

Jaycox, L. H., Stein, B. D., Paddock, S., Miles, J. N., Chandra, A., Meredith, L. S., et al. (2009). Impact of teen depression on academic, social, and physical functioning. *Pediatrics, 124*(4), e596–e605. doi:10.1542/peds.2008-3348.

Jee, Y., Haejung, L., Hwa, Y. U., & Eunyoung, Y. (2010). Factors influencing on depression among middle-school girls in South Korea. *Journal of Korean Academy of Nursing, 41*(4), 550–557. doi:10.4040/jkan.2011.41.4.550.

Jenson, J. M., Dieterich, W. A., Brisson, D., Bender, K. A., & Powell, A. (2010). Preventing childhood bullying: Findings and lessons from the Denver Public Schools trial. *Research on Social Work Practice, 20*(5), 509–517. doi:10.1177/1049731509359186.

Jepson, R. G., Harris, F. M., Platt, A., & Tannahill, C. (2010). The effectiveness of interventions to change six health behaviors: A review of reviews. *BMC Public Health, 10,* 538. doi:10.1186/1471-2458-10-538.

Jimba, K. T., & Sharma, M. (2012). Ethnic differences in susceptibility to smoking and intention to smoke on smoking behavior among adolescents. *Community Medicine & Health Education, 2*(4), 2–5. doi:10.4172/2161-0711.1000143.

Johnes, F. (2006). Didacticism and educational outcomes. *Educational Research and Reviews, 1*(2), 23–28. Retrieved from http://www.academicjournals.org/

Johnson, A. C., Cen, S., Gallaher, P., Palmer, P. H., Xian, L., Ritt-Olsen, A., et al. (2007). Why smoking prevention programs sometimes fail. Does effectiveness depend on sociocultural context and individual characteristics? *Cancer Epidemiology, Biomarkers & Prevention, 16*(6), 1043–1049. doi:10.1158/1055-9965.EPI-07-0067.

Johnson, C. A., Unger, J. B., Ritt-Olson, A., Palmer, P. H., Cen, S. Y., Gallaher, P., et al. (2005). Smoking prevention for ethnically diverse adolescents: 2-year outcomes of a multicultural, school-based smoking prevention curriculum in Southern California. *Preventive Medicine, 40*(6), 842–852. doi:10.1016/j.ypmed.2004.09.032.

Johnston, L. D., Bachman, J. G., O'Malley, P. M., & Schulenberg, J. E. (2010). *School bullying, family structure and socioeconomic status in the US from 1989–2009: Repetitive trends and persistent disadvantage.* Population Association of America 12th Annual Meeting, San Francisco.

Jones, K., Daley, D., Hitchings, J., Bywater, T., & Eames, C. (2007). Efficacy of the Incredible Years Programme as an early intervention for children with conduct problems and ADHD. *Child: Care, Health and Development, 34*(3), 380–390. doi:10.1111/j.1365-2214.2008.00817.x.

Jordan, G. B. (2010). A theory-based logic model for innovation policy and evaluation. *Research Evaluation, 19*(4), 263–273. doi:10.3152/095820210X12827366906445.

Joseph, G. E., & Strain, P. S. (2003). Comprehensive evidence-based social-emotional curricula for young children: An analysis of efficacious adoption potential. *Topics in Early Childhood Special Education, 23*(2), 65–76. doi:10.1177/02711214030230020201.

Jurecska, D., Hamilton, E. B., & Peterson, M. A. (2011). Effectiveness of the Coping Power Program in middle-school children with disruptive behaviours and hyperactivity difficulties. *Support for Learning, 26*(4), 168–172. doi:10.1111/j.1467-9604.2011.01499.x.

Juvonen, J., Graham, S., & Schuster, M. A. (2003). Bullying among young adolescents: The strong, the weak and the troubled. *Pediatrics, 112*(6), 1231–1237. doi:10.1542/peds.112.6.1231.

Kalibatseva, Z., & Leong, F. T. (2011). Depression among Asian Americans: Review and recommendations. *Depression Research and Treatment, 2011*(14), 1–9. doi:10.1155/2011/320902.

Kam, J. A., Cleveland, M. J., & Hecht, M. L. (2010). Applying general strain theory to examine perceived discrimination's indirect relation to Mexican-heritage youth's alcohol, cigarette, and marijuana use. *Prevention Science, 11*, 397–410. doi:10.1007/s11121-010-0180-7.

Kam, C., Greenberg, M. T., & Kusché, C. A. (2004). Sustained effects of the PATHS curriculum on the social and psychological adjustment of children in special education. *Journal of Emotional and Behavioral Disorders, 12*, 66–78. doi:10.1177/10634266040120020101.

Kaminski, J. W., Valle, L. A., Filene, J. H., & Boyle, C. L. (2008). A meta-analytic review of components associated with parent training program effectiveness. *Journal of Abnormal Child Psychology, 36*, 567–589. doi:10.1007/s10802-007-9201-9.

Kamphaus, R. W., & Reynolds, C. R. (2007). *BASC-2 Behavioral and Emotional Screening System (BESS) manual.* Circle Pines, MN: Pearson.

Karp, F. (2012). *The academic achievement of Latino students in Boston public schools.* Boston: The Mauricio Gastón Institute for Latino Community Development. Retrieved from http://www.umb.edu

Kataoka, S., Novins, D. K., & DeCarlo, S. C. (2010). The practice of evidence-based treatments in ethnic minority youth. *Child and Adolescent Psychiatric Clinics of North America, 19*(4), 775–789. doi:10.1016/j.chc.2010.07.008.

Kataoka, S., Zhang, L., & Wells, K. (2002). Unmet need for mental health care among U.S. children: Variation by ethnicity and insurance status. *The American Journal of Psychiatry, 159*(9), 1548–1555. doi:10.1176/appi.ajp.159.9.1548.

Keenan, K., Feng, X., Hipwell, A., & Klostermann, S. (2009). Depression begets depression: Comparing the predictive utility of depression and anxiety symptoms to later depression. *Journal of Child Psychology and Psychiatry, 50*(9), 1167–1175. doi:10.1111/j.1469-7610.2009.02080.x.

Keenan, K., & Hipwell, A. E. (2005). Preadolescent clues to understanding depression in girls. *Clinical Child and Family Psychology Review, 8*(5), 89–105. doi:10.1007/s10567-005-4750-3.

Keenan-Miller, D., Hammen, C. L., & Brennan, P. A. (2007). Health outcomes related to early adolescent depression. *Journal of Adolescent Health, 41*(3), 256–262. doi:10.1002/jts.20652.

Kelder, S. H., Murray, N. G., Orpinas, P., Prokhorov, A., McReynolds, L., Zhang, Q., et al. (2001). Depression and substance use in minority middle-school students. *American Journal of Public Health, 91*(5), 761–766. doi:10.2105/AJPH.91.5.761.

Keller-Margulis, M. A. (2012). Fidelity of implementation framework: A critical need for response to intervention models. *Psychology in the Schools, 49*(4), 342–352. doi:10.1002/pits.21602.

Kelly, M. S., Berzin, S. C., Frey, A., Alvarez, M., Shaffer, G., & O'Brien, K. (2010). The state of school social work: Findings from the National School Social Work Survey. *School Mental Health, 2*, 132–141. doi:10.1007/s12310010-9034-5.

Kendall, P. C. (1994). Treating anxiety disorders in children: Results of a randomized clinical trial. *Journal of Consulting and Clinical Psychology, 62*(1), 100–110. Retrieved from http://www.apa.org

Kendall, P. C., Brady, E. U., & Verduin, T. L. (2001). Comorbidity in childhood anxiety disorders and treatment outcome. *Journal of the American Academy of Child and Adolescent Psychiatry, 40*(7), 787–794. doi:10.1097/00004583-200107000-00013.

Kendall, P. C., Choudhury (Khanna), M., Hudson, J., & Webb, A. (2002). *The C.A.T. project therapist manual*. Ardmore, PA: Workbook Publishing.

Kendall, P. C., Flannery-Schroeder, E., Panichelli-Mindel, S. M., Southam-Gerow, M., Henin, A., & Warman, M. (1997). Therapy for youths with anxiety disorders: A second randomized clinical trial. *Journal of Consulting and Clinical Psychology, 65*(3), 366–380. Retrieved from http://www.apa.org

Kendall, P. C., Safford, S., Flannery-Schroeder, E., & Webb, A. (2004). Child anxiety treatment: Outcomes in adolescence and impact on substance use and depression at 7.4-year follow-up. *Journal of Consulting and Clinical Psychology, 72*(2), 276–287. doi:10.1037/0022-006X.72.2.276.

Kendall, P. C., & Southam-Gerow, M. A. (1996). Long-term follow-up of a cognitive-behavioral therapy for anxiety-disordered youth. *Journal of Consulting and Clinical Psychology, 64*(4), 724–730. doi:10.1037/0022-006X.64.4.724.

Kennard, B. D., Stewart, S. M., Hughes, J. L., Patel, P. G., & Emslie, G. J. (2006). Cognitions and depressive symptoms among ethnic minority adolescents. *Cultural Diversity and Ethnic Minority Psychology, 12*(3), 578–591. doi:10.1037/1099-9809.12.3.578.

Kennelly, L., & Monrad, M. (2007). *Approaches to dropout prevention: Heeding early warning signs with appropriate interventions*. Washington, DC: National High School Center at the American Institutes for Research. Retrieved from http://www.betterhighschools.org

Kerka, S. (Ed.). (2006). *What works: Evidence-based strategies for youth practitioners*. Dropout prevention. Columbus, OH: Learning Work Connection. Retrieved from http://cle.osu.edu/lwc-publications/what-works/downloads/WW-Dropout-Prevention.pdf

Kessler, R. C., Berglund, P., Demler, O., Jin, R., Merikangas, K. R., & Walters, E. E. (2005). Lifetime prevalence and age-of-onset distributions of DSM-IV disorders in the National Comorbidity Survey Replication. *Archives of General Psychiatry, 62*(6), 593–602. doi:10.1001/archpsyc.62.6.593.

Kessler, R., Demier, O., Frank, R. G., Olfson, M., Pincus, H. A., Walters, E. E., et al. (2005). Prevalence and treatment of mental disorders 1990–2003. *The New England Journal of Medicine, 352*, 2515–2523. doi:10.1056/NEJMsa043266.

Khan, K. S., & Coomarasamy, A. (2006). A hierarchy of effective teaching and learning to acquire competence in evidence-based medicine. *BMC Medical Education, 6*, 59. doi:10.1186/1472-6920-6-59.

Khanna, M. S., & Kendall, P. C. (2008). Computer-assisted CBT for child anxiety: The Coping Cat CD-ROM. *Cognitive and Behavioral Practice, 15*(2), 159–165. doi:10.1016/j.cbpra.2008.02.002.

Khanna, M. S., & Kendall, P. C. (2009). Exploring the role of parent training in the treatment of childhood anxiety. *Journal of Consulting and Clinical Psychology, 77*(5), 981–986. doi:10.1037/a0016920.

Kidd, P. S., & Parshall, M. B. (2000). Getting the focus and the group: Enhancing analytical rigor in focus group research. *Qualitative Health Research, 10*(3), 293–308. doi:10.1177/104973200129118453.

Kiesner, J. (2002). Depressive symptoms in early adolescence: Their relations with classroom problem behavior and peer status. *Journal of Research on Adolescence, 12*, 463–478. doi:10.1111/1532-7795.00042.

Kilbourne, M., Williams, M., Bauer, M. S., & Arean, P. (2012). Implementation research: Reducing the research-to-practice gap in depression treatment. *Depression Research and Treatment, 2012*, 2. doi:10.1155/2012/476027.

Kim, H. S., Sherman, D. K., & Taylor, S. E. (2008). Culture and social support. *American Psychologist, 63*(6), 518–526. doi:10.1037/0003-066X.

Kincaid, D., Childs, K., & George, H. (2010). *School-wide benchmarks of quality (revised).* Unpublished instrument, USF, Tampa, FL.

Kingery, J. N., Ginsburg, G. S., & Alfano, C. A. (2007). Somatic symptoms and anxiety among African American adolescents. *Journal of Black Psychology, 33*(4), 363–378. doi:10.1177/0095798407307041.

Kirby, S. N., Berends, M., & Naftel, S. (2001). *Implementation in a longitudinal sample of New American Schools: Four years into scale-up.* RAND Monograph reports (MR1413) (pp. 45–66). Retrieved from http://www.rand.org

Kiresuk, T. J., & Sherman, R. E. (1968). Goal attainment scaling: A general method for evaluating community health programs. *Community Mental Health Journal, 4*(6), 443–453. doi:10.1007/BF01530764.

Kleftaras, G., & Didaskalou, E. (2006). Incidence and teachers' perceived causation of depression in primary school children in Greece. *School Psychology International, 27*(3), 296–314. doi:10.1177/014303430606728.

Klem, A. M., & Connell, J. P. (2004). Relationships matter: Linking teacher support to student engagement and achievement. *Journal of School Health, 74*(7), 262–273. doi:10.1111/j.1746-1561.2004.tb08283.x.

Klima, T., Miller, M., & Nunlist, C. (2009). *What works? Targeted truancy and dropout programs in middle and high school.* Olympia, WA: Washington State Institute for Public Policy.

Knappe, S., Lieb, R., Beesdo, K., Fehm, L., Low, N. C., Gloster, A. T., et al. (2009). The role of parental psychopathology and family environment for social phobia in the first three decades of life. *Depression and Anxiety, 26*(4), 363–370. doi:10.1002/da.20527.

Knoff, H. M. (1996). The interface of school, community, and health care reform: Organizational directions toward effective services for children and youth. *School Psychology Review, 25*, 446–464. Retrieved from http://www.nasponline.org

Knoff, H. M., & Curtis, M. J. (1996). Introduction to mini-series: Organizational change and school reform: School psychology at a professional crossroad. *School Psychology Review, 25*(4), 406–408. Retrieved from http://www.nasponline.org

Knott, D., Muers, S., & Aldridge, S. (2008). *Achieving culture change.* The Prime Minister's Strategy Unit. London: Cabinet Office.

Koinson, C., Heron, J., Lewis, G., Croudace, T., & Araya, R. (2011). Timing of menarche and depressive symptoms in adolescent girls from a UK cohort. *The British Journal of Psychiatry, 198*, 17–23. doi:10.1192/bjp.bp.110.080861.

Komor, K. A., Perry, C. L., Veblen-Mortenson, A., Bosma, L. M., Dudovitz, B. S., Williams, C. L., et al. (2004). Brief report: The adaptation of Project Northland for urban youth. *Journal of Pediatric Psychology, 29*(6), 457–466. doi:10.1093/jpepsy/jsh049.

Komro, K. A., & Toomey, T. L. (2002). Strategies to prevent underage drinking. *Alcohol Research & Health, 26*, 5–14. Retrieved from http://pubs.niaaa.nih.gov/

Kong, G., Singh, N., & Krishnan-Sarin, S. (2012). A review of culturally targeted/tailored tobacco prevention and cessation interventions for minority adolescents. *Nicotine & Tobacco Research, 14*(12), 1394–1406. doi:10.1093/ntr/nts118.

Kosciw, J. G., & Diaz, E. M. (2008). *Involved, invisible ignored: The experiences of lesbian, gay, bisexual and transgender parents and their children in our nation's K-12 schools*. New York: GLSEN.

Kosunen, E., Kaltiala-Heino, R., Rimpelä, M., & Laippala, P. (2003). Risk-taking sexual behaviour and self-reported depression in middle adolescence—A school-based survey. *Child: Care, Health and Development, 29*(5), 337–344. doi:10.1046/j.1365-2214.2003.00357.x.

Kovacs, M., & Lopez-Duran, N. (2010). Prodromal symptoms and atypical affectivity as predictors of major depression in juveniles: Implications for prevention. *Journal of Child Psychology and Psychiatry, 51*(4), 472–496. doi:10.1111/j.1469-7610.2010.02230.x.

Kovaleski, J. F. (2007). Response to intervention: Considerations for research and systems change. *School Psychology Review, 36*(4), 638–646. Retrieved from http://www.nasponline.org

Kovaleski, J. F., & Pedersen, J. A. (2008). Best practices in data-analysis teaming. In A. Thomas & A. J. Grimes (Eds.), *Best practices in school psychology V* (Vol. 2, pp. 115–129). Bethesda, MD: National Association of School Psychologists.

Kramer, T. J., Caldarella, P., Christensen, L., & Shatzer, R. H. (2010). Social and emotional learning in the kindergarten classroom: Evaluation of the strong start curriculum. *Early Childhood Education Journal, 37*(4), 303–309. doi:10.1007/s10643-009-0354-8.

Kratochwill, T. R., McDonald, L., Levin, J. R., Bear-Tibbetts, H. Y., & Demaray, M. K. (2004). Families and Schools Together: An experimental analysis of a parent-mediated multi-family group program for American Indian children. *Journal of School Psychology, 42*(5), 359–383. doi:10.1016/j.jsp.2004.08.001.

Kratochwill, T. R., & Shernoff, E. S. (2004). Evidence-based practice: Promoting evidence-based interventions in school psychology. *School Psychology Review, 33*(1), 34–48. Retrieved from http://www.nasponline.org

Kratochwill, T. R., Volpiansky, P., Clements, M., & Ball, C. (2007). Professional development in implementing and sustaining multitier prevention models: Implications for response to intervention. *Schools Psychology Review, 36*(4), 618–631. Retrieved from http://www.nasponline.org

Kress, J. S., & Elias, M. J. (2006). School-based social and emotional learning programs. In K. A. Renninger & I. E. Sigel (Eds.), *Handbook of child psychology* (6th ed., pp. 592–618). New York: Wiley.

Kress, V. E., & Shoffner, M. F. (2007). Focus groups: A practical and applied research approach for counselors. *Journal of Counseling and Development, 85,* 189–195. doi:10.1002/j.1556-6678.2007.tb00462.x.

Kreuter, M. W., Lukwago, S. N., Bucholtz, D. C., Clark, E. M., & Sanders-Thompson, V. (2003). Achieving cultural appropriateness in health promotion programs: Targeted and tailored approaches. *Health Education & Behavior, 30,* 133–146. doi:10.1177/1090198102251021.

Kropski, J. A., Keckley, P. H., & Jensen, G. L. (2008). School-based obesity prevention programs: An evidence-based review. *Obesity, 16*(5), 1009–1018. doi:10.1038/oby.2008.29.

Kulis, S., Marsiglia, F. F., Elek, E., Dustman, P., Wagstaff, D., & Hecht, M. (2005). Mexican/Mexican American adolescents and keepin' it REAL: An evidence-based substance use prevention program. *Children and Schools, 27*(3), 133–145. doi:10.1093/cs/27.3.133.

Kulis, S., Yabikku, S., Marsiglia, F. F., Nieri, T., & Crossman, A. (2007). Differences by gender, ethnicity and acculturation in the efficacy of the keepin' it REAL model prevention program. *Journal of Drug Education, 37*(2), 23–144. Retrieved from http://www.baywood.com

Kumpfer, K. L., Alvarado, R., Smith, P., & Bellamy, N. (2002). Cultural sensitivity and adaptation in family-based prevention interventions. *Prevention Science, 3*(3), 241–246. doi:10.1023/A:1019902902119.

Kumpfer, K. K., Pinyuchon, M., de Melo, A. T., & Whiteside, H. O. (2008). Cultural adaptation process for international dissemination of the Strengthening Families program. *Evaluation & the Health Professions, 31*(2), 226–239. doi:10.1177/0163278708315926.

Kumpfer, K. L., & Tait, C. M. (2000). *Family skills training for parents and children.* OJJDP: Juvenile Justice Bulletin. Retrieved from https://www.ncjrs.gov/

Kumpfer, K. L., Whiteside, H. O., Greene, J. A., & Allen, K. C. (2010). Effectiveness outcomes of four age versions of the Strengthening Families Program in statewide field sites. *Group Dynamics: Theory, Research, and Practice, 14*(3), 211–229. doi:10.1037/a0020602.

Kuo, E. S., Stoep, A. V., Herting, J. R., Grupp, K., & McCauley, E. (2012). How to identify students for school-based depression intervention: Can school record review be substituted for universal depression screening? *Journal of Child and Adolescent Psychiatric Nursing, 26*(1), 42–52. doi:10.1111/jcap.12010.

Kusché, C. A., & Greenberg, M. T. (1994a). *The PATHS curriculum.* Seattle, WA: Developmental Research and Programs.

Kusché, C. A., & Greenberg, M. (1994b). *PATHS: Promoting Alternative Thinking Strategies.* South Deerfield, MA: Developmental Research Programs.

Kusché, C. A., & Greenberg, M. T. (2005). *PATHS (Promoting Alternative Thinking Strategies) evaluation kits.* South Deerfield, MA: Channing Bete.

Kushner, S. C., Tackett, J. L., & Bagby, R. M. (2012). The structure of internalizing disorders in middles childhood and evidence for personality correlates. *Journal of Psychopathology and Behavioral Assessment, 34*(1), 22–34. doi:10.1007/s10862-011-9263-4.

Kutash, K., Duchnowski, A. J., & Green, A. L. (2011). School-based mental health programs for students who have emotional disturbances: Academic and social–emotional outcomes. *School Mental Health, 3*, 191–208. doi:10.1007/s123108-011-9062-9.

Kutash, K., Duchnowski, A. J., & Lynn, N. (2006). *School-based mental health: An empirical guide for decision-makers.* Tampa, FL: Department of Child & Family Studies, Research and Training Center for Children's Mental Health, University of South Florida, The Louis de la Parte Florida Mental Health Institute.

Kykyri, V., Puutio, R., & Wahlstrom, J. (2010). Inviting participation in organizational change through ownership talk. *The Journal of Applied Behavioral Science, 46*(1), 92–118. doi:10.1177/002/886309357441.

La Roche, M. J., Batista, C., & D'Angelo, E. (2011). A culturally competent relaxation intervention for Latino/as: Assessing a culturally specific match model. *The American Journal of Orthopsychiatry, 81*(4), 535–542. doi:10.1111/j.1939-0025.2011.01124x.

Lam, A., Wong, B. P., Yang, H., & Liu, Y. (2012). Understanding student engagement with a contextual model. In S. L. Christenson, A. L. Reschly, & C. Wylie (Eds.), *Handbook of research on student engagement* (pp. 403–419). New York: Springer.

Lambert, S. F., Bradshaw, C. P., Cammack, N. L., & Ialongo, N. S. (2011). Examining the developmental process of risk for exposure to community violence among urban youth. *Journal of Prevention & Intervention in the Community, 39*(2), 98–113. doi:10.1080/10852352.2011.556558.

Landaeta, R. E., Mun, J. H., & Rabadi, G. (2008). Identifying sources of resistance to change in healthcare. *International Journal of Healthcare Technology and Management, 9*(1), 74–96. doi:10.1504/IJHTM.2008.016849.

Lane, K., Colan, V. L., & Reicher, S. R. (2011). *Achieving positive system outcomes: Building PBIS capacity using resource mapping.* Paper presented at the NASP 2011 Annual Convention, San Francisco.

Lane, K. L., Kalberg, J. R., Bruhn, A. L., Mahoney, M. E., & Driscoll, S. A. (2008). Primary prevention programs at the elementary level: Issues of treatment integrity, systematic screening, and reinforcement. *Education and Treatment of Children, 31*(4), 465–494.

Langford, L. (2010, March). *Adapting programs from the SPRC/AFSP best practices registry for diverse communities.* Suicide Prevention Grantee Meeting. American Foundation for Suicide Prevention. Retrieved from http://www.sprc.org

Langley, A. K., Nadeem, E., Kataoka, S. H., Stein, B. D., & Jacox, L. H. (2010). Evidence-based mental health programs in schools: Barriers and facilitators of successful implementation. *School Mental Health, 2*(3), 105–113. doi:10.1007/s12310-010-9038-1.

Lansford, J. E., Criss, M. M., Laird, R. D., Shaw, D. S., Pettit, G. S., Bates, J. E., et al. (2011). Reciprocal relations between parents' physical discipline and children's externalizing behavior during middle childhood and adolescence. *Developmental Psychopathology, 23*(1), 225–238. doi:10.1017/S0954579410000751.

Larson, K., Russ, S. A., Crall, J. J., & Halfon, N. (2008). Influence of multiple social risks on children's health. *Pediatrics, 12*(2), 337–344. doi:10.1542/peds.2007-0447.

Lau, A. S. (2006). Making the case for selective and directed cultural adaptations of evidence-based treatments: Examples from parent training. *Clinical Psychology: Science and Practice, 13*(4), 295–310. doi:10.1111/j.1468-2850.2006.00042.x.

Lau, E. X., & Rapee, R. M. (2011). Prevention of anxiety disorders. *Current Psychiatry Reports, 13*(4), 258–266. doi:10.1007/s11920-011-0199-x.

Lawson, M., Askell-Williams, H., Dix, K., Slee, P., Skrzypiec, G., & Spears, B. (2009). *Implementing a new initiative in mental health in Australian primary schools.* Paper presented at the Annual meeting of the Australian Association for Research in Education. Retrieved from https://www.flinders.edu.au

Lazarus, P. J., & Sulkowski, M. L. (2011). The emotional well-being of our nations' youth and the promise of social-emotional learning. *Communiqué, 40*(2), 16–17. Retrieved from http://www.nasponline.org

Leadbetter, B., & Sukhawathanakul, P. (2011). Multicomponent programs for reducing peer victimization in early elementary school: A longitudinal evaluation of the WITS primary program. *Journal of Community Psychology, 39*(5), 606–620. doi:10.1002/cop.20447.

LeBuffe, P. A., Shapiro, V. B., & Naglieri, J. A. (2009). *The DESSA: A new assessment of social-emotional competencies.* Mini-skills workshop presented at the Annual Meeting of the National Association of School Psychologists, Boston.

Lee, S. J., Altschul, I., & Mowbray, C. T. (2008). Using planned adaptation to implement evidence-based programs with new populations. *American Journal of Community Psychology, 41*(3–4), 290–303. doi:10.1007/s10464-008-9160-5.

Lee, T., & Cornell, D. (2010). Current validity of the Olweus Bully/Victim Questionnaire. *Journal of School Violence, 9*(1), 56–73. doi:10.1080/15388220903185613.

Leedy, A., Bates, P., & Safran, S. P. (2004). Bridging the research-to-practice gap: Improving hallway behavior using positive behavior supports. *Behavioral Disorders, 29*(2), 130–139.

Leerlooijer, J., James, S., Reinders, J., & Mullen, P. D. (2011). Using intervention mapping to adapt evidence-based programs to new setting and populations (Chapter 10). In L. K. Bartholomew, G. S. Parcel, G. Kok, N. H. Gottlieb, & M. E. Fernandez (Eds.), *Planning health promotion programs: An intervention mapping approach.* San Francisco: Jossey-Bass.

Leff, S. S., Angelucci, J., Goldstein, A. B., Cardaciotto, L., Paskewich, B., & Grossman, M. (2007). Using a participatory action research model to create a school-based intervention program for relationally aggressive girls: The Friend to Friend Program. In J. Zins, M. Elias, & C. Maher (Eds.), *Bullying, victimization, and peer harassment: Handbook of prevention and intervention* (pp. 199–218). New York: Haworth Press.

Leff, S. S., Kupersmidt, J. B., & Power, T. J. (2003). An initial examination of girls' cognitions of their relationally aggressive peers as a function of their own social standing. *Merrill-Palmer Quarterly, 49*, 28–54. doi:10.1353/mpq.2003.0003.

Leff, S. S., Power, T. J., Manz, P. H., Costigan, T. E., & Nabors, L. A. (2001). School-based aggression prevention programs for young children: Current status and implications for violence prevention. *School Psychology Review, 30*, 343–360. Retrieved from http://www.nasponline.org

Lehrer, J. A., Shrier, L. A., Gortmaker, S., & Buka, S. (2006). Depressive symptoms as a longitudinal predictor of sexual risk behaviors among U.S. middle and high school students. *Pediatrics, 118*(1), 189–200. doi:10.1542/peds.2005-1320.

Lehrt, C. A., Johnson, D. R., Bremer, C. D., Cosio, A., & Thompson, M. (2004). *Essential tools: Increasing rates of school completion: Moving from policy and research to practice. A manual for policymakers, administrators, and educators.* Minneapolis, MN: ICI Publications Office. Retrieved from http://www.ncset.org/publications/essentialtools/dropout/dropout.pdf

Letarte, M., Normandeau, S., & Allard, J. (2010). Effectiveness of a parent training program "Incredible Years" in a child protection service. *Child Abuse & Neglect, 34*, 253–261. doi:10.1016/j.chiabu.2009.06.003.

Leung, B., Wu, T., Questin, M., Staresnick, J., & Le, P. (2008). Communicating with Asian parents and families. *Communiqué, 37*(4). Retrieved from http://www.nasponline.org

Lewin, K. (1951). *Field theory in social science.* New York: Harper & Row.

Lewinsohn, P. M., Gotlib, I. H., Lewinsohn, M., Seeley, J. R., & Allen, N. B. (1998). Gender differences in anxiety disorders and anxiety symptoms in adolescents. *Journal of Abnormal Psychology, 107*(1), 109–117. doi:10.1037/0021-843X.107.1.109.

Lewis, T. J., Powers, L. J., Kely, M. J., & Newcomer, L. L. (2002). Reducing problem behaviors on the playground: An investigation of the application of schoolwide positive behavior supports. *Psychology in the Schools, 39*(2), 181–190. doi:10.1002/pits.10029.

Lezin, N., Rolleri, L. A., Wilson, M. M., Taylor, J., Fuller, T. R., Firpo-Triplett, R., et al. (2011). *Safer choices: Adaptation kit: Tools and resources for making informed adaptations to safer choices.* Scotts Valley, CA: ETR Associates. Retrieved from http://www.etr.org

Li, K., Washburn, I., DuBois, D. L., Vuchinich, S., Ji, P., Brechling, V., et al. (2009). *Effects of the Positive Action program on problem behaviors in elementary school students: A matched-pair randomized control trial in Chicago.* Unpublished manuscript, Oregon State University.

Li, Y., Zhang, W., Liu, J., Arbeit, M. R., Schwartz, S. J., Bowers, E. P., et al. (2011). The role of school engagement in preventing adolescent delinquency and substance use: A survival analysis. *Journal of Adolescence, 34*(6), 1181–1192. doi:10.1016/j.adolescence.2011.07.003.

Liew, J., & McTigue, E. M. (2010). Educating the whole child: The role of social and emotional development in achievement and school success. In L. E. Kattington (Ed.), *Handbook of curriculum development* (pp. 465–478). Hauppauge, NY: Nova Sciences.

Lillenstein, J. A. (2001). *Efficacy of a social skills training curriculum with early elementary students in four parochial schools.* Doctoral dissertation, Villanova University, Villanova, PA.

Lindsey, M. A., Joe, S., & Nebbitt, V. (2010). Family matters: The role of mental health stigma and social support on depressive symptoms and subsequent help seeking among African American boys. *Journal of Black Psychology, 36*(4), 458–482. doi:10.1177/0095798409355796.

Liu, J., Chen, X., & Lewis, G. (2011). Childhood internalizing behavior: Analysis and implications. *Journal of Psychiatric and Mental Health Nursing, 18*(10), 884–894. doi:10.1111/j.1365-2850.2011.01743.x.

Lo, C. C., & Prohaska, A. (2011). Creating an environment conducive to active and collaborative learning: Redesigning introduction to sociology at a large research university. *Journal on Excellence in College Teaching, 21*(4), 75–98. Retrieved from http://www.celt.muohio.edu/ject

Lochman, J. E. (2000). Parent and family skills training in targeted prevention programs for at-risk youth. *The Journal of Primary Prevention, 21*(2), 253–265. doi:10.1023/A:1007087304188.

Lochman, J. E. (2003). Commentary: School contextual influences on the dissemination of interventions. *School Psychology Review, 32*(2), 169–173. Retrieved from http://www.nasponline.org

Lochman, J. E., & Wells, K. C. (2002). The Coping Power Program at the middle school transition: Universal and indicated prevention effects. *Psychology of Addictive Behaviors, 16*(4S), S40–S54. doi:10.1037//0893-164X.16.4S.S40.

Lochman, J. E., & Wells, K. C. (2004). The Coping Power program for preadolescent aggressive boys and their parents: Outcome effects at the 1-year follow up. *Journal of Consulting and Clinical Psychology, 72*(4), 571–578. doi:10.1037/0022-006X.72.4.571.

Loeber, R., & Burke, J. D. (2011). Developmental pathways in juvenile externalizing and internalizing problems. *Journal of Research on Adolescence, 21*(1), 34–46. doi:10.1111/j.1532-7795.2010.00713.x.

Lohr, K. N. (2004). Rating the strength of scientific evidence: Relevance for quality improvement programs. *International Journal for Quality in Health Care, 16*(1), 9–18. doi:10.1093/intqhc/mzh005.

Lohrmann, S., Forman, S., Martin, S., & Palmieri, M. (2008). Understanding school personnel's resistance to adopting Schoolwide Positive Behavior Support at a universal level of intervention. *Journal of Positive Behavior Interventions, 10*(4),256–269. doi:10.1177/1098300708318963.

Lopez, S. J., Edwards, L. M., Teramoto Pedrotti, J., Ito, A., & Rasmussen, H. N. (2002). Culture counts: Examinations of recent applications of the Penn Resiliency Program or, toward a rubric for examining cultural appropriateness of prevention programming. *Prevention & Treatment, 5*(1), Article 12. doi:10.1037/1522-3736.5.1.512c

López, S. R., & Guarnaccia, P. J. (2008). Cultural dimensions of psychopathology: The social world's impact on mental disorders. In J. E. Maddux & B. A. Winstead (Eds.), *Psychopathology: Foundation for a contemporary understanding* (2nd ed., pp. 19–38). New York: Routledge.

López, I., Rivera, F., Ramirez, R., Guarnaccia, P. J., Canino, G., & Bird, H. R. (2009). Ataques de Nervios and their psychiatric correlates in Puerto Rican children from two different contexts. *Journal of Nervous & Mental Disorders, 197*(2), 923–929. doi:10.1097/NMD.0b013e3181c2997d.

Lorenzo, M., Crouch, C. H., & Mazur, E. (2006). Reducing the gender gap in the physics classroom. *American Journal of Physics, 74*(2), 118–122. doi:10.1119/1.2162549.

Lösel, F., & Bender, D. (2011). Emotional and antisocial outcomes of bullying and victimization at school: A follow-up from childhood to adolescence. *Journal of Aggression, Conflict and Peace Research, 3*(2), 89–96. doi:10.1108/17596591111132909.

Losen, D. J., & Martinez, T. E. (2013). *Out of school & off track: The overuse of suspensions in American middle and high schools.* Los Angeles: The Civil Rights Project.

Lubell, K. M., Lofton, R., & Singer, H. H. (2008). *Promoting healthy parenting practices across cultural groups: A CDC research brief.* Atlanta, GA: Centers for Disease Control and Prevention, National Center for Injury Prevention and Control.

Luk, J. W., Wang, J., & Simons-Morton, B. G. (2010). Bullying victimization and substance use among U.S. adolescents: Mediation by depression. *Prevention Science, 11*(4), 355–359. doi:10.1007/s11121-010-0179-0.

Lundahl, B., Risser, H. J., & Lovejoy, M. C. (2006). A meta-analysis of parenttraining: Moderators and follow-up effects. *Clinical Psychology Review, 26*(1), 86–104. doi:10.1016/j.cpr.2005.07.004.

Lynch, K. B., Geller, S. R., & Schmidt, M. G. (2004). Multi-year evaluation of the effectiveness of a resilience-based prevention program for young children. *The Journal of Primary Prevention, 24*(3), 335–353. doi:10.1023/B:JOPP.0000018052.12488.d1.

Mac Iver, M. A., & Mac Iver, D. J. (2009). *Beyond the indicators: An integrated school-level approach to dropout prevention.* Arlington, VA: The Mid-Atlantic Equity Center, The George Washington University Center for Equity and Excellence in Education.

Magalhaes, A. C., Holmes, K. D., Dale, L. B., Comps-Agrar, L., Lee, D., Yadav, P. N., et al. (2010). CRF receptor 1 regulates anxiety behavior via sensitization of 5-HT2 receptor signaling. *Nature Neuroscience, 13*(5), 622–629. doi:10.1038/nn.2529.

Magnuson, K., Meyers, M., Ruhm, C., & Waldfogel, J. (2004). Inequality in preschool education and school readiness. *American Education Research Journal, 41*, 115–157. doi:10.3102/00028312041001115.

Mahatmya, D., Lohman, B. J., Matjasko, J. L., & Farb, A. F. (2012). Engagement across developmental periods. In S. L. Christenson, A. L. Reschly, & C. Wylie (Eds.), *Handbook of research on student engagement* (pp. 45–63). New York: Springer.

Mance, G. A., Mendelson, T., Byrd, B., Jones, J., & Tandon, D. (2010). Utilizing community-based participatory research to adapt a mental health intervention for African American emerging adults. *Progress in Community Health Partnerships: Research, Education, and Action, 4*(2), 131–140. doi:10.1353/cpr.0.0112.

March, J. S., Silva, S., Petrycki, S., Curry, J., Wells, K., Fairbank, J., et al. (2007). The Treatment for Adolescents with Depression Study (TADS): Long-term effectiveness and safety outcomes. *Archives of General Psychiatry, 64*(10), 1132–1143. doi:10.1001/archpsyc.64.10.1132.

Margolis, J., & Nagel, L. (2006). Educational reform and the role of administrators in mediating teacher stress. *Teacher Education Quarterly, 33*(4), 143–159. Retrieved from http://www.teq-journal.org

Margulis, M. A. (2012). Fidelity of implementation framework: A critical need for response to intervention models. *Psychology in the Schools, 49*(4), 342–352. doi:10.1002/pits.21602.

Marshal, M. P., King, K. M., Stepp, S. D., Hipwell, A., Smith, H., Chung, T., et al. (2012). Trajectories of alcohol and cigarette use among sexual minority and heterosexual girls. *Journal of Adolescent Health, 50*(1), 97–99. doi:10.1016/j.jadohealth.2011.05.008.

Marsiglia, F. F. (2011). *To adapt or not to adapt, that is the question....* Powerpoint presentation. 13th Annual Conference: NHSN International Scientific Conference, Coral Gable, FL. Retrieved from http://www.nhsn.med.miami.edu

Marsiglia, F. F., Ayers, S., Gance-Cleveland, B., Mettler, K., & Booth, J. (2012). Beyond primary prevention of alcohol use: A culturally specific secondary prevention program for Mexican heritage adolescents. *Prevention Science, 13*, 241–251. doi:10.1007/s11121-011-0263-0.

Marsiglia, F. F., & Hecht, M. L. (2005). *Keepin' it REAL drug resistance strategies (curriculum manual).* Santa Cruz, CA: ETR Associates.

Marsiglia, F. F., Kulis, S., Wagstaff, D. A., Elek, E., & Dran, D. (2005). Acculturation status and substance use prevention with Mexican and Mexican American youth. *Journal of Social Work Practice in the Addictions, 5*(1/2), 85–111. doi:10.1300/J160v5n01_05.

Martinez, W., Polo, A. J., & Carter, J. S. (2012). Family orientation, language, and anxiety among low-income Latino youth. *Journal of Anxiety Disorders, 26*(4), 517–525. doi:10.1016/j.janxdis.2012.02.005.

Mason, M. J., & Korpela, K. (2009). Activity spaces and urban adolescent substance use and emotional health. *Journal of Adolescence, 32*(4), 925–939. doi:10.1016/j.adolescence.2008.08.004.

Mass-Galloway, R. L., Panyan, M. V., Smith, C. R., & Wessendorf, S. (2008). Systems change with school-wide Positive Behavior Supports: Iowa's work in progress. *Journal of Positive Behavior Interventions, 10*(2), 129–135. doi:10.1177/1098300707312545.

Masten, A. S. (2003). Commentary: Developmental psychopathology as a unifying context for mental health and education models, research, and practice in schools. *School Psychology Review, 32*(2), 169–173. Retrieved from http://www.nasponline.org/

Maughan, D. R., Christiansen, E., Jenson, W. R., Olympia, D., & Clark, E. (2005). Behavioral parent training as a treatment for externalizing behaviors and disruptive behavior disorders: A meta-analysis. *School Psychology Review, 34*(3), 267–286. Retrieved from http://www.nasponline.org/

Mauriello, L. M., Driskell, M. M., Sherman, K. J., Johnson, S. S., Prochaska, J. M., & Prochaska, J. O. (2006). Acceptability of a school-based intervention for the prevention of adolescent obesity. *The Journal of School Nursing, 22*, 269–277. doi:10.1177/10598405060220050501.

Mauriello, L. M., Sherman, K. J., Driskell, M. M., & Prochaska, J. M. (2007). Using interactive behavior change technology to intervene on physical activity and nutrition with adolescents. *Adolescent Medicine: State of the Art Reviews, 18*, 383–399. Retrieved from https://www.nfaap.org/

Mazza, J. J., Abbott, R. D., Fleming, C. B., Harachi, T. W., Cortes, R. C., Park, J., et al. (2009). Early predictors of adolescent depression: A 7-year longitudinal study. *Journal of Early Adolescence, 29*(5), 664–692. doi:10.1177/0272431608324193.

Mazza, J. J., Fleming, C. B., Abbott, R. D., Haggerty, K. P., & Catalano, R. F. (2010). Identifying trajectories of adolescents' depressive phenomena: An examination of early risk factors. *Journal of Youth and Adolescence, 39*(6), 579–593. doi:10.1007/s10964-009-9406-z.

Mazzone, L., Ducci, F., Scoto, M. C., Passaniti, E., D'Arrigo, V. G., & Vitiello, B. (2007). The role of anxiety symptoms in school performance in a community sample of children and adolescents. *BMC Public Health, 7*, 347. doi:10.1186/1471-2458-7-347.

McCabe, N., Ricciardelli, L., & Banfield, S. (2011). Depressive symptoms and psychosocial functioning in preadolescent children. *Depression Research and Treatment*, Article ID 548034. doi:10.1155/2011/548034

McCabe, K. M., Yeh, M., Garland, A. F., Lau, A. S., & Chavez, G. (2005). The GANA program: A tailoring approach to adapting parent child interaction therapy for Mexican Americans. *Education and Treatment of Children, 28*(2), 111–129. Retrieved from http://www.highbeam.com

McCall, R. B. (2009). Evidence-based programming in the context of practice and policy. *Social Policy Report, 23*(3), 3–16. Retrieved from http://www.nationalcac.org

McCarty, C. A., Violette, H. D., & McCauley, E. (2011). Feasibility of the positive thoughts and actions prevention program for middle schoolers at risk for depression. *Depression Research and Treatment, 2011,* 9. doi:10.1155/2011/241386.

McCay, C. E. (2007). Evidence based practices in mental health: Advantages, disadvantages, and research considerations. *Center for Mental Health Services Research, 4*(5), 1–2. Worcester, MA: University of Massachusetts Medical School.

McConnachie, G., & Carr, E. (1997). The effects of child behavior problems on the maintenance of intervention fidelity. *Behavior Modification, 21*(2), 123–158. doi:10.1177/01454455970212001.

McDougal, J., Bardos, A. N., & Meier, S. T. (2007). *RTI and behavior: Measuring response to behavioral and social/emotional interventions.* Retrieved from www.docstoc.com/

McDougal, J. L., Bardos, A. N., & Meier, S. T. (2011). *Introduction to BIMAS: Behavior Intervention Monitoring Assessment System.* MHS. Retrieved from http://www.mhs.com

McEwan, K., Waddell, C., & Barker, J. (2007). Bringing children's mental health "out of the shadows". *Canadian Medical Association Journal, 176,* 471–472. doi:10.1503/cmaj.061028.

McGarvey, E. L., Collie, K. R., Fraser, G., Shufflebarger, C., Lloyd, B., & Norman Oliver, M. (2006). Using focus group results to inform preschool childhood obesity prevention programming. *Ethnicity & Health, 11*(3), 265–285. doi:10.1080/13557850600565707.

McGilloway, S., Mhaille, G. N., Bywater, T., Furlong, M., Leckey, Y., Kelly, P., et al. (2012). A parenting intervention for childhood behavioral problems: A randomized controlled trial in disadvantaged community-based settings. *Journal of Consulting and Clinical Psychology, 80*(1), 116–127. doi:10.1037/a0026304.

McKown, C., Gumbiner, L. M., Russo, N. M., & Lipton, M. (2009). Social-emotional learning skill, self-regulation, and social competence in typically developing and clinic-referred children. *Journal of Clinical Child and Adolescent Psychology, 38*(6), 858–871. doi:10.1080/15374410903258934.

McMahon, S. D., Washburn, J., Felix, E. D., Yakin, J., & Childrey, G. (2000). Violence prevention: Program effects on urban preschool and kindergarten children. *Applied and Preventive Psychology, 9,* 271–281. doi:10.1016/S0962-1849(00)80004-9.

Meehan, M., Wood, C., Hughes, G., Cowley, K., & Thompson, J. (2004). *Measuring treatment integrity: Testing a multiple-component, multiple-method intervention implementation evaluation model* (ED484856). Paper presented at Evaluation, 2004, the 18th Annual Conference of the American Evaluation Association, Atlanta, GA.

Meier, S. T. (1997). Nomothetic item selection rules for tests of psychological interventions. *Psychotherapy Research, 7*(4), 419–427. doi:10.1080/10503309712331332113.

Meier, S. T., McDougal, J. L., & Bardos, A. (2008). Development of a change-sensitive outcome measure for children receiving counseling. *Canadian Journal of School Psychology, 23*(2), 148–160. doi:10.1177/0829573507307693.

Meir, S. T. (2004). Improving design sensitivity through intervention-sensitive measures. *American Journal of Evaluation, 25*(3), 321–334. doi:10.1177/109821400402500304.

Mellin, E. A., & Weist, M. D. (2011). Exploring school mental health collaboration in an urban community: A social capital perspective. *School Mental Health, 3,* 81–92. doi:10.1007/s12310-011-9049-6.

Mereish, E. H., Liu, M. M., & Helms, J. E. (2012). Effects of discrimination on Chinese, Pilipino, and Vietnamese Americans' mental and physical health. *Asian American Journal of Psychology, 3*(2), 91–103. doi:10.1037/a0025876.

Merikangas, K. R., He, J., Brody, D., Fisher, P. W., Bourdon, K., & Koretz, D. S. (2010). Prevalence and treatment of mental disorders among US children in the 2001–2004 NHANES. *Pediatrics, 125*(1), 75–81. doi:10.1542/peds.2008-2598.

Merrell, K. W. (2002). Social-emotional intervention in schools: Current status, progress, and promise. *School Psychology Review, 31*(2), 143–147. Retrieved from http://www.nasponline.org

Merrell, K. W. (2011). *Social and emotional assets and resilience scales (SEARS).* Lutz, FL: Psychological Assessment Resources.

Merrell, K. W., Carrizales, D. C., Feuerborn, L., Gueldner, B. A., & Tran, O. K. (2007a). *Strong Teens A social-emotional learning curriculum for students in grades 9–12*. Baltimore: Paul H. Brookes Publishing.

Merrell, K. W., Carrizales, D. C., Feuerborn, L., Gueldner, B. A., & Tran, O. K. (2007b). *Strong Teens—Grades 9–12: A social-emotional learning curriculum*. Baltimore: Paul H. Brookes Publishing.

Merrell, K. M., Carrizales, D., Feurborn, L., Gueldner, B. A., & Tran, O. K. (2007). *Strong Kids— Grades 3–5: A social and emotional learning curriculum*. Baltimore: Paul H. Brookes Publishing.

Merrell, K. W., Gueldner, B. A., Ross, S. W., & Isava, D. M. (2008). How effective are school bullying intervention programs? A meta-analysis of intervention research. *School Psychology Quarterly, 23*(1), 26–42. doi:10.1037/1045-3830.23.1.26.

Merrell, K. W., Juskelis, M. P., Tran, O. K., & Buchanan, R. (2008). Social and emotional learning in the classroom: Impact of Strong Kids and Strong Teens on student's social-emotional knowledge and symptoms. *Journal of Applied School Psychology, 24*(2), 209–224. doi:10.1080/15377900802089981.

Merrell, K. W., Parisi, D., & Whitcomb, S. A. (2007). *Strong Start—Grades K-2: A social-emotional learning curriculum*. Baltimore: Paul H. Brookes Publishing.

Merrell, K. W., Whitcomb, S. A., & Parisi, D. M. (2009). *Strong Start pre-K: A social & emotional learning curriculum*. Baltimore: Paul H. Brookes Publishing.

Merry, S., McDowell, H., Wild, C. J., Bir, J., & Cunliffe, R. (2004). A randomized placebo controlled trial of a school-based depression prevention program. *Journal of the American Academy of Child and Adolescent Psychiatry, 43*, 538–547. doi:10.1097/00004583-200405000-00007.

Merry, S. N., & Spence, S. H. (2007). Attempting to prevent depression in youth: A systematic review of the evidence. *Early Intervention in Psychiatry, 1*(2), 128–137. doi:10.1111/j.1751-7893.2007.00030.x.

Meusel, D., Höger, C., Pérez-Rodrigo, C., Aranceta, J., Cavill, N., Armstrong, T., et al. (2008). *A framework to monitor and evaluate implementation*. Geneva, Switzerland: World Health Organization.

Meyers, A. B., Meyers, J., Graybill, E. C., Proctor, S. L., & Huddleston, L. (2012). Ecological approaches to organizational consultation and systems change in educational settings. *Journal of Educational and Psychological Consultation, 22*, 106–124. doi:10.1080/10474412.2011.64 9649.

Michael, J. (2006). Where's the evidence that active learning works. *Advances in Physiology Education, 30*(4), 159–167. doi:10.1152/advan.00053.2006.

Michael, S., Dittus, P., & Epstein, J. (2007). Family and community involvement in schools: Results from the school health policies and programs study 2006. *Journal of School Health, 77*(8), 567–587. doi:10.1111/j.1746-1561.2007.00236.x.

Michie, S., & Johnston, M. (2012). Theories and techniques of behavior change: Developing a cumulative science of behavior change. *Health Psychology Review, 6*(1), 1–6. doi:10.1080/174 37199.2012.654964.

Mier, N., Ory, M. G., Toobert, D. J., Smith, M. L., Osuna, D., McKay, J. R., et al. (2010). A qualitative case study examining intervention tailoring for minorities. *American Journal of Health Behavior, 34*(6), 822–832. doi:10.5993/AJHB.34.6.16.

Mihalic, S., & Aultman-Bettridge, T. (2004). A guide to effective school-based prevention programs: Environmentally focused programs. In W. L. Turk (Ed.), *School crime and policing*. NJ: Prentice Hall.

Mihalic, S. F., Fagan, A. A., & Argamaso, S. (2008). Implementing the LifeSkills training drug prevention program: Factors related to implementation fidelity. *Implementation Science, 3*, 5. doi:10.1186/1748-5908-3-5.

Mihalic, S. F., & Irwin, K. (2003). Blueprints for violence prevention: From research to real-world settings-factors influencing the successful implementation of model programs. *Youth Violence and Juvenile Justice, 1*(4), 307–329. doi:10.1177/1541204003255841.

Mikolajczyk, R. T., Bredehorst, M., Khelaifat, N., Maier, C., & Maxwell, A. E. (2007). Correlates of depressive symptoms among Latino and Non-Latino White adolescents: Findings from the 2003 California Health Interview Survey. *BMC Public Health, 7,* 21. doi:10.1186/1471-2458-7-21.

Miller, G. E., Arthur-Stanley, A., & Lines, C. (2012). Family-school collaboration services: Beliefs into action. *Communiqué, 40*(5), 12–14. Retrieved from http://www.nasponline.org

Miller, K., & Cloverdale, G. (2010, November). Exploring views on primary prevention of eating disorders. *British Journal of School Nursing, 5*(9), 441–448. Retrieved from http://www.school-nursing.co.uk/

Miller, N. E., & Dollard, J. (1941). *Social learning and imitation.* New Haven, CT: Yale University Press.

Miller, D. N., Eckert, T. L., & Mazza, J. J. (2009). Suicide prevention programs in the schools: A review and public health perspective. *School Psychology Review, 38*(2), 168–188. Retrieved from http://www.nasponline.org/publications/

Miller, M. J., Yang, M., Farrell, J. A., & Lin, L. (2011). Racial and cultural factors affecting the mental health of Asian Americans. *The American Journal of Orthopsychiatry, 81*(4), 489–497. doi:10.1111/j.1939-0025.2011.01118.x.

Miranda, J., Bernal, G., Lau, A., Kohn, L., Hwang, W., & LaFromboise, T. (2005). State of the science on psychosocial interventions for ethnic minorities. *Annual Review of Clinical Psychology, 1,* 113–142. doi:10.1146/annurev.clinpsy.1.102803.143822.

Moher, D., Hopewell, S., Schulz, K. F., Montori, V., Gøtzsche, P. C., Devereaux, P. J., et al. (2010). CONSORT 2010 explanation and elaboration: Updated guidelines for reporting parallel group randomised trials. *British Medical Journal, 340,* c869. doi:10.1136/bmj.c869.

Monshouwer, K., Harakeh, Z., Lugtig, P., Huizink, A., Creemers, H. E., Reijneveld, S. A., et al. (2012). Predicting transitions in low and high levels of risk behavior from early to middle adolescence: The TRAILS study. *Journal of Abnormal Child Psychology, 40*(6), 923–931. doi:10.1007/s10802-012-9624-9.

Montano, D. E., & Kasprzyk, D. (2008). Theory of reasoned action, theory of planned behavior, and the integrated behavioral model. In K. Glanz, B. K. Rimer, & K. Viswanath (Eds.), *Health behavior and health education: Theory, research, and practice* (4th ed., pp. 67–96). San Francisco: Jossey-Bass.

Morawska, A., Sanders, M., Goadby, E., Headley, C., Hodge, L., McAuliffe, C., et al. (2011). Is the Triple-P-Positive Parenting Program acceptable to parents from culturally diverse backgrounds? *Journal of Child and Family Studies, 20,* 614–622. doi:10.1007/s10826-010-9436-x.

Morgan, D. L., & Krueger, R. A. (1993). When to use focus groups and why. In D. L. Morgan (Ed.), *Successful focus groups: Advancing the state of the art* (pp. 3–19). Newbury Park, CA: Sage.

Mrazek, P. J., & Haggerty, R. J. (Eds.). (1994). *Reducing risks for mental disorders: Frontiers for preventive intervention research.* Washington, DC: National Academy Press.

Mrug, S., & Windle, M. (2008). Moderators of negative peer influence on early adolescent externalizing behaviors: Individual behavior, parenting, and school connectedness. *The Journal of Early Adolescence, 29*(4), 518–540. doi:10.1177/0272431608324473.

Muijs, D. (2004). Designing non-experimental studies. In D. Muijs (Ed.), *Doing qualitative research in education with SPSS* (2nd ed., pp. 30–55). Thousand, Oaks, CA: Sage. doi:10.4135/9781849209014.

Munford, M. B. (1994). Relationship of gender, self-esteem, social class, and racial identity to depression in Blacks. *Journal of Black Psychology, 20*(2), 157–174. doi:10.1177/00957984940202005.

Muñoz, R. F., & Mendelson, T. (2005). Toward evidence-based interventions for diverse populations: The San Francisco General Hospital prevention and treatment manuals. *Journal of Consulting and Clinical Psychology, 73*(5), 790–799. doi:10.1037/0022-006X.73.5.790.

Muris, P., Steerneman, P., Merckelbach, H., Holdrinet, I., & Meesters, C. (1998). Comorbid anxiety symptoms in children with pervasive developmental disorders. *Journal of Anxiety Disorders, 12*(4), 387–393. doi:10.1016/S0887-6185(98)00022-X.

Murphey, D., Barry, M., & Vaughn, B. (2013). Mental health disorders. *Child trends: Adolescent health highlight* (Publication No. 2013-1). Retrieved from http://www.childtrends.org

Murphey, D., Vaughn, B., & Barry, M. (2013). Access to mental health care. *Child trends: Adolescent health highlight* (Publication #2013-2). Retrieved from http://www.childtrends.org

Muscott, H. S., Mann, E. L., & LeBrun, M. R. (2008). Positive behavioral interventions and supports in New Hampshire: Effects of large-scale implementation of Schoolwide Positive Behavior Support on student discipline and academic achievement. *Journal of Positive Behavior Interventions, 10*(3), 190–205. doi:10.1177/1098300708316258.

Mychailyszyn, M. P., Brodman, D. M., Read, K. L., & Kendall, P. C. (2012). Cognitive-behavioral school-based interventions for anxious and depressed youth: A meta-analysis of outcomes. *Clinical Psychology: Science and Practice, 19*(2), 129–153. doi:10.1111/j.1468-2850.2012.01279.x.

NAEYC Pathways to Cultural Competence Project. (2010). Retrieved from http://www.ecementor. org/

Nagel, R. J., & Gagnon, S. G. (2008). Best practices in planning and conducting needs assessment. In A. Thomas & A. J. Grimes (Eds.), *Best practices in school psychology V* (Vol. 6, pp. 2207–2224). Bethesda, MD: National Association of School Psychologists.

Naglieri, J. A., LeBuffe, P., & Shapiro, V. B. (2011). Universal screening for social-emotional competencies: A study of the reliability and validity of the DESSA-MINI. *Psychology in the Schools, 48*(7), 660–671. doi:10.1002/pits.20586.

Najaka, S. S., Gottfredson, D. C., & Wilson, D. B. (2001). A meta-analytic inquiry into the relationship between selected risk factors and problem behavior. *Prevention Science, 2*(4), 257–271. doi:10.1023/A:1013610115351.

Nansel, T. R., Overpeck, M., Pilla, R. S., Ruan, W. J., Simons-Morton, B., & Scheidt, P. (2001). Bullying behaviors among US youth: Prevalence and association with psychosocial adjustment. *Journal of the American Medical Association, 285*(16), 2094–2100. doi:10.1001/jama.285.16.2094.

Nastasi, B. K., & Varjas, K. (2008). Best practices in developing exemplary mental health programs in schools. In A. Thomas & J. Grimes (Eds.), *Best practices in school psychology* (Vol. 4, pp. 1349–1360). Bethesda, MD: National Association of School Psychologists.

Nation, M., Crusto, C., Wandersman, A., Kumpfer, K. L., Seybolt, D., Morrissey-Kane, E., et al. (2003). What works in prevention: Principles of effective prevention programs. *American Psychologist, 58*(6/7), 449–456. doi:10.1037/0003-066X.58.6-7.449.

National Advisory Mental Health Council. (1990). *National plan for research on child and adolescent mental disorders* (DHHS Publication No. 90-1683). Washington, DC: U.S. Government Printing Office.

National Association of School Psychologists (NASP). (2010). *Model for comprehensive and integrated school psychological services*. Bethesda, MD: Author.

National Institute of Mental Health (NIMH). (1993). *The prevention of mental disorders: A national research agenda*. Bethesda, MD: NMHA.

National Institute of Mental Health (NIMH). (1998). *Priorities for prevention research* (NIMH Publication No. 98-4321). Bethesda, MD: NIMH.

National Scientific Council on the Developing Child. (2008/2012). *Establishing a level foundation for life: Mental health begins in early childhood: Working paper 6*. Updated edition. Retrieved from http://www.developingchild.harvard.edu

National Scientific Council on the Developing Child. (2008). *Mental health problems in early childhood can impair learning and behavior for life: Working paper #6*. Retrieved from http://www.developingchild.net

Neace, W. P., & Munoz, M. A. (2012). Pushing the boundaries of education: Evaluating the "Impact of Second Step[R]—A Violence Prevention Curriculum" with psychosocial and non-cognitive measures. *Child & Youth Services, 33*(1), 46–69. doi:10.1080/0145935X.2012.665324.

Nehmy, T. J. (2010). School-based prevention of depression and anxiety in Australia: Current state and future directions. *Clinical Psychologist, 14*(3), 74–83. doi:10.1080/13284207.2010.524884.

Neil, A. L., & Christensen, H. (2009). Efficacy and effectiveness of school-based prevention and early intervention programs for anxiety. *Clinical Psychology Review, 29*(3), 208–215. doi:10.1016/j.cpr.2009.01.002.

Nelson, G., Westhues, A., & MacLeod, J. (2003). A meta-analysis of longitudinal research on preschool prevention programs for children. *Prevention & Treatment, 6*(1), Article 31a. doi:10.1037/1522-3736.6.1.631a

Newell, M. L., Nastasi, B. K., Hatzichristou, C., Jones, J. M., Schanding, G. T., Jr., & Yetter, G. (2010). Evidence on multicultural training in school psychology: Recommendations for future directions. *School Psychology Quarterly, 25*(4), 249–278. doi:10.1037/a0021542.

Nichols, T. R., Mahadeo, M., Bryant, K., & Botvin, G. J. (2008). Examining anger as a predictor of drug use among multiethnic middle school students. *Journal of School Health, 78*(9), 480–486. doi:10.1111/j.1746-1561.2008.00333.x.

Nicolas, G., Arntz, D. L., Hirsch, B., & Schmiedigen, A. (2009). Cultural adaptation of a group treatment for Haitian American adolescents. *Professional Psychology: Research and Practice, 40*(4), 378–384. doi:10.1037/a0016307.

Nilsson, M., & Emmelin, M. (2010). "Immortal but frightened"-smoking adolescents' perceptions on smoking uptake and prevention. *BMC Public Health, 10*, 776. doi:10.1186/1471-2458-10-776.

Nix, R. (2004/2005, Winter). Improving parental involvement: Evaluating treatment effects in the Fast Track Program. *The Evaluation Exchange, X*(4). Retrieved from http://www.hfrp.org

No Child Left Behind Act of 2001. (2002). Pub. L. No. 117-110, 115 Stat. 1425. Retrieved from http://www.ed.gov/policy/elsec/leg/esea02/107-110.pdf

Norcross, J. C., Krebs, P. M., & Prochaska, J. O. (2011). Stages of change. *Journal of Clinical Psychology, 67*(2), 143–154. doi:10.1002/jclp.20758.

Northeast Foundation for Children. (2006). *Responsive Classroom principles and practices.* Retrieved from https://www.responsiveclassroom.org

O'Connor, E. P., & Freeman, E. W. (2012). District-level considerations in supporting and sustaining RTI implementation. *Psychology in the Schools, 49*(3), 297–310. doi:10.1002/pits.21598.

O'Connor, C., Small, S. A., & Cooney, S. M. (2007). Program fidelity and adaptation: Meeting local needs without compromising program effectiveness. *What works, Wisconsin research to practice series,* 4. Madison, WI: University of Wisconsin—Madison/Extension. Retrieved from http://whatworks.uwex.edu

O'Donnell, J., Hawkins, D., Catalano, R. F., Abbott, R. D., & Day, L. E. (1997). Seattle Social Development Project: Preventing delinquency among low-income children. *The Prevention Researcher, 4*(2), 7–9. Retrieved from http://www.tpronline.org

O'Keeffe, B., Fallon, L., & Sugai, G. (2011). *SWPBS: Examination of cultural relevance.* University of Connecticut, Center for Behavioral Education & Research, Storrs, CT.

Oakley, A., Strange, V., Bonell, C., Allen, E., Stephenson, J., & RIPPLE Study Team. (2008). Process evaluation in randomised controlled trials of complex interventions. *British Medical Journal, 332*(7538), 413–416. doi:10.1136/bmj.332.7538.413.

Oesterle, S., Hawkins, J. D., Fagan, A. A., Abbott, R. D., & Catalano, R. F. (2010). Testing the universality of the effects of the communities that care prevention system for preventing adolescent drug use and delinquency. *Prevention Science, 11*(4), 411–423. doi:10.1007/s11121-010-0178-1.

Ogletree, Q., & Larke, P. J. (2010). Implementing multicultural practice in early childhood education. *National Forum of Multicultural Issues Journal, 7*(1), 1–9. Retrieved from http://www.nationalforum.com

Oh, W., Rubin, K. H., Bowker, J. C., Booth-LaForce, C., Rose-Krasnor, L., & Laursen, B. (2008). Trajectories of social withdrawal from middle childhood to early adolescence. *Journal of Abnormal Child Psychology, 36*, 553–566. doi:10.1007/s10802-007-9199-z.

Oldenburg, B., & Glanz, K. (2008). Diffusion of innovations. In K. Glanz, B. K. Rimer, & K. Viswanath (Eds.), *Health behavior and health education: Theory, research, and practice* (4th ed., pp. 313–334). San Francisco: Jossey-Bass.

Olds, D. (2003). What can we conclude from meta-analyses of early interventions? *Prevention & Treatment, 6*(1), Article 34. doi:10.1037/1522-3736.6.1.634c.

Ollendick, T. H., Shortt, A. L., & Sander, J. B. (2008). Internalizing disorders in children and adolescents. In J. E. Maddux & B. A. Winstead (Eds.), *Psychopathology: Foundations for a contemporary understanding* (2nd ed., pp. 375–399). New York: Routledge.

Olweus, D. (1993). *Bullying at school: What we know and what we can do.* Oxford: Blackwell.

Olweus, D. (1994). Bullying at school: Long term outcomes for the victims and an effective school-based intervention program. In L. R. Huesmann (Ed.), *Aggressive behavior: Current perspectives* (pp. 97–130). New York: Plenum Press.

Olweus, D. (1996). *The Revised Olweus Bully/Victim Questionnaire.* Mimeo Research Center for Health Promotion (HEMIL). Bergen, Norway: University of Bergen.

Olweus, D. (2012). Cyberbullying: An overrated phenomenon? *The European Journal of Developmental Psychology, 9*(5), 520–538. doi:10.1080/17405629.2012.682358.

Olweus, D., & Limber, S. P. (2010). The Olweus Bullying Prevention Program: Implementation and evaluation over two decades. In S. R. Jimerson, S. M. Swearer, & D. L. Espelage (Eds.), *The handbook of bullying in schools: An international perspective* (pp. 377–402). New York: Routledge.

Opler, M., Sodhi, D., Zaveri, D., & Madhusoodanan, S. (2010). Primary psychiatric prevention in children and adolescents. *Annals of Clinical Psychiatry, 22*(4), 220–234. Retrieved from http://www.aacp.com

Ormiston, J., Shure, L., & Brentano, M. (2011). *PBIS Indiana: Applying culturally responsive practice to positive behavior supports.* APBS Conference, Denver, CO.

Orthner, D. K., Akos, P., Rose, R., Jones-Sanpei, H., Mercado, M., & Woolley, M. E. (2010). CareerStart: A middle school student engagement and academic achievement program. *Children and Schools, 32*(4), 223–234. doi:10.1093/cs/32.4.223.

Ozer, E. J., Wanis, M. G., & Bazell, N. (2010). Diffusion of school-based prevention programs in two urban districts: Adaptation, rationales, and suggestions for change. *Prevention Science, 11*, 42–55. doi:10.1007/s11121-009-0148-7.

Pabayo, R., O'Loughlin, J., Barnett, T. A., Cohen, J. E., & Gauvin, L. (2012). Does intolerance of smoking at school, or in restaurants or corner stores decrease cigarette use initiation in adolescents? *Nicotine & Tobacco Research, 14*(10), 1154–1160. doi:10.1093/ntr/ntr326.

Parcel, G. (1995). Diffusion research: The SMART choices project. *Health Education Research, 10*(3), 279–281. doi:10.1093/her/10.3.279.

Park-Higgerson, H. K., Perumean-Chaney, S. E., Bartolucci, A. A., Grimley, D. M., & Singh, K. P. (2008). The evaluation of school-based violence prevention programs: A meta-analysis. *Journal of School Health, 78*(9), 465–479. doi:10.1111/j.1746-1561.2008.00332.x.

Passel, J. S. (2011). Demography of immigrant youth: Past present and future. *Future Child, 21*(1), 19–41. Retrieved from http://www.futureofchildren.org

Pate, L. R. (2010). *Mexican American parents' beliefs about their adolescent's mental health and parental use of alternative interventions.* Unpublished doctoral dissertation, The University of Texas at Austin, Austin, TX.

Patient Protection and Affordable Care Act (PPACA). (2010). Pub. L. No. 111-148, §2702, 124 Stat. 119, 318–319.

Patnode, C. D., O'Connor, E., Whitlock, E. P., Perdue, L. A., Soh, C., & Hollis, J. (2013). Primary care-relevant interventions for tobacco use prevention and cessation in children and adolescents: A systematic evidence review for the U.S. Preventive Services Task Force. *Annals of Internal Medicine, 158*(4), 253–260. doi:10.7326/0003-4819-158-4-201302190-00580.

Pattison, C., & Lynd-Stevenson, R. M. (2001). The prevention of depressive symptoms in children: Immediate and long-term outcomes of a school-based program. *Behavior Change, 18*, 92–102. doi:10.1375/bech.18.2.92.

Patton, A. (2012). *Work that matters: The teacher's guide to project-based learning.* San Diego, CA: Paul Hamlyn Foundation.

Paulson, C. A., & Dailey, D. (2002). *A guide for education personnel: Evaluating a programs or intervention.* Washington, DC: American Institutes for Research.

Payton, J. W., Wardlaw, D. M., Graczyk, P. A., Bloodworth, M. R., Tompsett, C. J., & Weissberg, R. P. (2000). Social and emotional learning: A framework for promoting mental health and reducing risk behavior in children and youth. *Journal of School Health, 70*(5), 179–185. doi:10.1111/j.1746-1561.2000.tb06468.x.

Payton, J., Weissberg, R. P., Durlak, J. A., Dymnicki, A. B., Taylor, R. D., Schellinger, K. B., et al. (2008). *The positive impact of social and emotional learning for kindergarten to eighth-grade students: Findings from three scientific reviews.* Chicago: Collaborative for Academic, Social, and Emotional Learning.

Peguero, A. A., Popp, A. M., Latimore, L., Shekarkhar, Z., & Koo, D. J. (2011). Social control theory and school misbehavior: Examining the role of race and ethnicity. *Youth Violence and Juvenile Justice, 9*(3), 259–275. doi:10.1177/1541204010389197.

Peirson, L. J., Boydell, K. M., Ferguson, H. B., & Ferris, L. E. (2011). An ecological process model of systems change. *American Journal of Community Psychology, 47*, 307–321. doi:10.1007/s10464-010-9405-y.

Peña, A. M., Silvan, A., Claro, C., Gamarra, A., & Parra, E. (2008). Communicating with Latino parents and families. *Communiqué, 37*(4). Retrieved from http://www.nasponline.org

Penna, R., & Phillips, W. (2005). Eight outcome models. *The Evaluation Exchange, 11*(2), 5. Retrieved from http://www.hfrp.org

Pentz, M. A., Dwyer, J. H., MacKinnon, D. P., Flay, B. R., Hansen, W. B., Wang, E. U., et al. (1989). A multicommunity trial for primary prevention of adolescent drug abuse. Effects on drug use prevalence. *Journal of the American Medical Association, 261*, 3259–3266. doi:10.1001/jama.1989.03420220073030.

Pentz, M. A., Trebow, E. A., Hansen, W. B., MacKinnon, D. P., Dwyer, J. H., Johnson, C. A., et al. (1990). Effects of a program implementation on adolescent drug use behavior: The Midwestern Prevention Project (MPP). *Evaluation Review, 14*(3), 264–289. doi:10.1177/01938 41X9001400303.

Pérez-Edgar, K., Bar-Haim, Y., McDermott, J. M., Chronis-Tuscano, A., Pine, D. S., & Fox, N. A. (2010). Attention biases to threat and behavioral inhibition in early child-hood shape adolescent social withdrawal. *Emotion, 10*(3), 349–357. doi:10.1037/a0018486.

Perez-Johnson, I., Walters, K., Puma, M., Herman, R., Garet, M., Heppen, J., Burghardt, J. (2011). *Evaluating AARA programs and other educational reforms: A guide for states.* American Institutes for Research and Mathematica Policy Research.

Perkins, H. W., Craig, D. W., & Perkins, J. M. (2011). Using social norms to reduce bullying: A research intervention among adolescents in five middle schools. *Group Process & Intergroup Relations, 14*(5), 703–722. doi:10.1177/1368430210398004.

Perrin, E. C., Siegel, B. S., & The Committee on Psychosocial Aspects of Child and Family Health. (2013). Promoting the well-being of children whose parents are gay or lesbian. *Pediatrics, 131*(4), 827–830. doi:10.1542/peds.2013-0377.

Perry, D. F., Holland, C., Darling-Kuria, N., & Nadiv, S. (2011). Challenging behavior and expulsion from child care. *Zero to Three, 32*(2), 4–11. Retrieved from http://www.zerotothree.org

Perry, C. L., Williams, C. L., Komro, K. A., Veblen-Mortenson, S., Stigler, M. H., Munson, K. A., et al. (2002). Project Northland. Long-term outcomes of community action to reduce adolescent alcohol use. *Health Education Research, 17*(1), 117–132. doi:10.1093/her/17.1.117.

Perry, C. L., Williams, C. L., Veblen-Mortenson, S., Toomey, T. L., Komro, K. A., Anstine, P. S., et al. (1996). Project Northland: Outcomes of a communitywide alcohol use prevention program during early adolescence. *American Journal of Public Health, 86*(7), 956–965. doi:10.2105/AJPH.86.7.956.

Petticrew, M., & Roberts, H. (2003). Evidence, hierarchies, and typologies: Horses for courses. *Journal of Epidemiology and Community Health, 57*, 527–529. doi:10.1136/jech.57.7.527.

Pickens, J. (2009). Socio-emotional programme promotes positive behaviour in preschoolers. *Child Care in Practice, 15*(4), 261–278. doi:10.1080/13575270903149323.

Pina, A. A., Zerr, A. A., Villalta, I. K., & Gonzales, N. A. (2012). Indicated prevention and early intervention for childhood anxiety: A randomized trial with Caucasian and Latino youth. *Journal of Consulting and Clinical Psychology, 80*(5), 940–946. doi:10.1037/a0029460.

Pirkis, J., Hickie, I., Young, L., Burns, J., Highet, N., & Davenport, T. (2005). An evaluation of *beyondblue*, Australia's National Depression Initiative. *The International Journal of Mental Health Promotion, 7*(2), 35–53. Retrieved from http://www.ijmhp.co.uk/

Podell, J., Mychailyszyn, M., Edmunds, J., Puleo, C., & Kendall, P. C. (2010). *The Coping Cat Program* for anxious youth: The FEAR plan comes to life. *Cognitive and Behavioral Practice, 17*, 132–141. doi:10.1016/j.cbpra.2009.11.001.

Polanin, J. R., Espelage, D. L., & Pigott, T. D. (2012). A meta-analysis of school-based bullying prevention programs' effects on bystander intervention behavior. *School Psychology Review, 41*(1), 47–65. Retrieved from http://www.nasponline.org/publications/

Polo, A. J., & López, S. R. (2009). Culture, context and the internalizing of Mexican American youth. *Journal of Clinical Child and Adolescent Psychology, 38*(2), 273–285. doi:10.1080/15374410802698370.

Pössel, P. (2005). Strategies for universal prevention of depression in adolescents. *Journal of Indian Association for Child and Adolescent, Mental Health, 1*(1). Article 5. Retrieved from http://cogprints.org/4209/

Poteat, V. P., & Espelage, D. L. (2007). Predicting psychosocial consequences of homophobic victimization in Middle school students. *Journal of Early Adolescence, 27*(2), 175–191. doi: 10.1177/0272431606294839.

Powell, D., & Dunlap, G. (2009). *Evidence-based social emotional curricula and intervention packages for children 0–5 years and their families* (Roadmap to Effective Intervention Practices). Tampa, FL: University of South Florida.

Powell, D., Dunlop, G., & Fox, L. (2006). Prevention and intervention for the challenging behaviors of toddlers and preschoolers. *Infants & Young Children, 19*(1), 25–35. Retrieved from http://journals.lww.com

President's New Freedom Commission on Mental Health. (2003). *Achieving the promise: Transforming mental health care in America.* Final report (DHHS Publication No. SMA-03-3832). Rockville, MD: U.S. Department of Health and Human Services.

Prince, M. (2004). Does active learning work? A review of the research. *Journal of Engineering Education, 93*(3), 223–231. Retrieved from http://www.asee.org

Prinz, R. J., Sanders, M. R., Shapiro, C. J., Whitaker, D. J., & Lutzker, J. R. (2009). Population-based prevention of child maltreatment: The U.S. Triple P System Population Trial. *Prevention Science, 10*(1), 1–12. doi:10.1007/s11121-009-0123-3.

Prochaska, J. O., & DiClemente, C. C. (1983). Stages and processes of self-change of smoking: Toward an integrative model of change. *Journal of Consulting and Clinical Psychology, 51*, 390–395. doi:10.1037/0022-006X.51.3.390.

Prochaska, J. O., Evers, K. E., Prochaska, J. M., Van Marter, D., & Johnson, J. L. (2007). Efficacy and effectiveness trials: Examples from smoking cessation and bullying prevention. *Journal of Health Psychology, 12*(1), 170–178. doi:10.1177/1359105307071751.

Prochaska, J. O., Redding, C. A., & Evers, K. E. (2008). The transtheoretical model and stages of change. In K. Glanz, K. B. Rimer, & K. Viswanath (Eds.), *Health behavior and health education: Theory, research, and practice* (4th ed., pp. 97–122). San Francisco: Jossey-Bass.

Protection of Pupil Rights Amendment (PPRA) (20 U.S.C. § 1232h; 34 CFR Part 98) (2002). Retrieved from (http://www2.ed.gov/policy/gen/guid/fpco/ppra/index.html).

Prothrow-Stith, D. (2007). A major step forward in violence prevention. *American Journal of Preventive Medicine, 33*(2S), S109–S111. doi:10.1016/j.amepre.2007.04.025.

Puddy, R. W., & Wilkins, N. (2011). *Understanding evidence part 1: Best available research evidence. A guide to the continuum of evidence of effectiveness.* Atlanta, GA: Centers for Disease Control and Prevention.

Pumariega, A. J., & Rothe, E. (2010). Leaving no children or families outside: The challenges of immigration. *The American Journal of Orthopsychiatry, 80*(4), 505–515. doi:10.1111/j.1939-0025.2010.01053.x.

Putnam, S. P., Samson, A. V., & Rothbart, M. K. (2002). Child temperament and parenting. In M. H. Bornstein (Ed.), *Handbook of parenting* (2nd ed., pp. 225–278). Mahwah, NJ: Lawrence Erlbaum Associates.

Raferty, J. N., Grolnick, W. S., & Flamm, E. S. (2012). Families as facilitators of student engagement: Toward a home-school partnership model. In S. L. Christenson, A. L. Reschly, & C. Wylie (Eds.), *Handbook of research on student engagement* (pp. 343–364). New York: Springer.

Ramos, D., & Perkins, D. F. (2006). Goodness of fit assessment of an alcohol intervention program and the underlying theories of change. *Journal of American College Health, 55*(1), 57–64. doi:10.3200/JACH.55.1.57-64.

Ransford, C. R., Greenberg, M. T., Domitrovich, C. E., Small, M., & Jacobson, L. (2009). The role of teachers' psychological experiences and perceptions of curriculum supports on the implementation of a social and emotional learning curriculum. *School Psychology Review, 38*(4), 510–532. Retrieved from http://www.nasponline.org/

Rapee, R. M., Kennedy, S., Ingram, M., Edwards, S., & Sweeney, L. (2005). Prevention and early intervention of anxiety disorders in inhibited preschool children. *Journal of Consulting and Clinical Psychology, 73*(3), 488–497. doi:10.1037/0022-006X.73.3.488.

Rapee, R. M., Kennedy, S. J., Ingram, M., Edwards, S. L., & Sweeney, L. (2010). Altering the trajectory of anxiety in at-risk young children. *The American Journal of Psychiatry, 167*(12), 1518–1525. doi:10.1176/appi.ajp.2010.09111619.

Rappaport, N., & Thomas, C. (2004). Recent research findings on aggressive and violent behavior in youth: Implications for clinical assessment and intervention. *Journal of Adolescent Health, 35*, 260–277. doi:10.1016/j.jadohealth. 2003.10.009.

Ratiani, M., Kitiashvili, A., Labartkava, N., Sadunishvili, P., Tsereteli, E., & Gvetadze, N. (2011). *Teaching disaster risk reduction with interactive methods: Book for head of class teachers* (Grades V-IX) (UNICEF). Tbilisi, GA: National Curriculum and Assessment Centre.

Redding, S. (2009). *Framework for an effective statewide system of support.* Lincoln, IL: Center on Innovations & Improvement. Retrieved from http://www.michigan.gov

Redding, C. A., Rossi, J. S., Rossi, S. R., Velicer, W. F., & Prochaska, J. O. (2000). Health behavior models. *The international Electronic Journal of Health Education, 3*, 180–193. Retrieved from http://www.aahperd.org

Reed, J. G. (2004). *An examination of treatment integrity practices and behavioral outcomes when utilizing the Second Step curriculum.* Unpublished doctoral dissertation, University of Maryland, College Park, MD.

Reeve, J. (2012). A self-determination theory perspective on student engagement. In S. L. Christenson, A. L. Reschly, & C. Wylie (Eds.), *Handbook of research on student engagement* (pp. 149–172). New York: Springer.

Reeves, T. (2011). Can educational research be both rigorous and relevant? *Journal of the International Society for Design and Development in Education, 1*(4), 1–24. Retrieved from http://www.isdde.org

Reid, M. J., Webster-Stratton, C., & Hammond, M. (2007). Enhancing a classroom social competence and problem-solving curriculum by offering parent training to families of moderate- to high-risk elementary school children. *Journal of Clinical Child and Adolescent Psychology, 36*(4), 605–620. doi:10.1080/15374410701662741.

Reinke, W. M., Lewis-Palmer, T., & Merrell, K. (2008). The classroom check-up: A classwide teacher consultation model for increasing praise and decreasing disruptive behavior. *School Psychology Review, 37*(3), 315–332. Retrieved from http://www.nasponline.org

Reinke, W. M., Stormont, M., Herman, K. C., Puri, R., & Goel, N. (2011). Supporting children's mental health in schools: Teacher perceptions of needs, roles, and barriers. *School Psychology Quarterly, 26*(1), 1–13. doi:10.1037/a0022714.

Renger, R., & Titcomb, A. (2002). A three-step approach to teaching logic models. *American Journal of Evaluation, 23*(4), 493–503. doi:10.1177/109821400202300409.

Report of the Committee on the Prevention of Mental Disorders and Substance Abuse. (2009, March 25). *Preventing mental, emotional, and behavioral disorders among young people. Public briefing.* Washington, DC: The National Academies.

Reschly, A., & Christenson, S. L. (2006). Promoting successful school completion. In G. Bear & K. Minki (Eds.), *Children's needs-III: Development, prevention, and intervention* (pp. 103–113). Bethesda, MD: National Association of School Psychologists.

Reschly, A. L., & Christenson, S. L. (2012a). Moving from 'context matters' to engage partnerships with families. *Journal of Educational and Psychological Consultation, 22,* 62–78. doi:1 0.1080/10474412.2011.649650.

Reschly, A. L., & Christenson, S. L. (2012b). Jingle, jangle, and conceptual haziness: Evolution and future directions of the engagement construct. In S. L. Christenson, A. L. Reschly, & C. Wylie (Eds.), *Handbook of research on student engagement* (pp. 3–19). New York: Springer.

Resnicow, K., Soler, R., Braithwaite, R. L., Ahluwalia, J. S., & Butler, J. (2000). Cultural sensitivity in substance use prevention. *Journal of Community Psychology, 28,* 271–290. doi:10.1002/(SICI)1520-6629(200005)28:3<271::AID-JCOP4>3.0.CO;2-I.

Reynolds, S., Wilson, C., Austin, J., & Hooper, L. (2012). Effects of psychotherapy for anxiety in children and adolescents: A meta-analytic review. *Clinical Psychology Review, 32*(4), 251–262. doi:10.1016/j.cpr.2012.01.005.

Rhew, I. C., Simpson, K., Tracy, M., Lymp, J., McCauley, E., Tsuang, D., et al. (2010). Criterion validity of the Short Mood and Feelings Questionnaire and one- and two-item depression screens in young adolescents. *Child and Adolescent Psychiatry and Mental Health, 4,* 8. doi:10.1186/1753-20000-4-8.

Richard, L., Gauvin, L., & Raine, K. (2011). Ecological models revisited: Their uses and evolution in health promotion over two decades. *Annual Review of Public Health, 32,* 307–326. doi:10.1146/annurev-publhealth-031210-101141.

Riggs, N. R., Greenberg, M. T., Kusché, C. A., & Pentz, M. A. (2006). The meditational role of neurocognition in the behavioral outcomes of a social-emotional prevention program in elementary school students: Effects of the PATHS curriculum. *Prevention Science, 7*(1), 91–102. doi:10.1007/s11121-00500221.

Rimer, B., & Glanz, K. (2005). *Theory at a glance: A guide for health promotion practice* (2nd ed.). Washington, DC: U.S. Department of Health and Human Services.

Rimm-Kaufman, S. E. (2006). *Social and academic learning study on the contribution of the Responsive Classroom approach.* Turners Falls, MA: Northeast Foundation for Children.

Ringeisen, H., Henderson, K., & Hoagwood, K. (2003). Context matters: Schools and the "research to practice gap" in children's mental health. *School Psychology Review, 322,* 153–168. Retrieved from http://www.nasponline.org/publications/spr/about.aspx

Ringwalt, C. L., Ennett, S., Johnson, R., Rohrbach, L. A., Simons-Rudolph, A., Vincus, A., et al. (2003). Factors associated with fidelity to substance use prevention curriculum guides in the nation's middle schools. *Health Education & Behavior, 30*(3), 375–391. doi:10.1177/1090198103253627.

Ringwalt, C., Ennett, S., Vincus, A., & Simons-Rudolph, A. (2004). Students' special needs and problems as reasons for the adaptation of substance abuse prevention curricula in the nation's middle schools. *Prevention Science, 5*(3), 197–206. doi:10.1023/B:PREV.0000037642.40783.95.

Ringwalt, C. L., Ennett, S., Vincus, A., Thorne, J., Rohrbach, L. A., & Simmons-Rudolph, A. (2002). The prevalence of effective substance use prevention curricula in U.S. middle schools. *Prevention Science, 3*(4), 257–265. doi:10.1023/A:1020872424136.

Ringwalt, C. L., Vincus, A., Ennett, S., Johnson, R., & Rohrbach, L. A. (2004). Reasons for teachers' adaptation of substance use prevention curricula in schools with non-White student populations. *Journal of Prevention Science, 5*(1), 61–67. doi:10.1023/B:PREV.0000013983.87069.a0.

Rishel, C. (2007). Evidence-based prevention practice in mental health: What is it and how do we get there? *The American Journal of Orthopsychiatry, 77*(1), 153–164. doi:10.1037/0002-9432.77.1.153.

Roberts, R. E., Roberts, C. R., & Chen, Y. R. (1997). Ethnocultural differences in prevalence of adolescent depression. *American Journal of Community Psychology, 25*(1), 95–110. doi:10.10 23/A:1024649925737.

Robles-Piña, R. A., Defrance, E., & Cox, D. L. (2008). Self-concept, early childhood depression and school retention as predictors of adolescent depression in urban Hispanic adolescents. *School Psychology International, 29*(4), 426–441. doi:10.1177/0143034308096434.

Rodney, L. W., Johnson, D. L., & Srivastava, R. P. (2005). The impact of culturally relevant violence prevention models on school-age youth. *The Journal of Primary Prevention, 26*(5), 439–454. doi:10.1007/s10935-005-0003-y.

Rodríguez, M. M., Baumann, A. A., & Schwartz, A. L. (2011). Cultural adaptation of an evidence based intervention: From theory to practice in a Latino/a community context. *American Journal of Community Psychology, 47*(1–2), 170–186. doi:10.1007/s10464-010-9371-4.

Rodriguez, J., McKay, M. M., & Bannon, W. M., Jr. (2008). The role of racial socialization in relation to parenting practices and youth behavior: An exploratory analysis. *Social Work in Mental Health, 6*(4), 30–54. doi:10.1080/15332980802032409.

Rogers, E. M. (1976). New product adoption and diffusion. *Journal of Consumer Research, 2*(4), 290–301. Retrieved from http://www.jstor.org

Rogers, E. M. (2002). Diffusion of preventive innovations. *Addictive Behaviors, 27*(6), 989–993. doi:10.1016/S0306-4603(02)00300-3.

Rogers, E. M. (2003). *Diffusion of innovations* (5th ed.). New York: Simon & Shuster.

Rogler, L. H., Malgady, R. G., Costantino, G., & Blumenthal, R. (1987). What do culturally sensitive mental health services mean? *American Psychologist, 42*(6), 565–570. doi:10.1037/0003-066X.42.6.565.

Romano, J. L., & Hage, S. M. (2000). Prevention: A call to action. *The Counseling Psychologist, 28*(6), 854–856. doi:10.1177/0011000000286007.

Romer, N., Ravitch, N. K., Tom, K., & Merrell, K. W. (2011). Gender differences in positive social-emotional functioning. *Psychology in the Schools, 48*(10), 958–970. doi:10.1002/pits.20604.

Rones, M., & Hoagwood, K. (2000). School-based mental health services: A research review. *Clinical Child and Family Psychology Review, 34*, 223–241. doi:10.1023/A:1026425104386.

Roona, M. R., Streke, A. V., & Marshall, D. G. (2003). Substances, adolescence (meta-analysis). In T. P. Gulotta & M. Bloom (Eds.), *Encyclopedia of primary prevention and health promotion* (pp. 1065–1079). New York: Kluwer Academic/Plenum Press.

Roosa, M. W., & Gonzales, N. A. (2000). Minority issues in prevention: Introduction to the special issue. *American Journal of Community Psychology, 28*(2), 145–148. doi:10.1023/A:1005131116540.

Rosen, L., Rosenberg, E., McKee, M., Gan-Noy, S., Levin, D., Mayshar, E., et al. (2010). A framework for developing an evidence-based comprehensive tobacco control program. *Health Research Policy and Systems, 8*, 17. doi:10.1186/1478-4505-8-17.

Rosenblatt, J. L., & Elias, M. J. (2008). Dosage effects of a preventive social-emotional learning intervention on achievement loss associated with middle school transition. *The Journal of Primary Prevention, 29*(6), 535–555. doi:10.1007/s10935-008-0153-9.

Rosenstock, I. (1974). Historical origins of the health belief model. *Health Education Monographs, 2*(4). Retrieved from http://ajph.aphapublications.org

Rosenstock, I. M. (1966). Why people use health services. *Milbank Memorial Fund Quarterly, 44*, 92–107. Retrieved from http://www.milbank.org.

Roza, S. J., Hofstra, M. B., van der Ende, J., & Verhulst, F. C. (2003). Stable prediction of mood and anxiety disorders based on behavioral and emotional problems in childhood: A 14-year follow-up during childhood, adolescence, and young adulthood. *The American Journal of Psychiatry, 160*, 2116–2121. doi:10.1176/appi.ajp.160.12.2116.

Rubin, A., & Parrish, D. (2007). Problematic phrases in the conclusions of published outcome studies: Implications of evidence-based practice. *Research on Social Work Practice, 16*, 334–347. doi:10.1177/1049731506293726.

Ruby, A., & Doolittle, E. (2010). *Efficacy of schoolwide programs to promote social and character development and reduce problem behavior in elementary school children: Report from the social and character development research program* (NCER 2011-2001). Washington, DC: National Center for Educational Research, Institute of Education Sciences, U.S. Department of Education.

Rumberger, R. W., & Larson, K. A. (1994). Keeping high-risk Chicano students in school: Lessons from a Los Angeles junior high school dropout prevention program. In R. J. Rossi (Ed.), *Educational reforms for at-risk students* (pp. 141–162). New York: Teachers College Press.

Ryan, C. S., Casas, J. F., Kelly-Vance, L., & Ryalls, B. O. (2010). Parent involvement and views of school success: The role of parents' Latino and White American cultural orientations. *Psychology in the Schools, 47*(4), 391–405. doi:10.1002/pits.20477.

Ryan, K. E., Chandler, M., & Samuels, M. (2007). What should school-based evaluation look like? *Studies in Educational Evaluation, 33*, 197–202. doi:10.1016/j.stueduc.2007.07.001.

Ryan, B., & Gross, N. C. (1943). The diffusion of hybrid seed corn in two Iowa communities. *Rural Sociology, 8*(1), 15–24. Retrieved from http://onlinelibrary.wiley.com

Ryan, D., & Martin, A. (2000). Lesbian, gay, bisexual, and transgender parents in the school systems. *School Psychology Review, 29*(2), 207–216. Retrieved from http://www.nasponline.org/publications/

Ryba, M. M., & Hopko, D. R. (2012). Gender differences in depression: Assessing mediational effects of overt behaviors and environmental reward through daily diary monitoring. *Depression Research and Treatment,* Article ID 865679. doi:10.1155/2012/865679.

Saeki, E., & Quirk, M. (2012). *Student engagement and motivation: Their relations to social-emotional and behavioral functioning.* Participant Information Exchange Session. National Association of School Psychologists Annual Conference, Philadelphia.

Saluja, G., Iachan, R., Scheidt, P. C., Overpeck, M. D., Sun, W., & Giedd, J. N. (2004). Prevalence of and risk factors for depressive symptoms among young adolescents. *Archives of Pediatric Adolescent Medicine, 158*(4), 760–765. doi:10.1001/archpedi.158.8.760.

Salvador, S. K. (2012). *Research-informed dropout prevention programs.* Charlotte, NC: The Larry King Center of the Council for Children's Rights.

Samuels, M., & Ryan, K. (2011). Grounding evaluations in culture. *American Journal of Evaluation, 32*(2), 183–198. doi:10.1177/1098214010387657.

Sanders, M. R., Ralph, A., Sofronoff, K., Gardiner, P., Thompson, R., Dwyer, S., et al. (2008). Every family: A population approach to reducing behavioral and emotional problems in children making the transition to school. *The Journal of Primary Prevention, 29*(3), 197–222. doi:10.1007/s10935-008-0139-7.

Sandhu, S., Afifi, T. O., & Amara, F. M. (2012). Theories and practical steps for delivering effective lectures. *Journal of Community Medicine & Health Education, 2,* 158. doi:10.4172/2161-0711.1000158.

Sanetti, L. M., Dobey, L. M., & Gritter, K. L. (2012). Treatment integrity of interventions with children in the *Journal of Positive Behavior Interventions* from 1999 to 2009. *Journal of Positive Behavior Interventions, 14*(1), 29–46. doi:10.1177/1098300711405853.

Sanetti, L. M., Fallon, L. M., & Collier-Meeka, M. A. (2011). Treatment integrity assessment and intervention by school-based personnel: Practical applications based on a preliminary study. *School Psychology Forum: Research in Practice, 5*(3), 87–102. Retrieved from http://www.nasponline.org

Sanetti, L. M., Gritter, K. L., & Dobey, L. M. (2011). Treatment integrity of interventions with children in the school psychology literature from 1995 to 2008. *School Psychology Review, 40*(1), 72–84. Retrieved from http://www.nasponline.org/

Sanetti, L. M., & Kratochwill, T. R. (2009). Toward developing a science of treatment integrity: Introduction to the special series. *School Psychology Review, 38*(4), 445–459. Retrieved from http://www.nasponline.org

Sanetti, L. H., Kratochwill, T. R., Volpiansky, P., & Ring, M. (2011). *Resource mapping: A toolkit for Education Communities. Enacting the EOCA vision for school success.* Wisconsin Department of Public Instruction.

Savaya, R., & Waysman, M. (2005). The logic model: A tool for incorporating theory in development and evaluation of programs. *Administration in Social Work, 29*(2), 85–103. doi:10.1300/J147v29n02_06.

Sawyer, M. G., Harchak, T. F., Spence, S. H., Bond, L., Graetz, B., Kay, D., et al. (2010). School-based prevention of depression: A 2-year follow-up of a randomized controlled trial of the beyondblue schools research initiative. *Journal of Adolescent Health, 47*(3), 297–304. doi:10.1016/j.jadohealth.2010.02.007.

Saxena, S., & Maulik, P. K. (2002). *Prevention and promotion in mental health.* Geneva, Switzerland: World Health Organization.

Schaeffer, C. M., Bruns, E., Weist, M., Stephan, S. H., Goldstrin, J., & Simpson, Y. (2005). Overcoming challenges to evidence-based interventions in schools. *Journal of Youth and Adolescence, 34*(1), 15–22. doi:10.1007/s10964-005-1332-0.

Schaeller, C. (2002). *Empirically-supported interventions in school mental health: Empirically-supported interventions resource packet.* Baltimore: Center for School Mental Health.

Schlosser, R. W. (2007). Appraising the quality of systematic reviews. Technical Brief No. 17. *FOCUS: A publication of the National Center for the Dissemination of Disability Research.* Retrieved from http://www.ncddr.org.

Schmidt, F. (1993). *Peacemaking skills for little kids* (2nd ed.). Miami, FL: Peace Education Foundation, Inc.

Schmidt, F., & Friedman, A. (1988). *Peacemaking skills for little kids.* Miami, FL: Grace Contrino Abrams Peace Education Foundation.

Schneider, S. K., O'Donnell, L., Stueve, A., & Coulter, R. W. (2012). Cyberbullying, school bullying, and psychological distress: A regional census of high school students. *American Journal of Public Health, 102*(1), 171–177. doi:10.2105/AJPH.2011.300308.

Schoenfeld, N. A., Rutherford, R. B., Gable, R. A., & Rock, M. L. (2008). ENGAGE: A blueprint for incorporating social skills training into daily academic instruction. *Preventing School Failure, 52*(3), 17–28. doi:10.3200/PSFL.52.3.17-28.

Schrag, J. A. (1996). Systems change leading to better integration of services for students with special needs. *School Psychology Review, 25*(4), 489–495. Retrieved from http://www.nasponline.org

Schroeder, B. A., Messina, A., Schroeder, D., Good, K., Barto, S., Saylor, J., et al. (2011). The implementation of a statewide bullying prevention program: Preliminary findings from the field and the importance of coalitions. *Health Promotion Practice, 13*(4), 489–495. doi:10.1177/1524839910386887.

Schulte, A. C., Easton, J. E., & Parker, J. (2009). Advances in treatment integrity research: Multidisciplinary perspectives on the conceptualization, measurement, and enhancement of treatment integrity. *School Psychology Review, 38*(4), 460–475. Retrieved from http://www.nasponline.org

Schultz, D., Barnes-Proby, D., Chandra, A., Jaycox, L. H., Maher, E., & Pecora, P. (2010). *Toolkit for adapting Cognitive Behavioral Intervention for Trauma in Schools (CBITS) or Supporting Students Exposed to Trauma (SSET) for implementation with youth in foster care.* Santa Monica, CA: The Rand Corporation.

Schultz, J. L., & Mueller, D. (2007). *Effective interventions for the prevention and treatment of depression in adolescent girls.* St. Paul, MN: Wilder Research.

Schweinhart, L. J., Weikart, D. P., & Larner, M. B. (1986). Consequences of three preschool curriculum models through age 15. *Early Child Research Quarterly, 1*(1), 15–45. doi:10.1016/0885-2006(86)90005-0.

Scime, M., Cook-Cottone, C., Kane, L., & Watson, T. (2006). Group prevention of eating disorders with fifth-grade females: Impact on body dissatisfaction, drive for thinness, and media influence. *Eating Disorders, 14*, 143–155. doi:10.1080/10640260500403881.

Seigle, P. (2001). Reach out to schools: A social competency program. In J. Cohen (Ed.), *Caring classrooms/intelligent schools: The social and emotional education of young children* (pp. 108–121). New York: Teachers College Press.

Self-Brown, S., Frederick, K., Binder, S., Whitaker, D., Lutzker, J., Edwards, A., et al. (2011). Examining the need for cultural adaptations to an evidence-based parent training program targeting the prevention of child maltreatment. *Children and Youth Services Review, 33*(7), 1166–1172. doi:10.1016/j.childyouth.2011.02.010.

Serwacki, M., & Nickerson, A. B. (2012). *Guide to school-wide bullying prevention programs.* Buffalo, NY: Alberti Center for Bullying Abuse Prevention.

Seymour, K. E. (2010). *Emotion regulation mediates the relationship between ADHD and depressive symptoms in youth.* Unpublished doctoral dissertation, University of Maryland, College Park, MD.

Shahar, G., Henrich, C. C., Winokur, A., Blatt, S. J., Kuperminc, G. P., & Leadbeater, B. J. (2006). Self-criticism and depressive symptomatology interact to predict middle school academic achievement. *Journal of Clinical Psychology, 62*(1), 147–155. doi:10.1002/jclp.20210.

Sharkey, J. D., You, S., & Schnoebelen, K. (2008). Relations among school assets, individual resilience, and student engagement for youth grouped by level of family functioning. *Psychology in the Schools, 45*(5), 402–418. doi:10.1002/pits.20305.

Sharma, M., & Kanekar, A. (2008). Diffusion of innovations theory for alcohol, tobacco, and drugs. *Journal of Alcohol & Drug Education, 52*(1). Retrieved from http://www.jadejournal.com

Sharp, C., Goodyer, I. M., & Croudace, T. (2006). The Short Mood and Feelings Questionnaire (SMFQ): A unidimensional item response theory and categorical data factor analysis of self-report ratings from a community sample of 7- through 11-year-old children. *Journal of Abnormal Child Psychology, 34*(3), 365–377. doi:10.1007/s10802-006-9027-x.

Shaw, A. L. (n.d.). *Strengthening Families program: Outcomes for African-American vs non African-American families.* Retrieved from http://people.westminstercollege.edu/staff/mjhinsdale/.../aliesha_paper.doc

Sheridan, S. M., Knoche, L., Edwards, C. P., Bovaird, J. A., & Kupzyk, K. A. (2010). Parent engagement and school readiness: Effects of the getting ready intervention on preschool children's social-emotional competencies. *Faculty Publications from Children, Youth, Families, & Schools*, Paper 12, Lincoln, NE.

Sherman, D. (2010). A paradigm shift in selecting evidence-based approaches for substance abuse prevention. *Prevention Tactics, 9*(6), 7–11. Retrieved from http://www.cars-rp.org

Sherman, L. W., Gottfredson, D. C., MacKenzie, D. L., Eck, J., Reuter, P., & Bushway, S. D. (1997). *Preventing crime: What works, what doesn't, what's promising. A report to the United States Congress* (NCJ 171676). Washington, DC: U.S. Department of Justice, Office of Justice Programs.

Shih, R. A., Miles, J. N. V., Tucker, J. S., Zhou, A. J., & D'Amico, E. J. (2010). Racial/ethnic differences in adolescent substance use: Mediation by individual, family, and school factors. *Journal of Studies on Alcohol and Drugs, 71*(5), 640–651. Retrieved from http://www.jsad.com

Shirk, S. R., Kaplinski, H., & Gudmundsen, G. (2009). School-based cognitive-behavioral therapy for adolescent depression: A benchmarking study. *Journal of Emotional and Behavioral Disorders, 17*(2), 106–117. doi:10.1177/1063426608326202.

Shlay, A. B. (2010). African American, White and Hispanic child care preferences: A factorial survey analysis of welfare leavers by race and ethnicity. *Social Science Research, 39*(1), 125–141. doi:10.1016/j.ssresearch.2009.07.005.

Shlonsky, A., & Gibbs, L. (2004). Will the real evidence-based practice please stand up? Teaching the process of evidence-based practice to the helping professions. *Brief Treatment and Crisis Intervention, 4*(2), 137–153. doi:10.1093/brief-treatment/mhh011.

Shochet, I. M., Dadds, M. R., Holland, D., Whitefield, K., Harnett, P. H., & Osgarby, S. M. (2001). The efficacy of a universal school-based program to prevent adolescent depression. *Journal of Clinical Child Psychology, 30*(3), 303–315. doi:10.1207/S15374424JCCP3003_3.

Short, R. J. (2003). Commentary: School psychology, context, and population-based practice. *School Psychology Review, 32*(2), 169–173. Retrieved from http://www.nasponline.org/

Shortt, A. L., Barrett, P. M., & Fox, T. L. (2001). Evaluating the FRIENDS program: A cognitive-behavioral group treatment for anxious children and their parents. *Journal of Clinical Child Psychology, 30*(4), 525–535. doi:10.1207/S15374424JCCP3004_09.

Shure, M. B., & Spivack, G. (1980). Interpersonal problem solving as a mediator of personal adjustment in preschool and kindergarten children. *Journal of Applied Developmental Psychology, 1*(1), 29–44. doi:10.1016/0193-3973(80)90060-X.

Shure, M. B., & Spivack, G. (1982). Interpersonal problem solving in young children: A cognitive approach to prevention. *American Journal of Community Psychology, 10*(3), 341–356. doi:10.1007/BF00896500.

Shure, M. B., & Spivack, G. (1988). Interpersonal cognitive problem solving. In R. Price, E. L. Cowen, R. P. Lorion, & J. Ramos-McKay (Eds.), *14 ounces of prevention: A casebook for practitioners* (pp. 69–82). Washington, DC: American Psychological Association.

Shure, M. B., Spivack, G., & Jaeger, M. (1971). Problem-solving, thinking and adjustment among disadvantaged preschool children. *Child Development, 42*, 1791–1803. doi:10.2307/1127585.

Sibbald, B., & Roland, M. (1998). Understanding controlled trials: Why are randomised controlled trials important? *British Medical Journal, 316*, 201. doi:10.1136/bmj.316.7126.201.

Silk, J. S., Davis, S., McMakin, D. L., Dahl, R. E., & Forbes, E. E. (2012). Why do anxious children become depressed teenagers? The role of social evaluative threat and reward processing. *Psychological Medicine, 42*(10), 2095–2107. doi:10.1017/S0033291712000207.

Silver, R. B., Measelle, J. R., Armstrong, J. M., & Essex, M. J. (2005). Trajectories of classroom externalizing behavior: Contributions of child characteristics, family characteristics, and the teacher–child relationship during the school transition. *Journal of School Psychology, 43*(1), 39–60. doi:10.1016/j.jsp.2004.11.003.

Simonsen, B., Eber, L., Black, A. C., Sugai, G., Lewandowski, H., Sims, B., et al. (2012). Illinois Statewide Positive Behavioral Interventions and Supports: Evolution and impact on student outcomes across years. *Journal of Positive Behavior Interventions, 14*(1), 5–16. doi:10.1177/1098300711412601.

Simonsen, B., & Sugai, G. (2007). Using school-wide data systems to make decisions efficiently an effectively. *School Psychology Forum: Research in Practice, 1*(2), 46–58. doi:10.1016/j.jsp.2004.11.003.

Simonsen, B., Sugai, G., & Negron, M. (2008). Schoolwide Positive Behavior Support: Primary systems and practices. *Teaching Exceptional Children, 40*(6), 32–40. Retrieved from http://www.cec.sped.org

Sinclair, M. F., Christenson, S. L., Evelo, D. L., & Hurley, C. M. (1998). Dropout prevention for youth with disabilities: Efficacy of a sustained school engagement procedure. *Exceptional Children, 65*(1), 7–21. Retrieved from http://www.cec.sped.org

Sinclair, M., & Kaibel, C. (2002). *Dakota County: School Success Check and Connect Program evaluation, 2002 final summary report.* Minneapolis, MN: University of Minnesota, Institute on Community Integration.

Siu, S. (1996). *Asian American students at-risk.* Report No. 8. Baltimore: Center for Research on the Education of Students Placed at Risk. Retrieved from http://www.csos.jhu.edu/crespar/

Skiba, R. J., Poloni-Staudinger, L., Simmons, A. B., Feggins-Aziz, R., & Chung, C. (2005). Unproven links: Can poverty explain ethnic disproportionality in special education? *Journal of Special Education, 39*(3), 130–144. doi:10.1177/00224669050390030101.

Skinner, E. A., & Pitzer, J. R. (2012). Developmental dynamics of student engagement coping and everyday resilience. In S. L. Christenson, A. L. Reschly, & C. Wylie (Eds.), *Handbook of research on student engagement* (pp. 21–44). New York: Springer.

Sklad, M., Diekstra, R., Ritter, M., Ben, J., & Gravesteijn, C. (2012). Effectiveness of school-based universal social, emotional and behavioral programs: Do they enhance students' development in the area of skills, behavior, and adjustment? *Psychology in the Schools, 49*(9), 892–909. doi:10.1002/pits.21641.

Small, S. A., Cooney, S. M., Eastman, G., & O'Connor, C. (2007). *Guidelines for selecting an evidence-based program: Balancing community needs, program quality, and organizational resources.* What works, Wisconsin—Research to practice series, Madison, WI.

Smith, E., & Caldwell, L. (2007). Adapting evidence-based programs to new contexts: What needs to be changed? *The Journal of Rural Health, 23*(Suppl. 1), 37–41. doi:10.1111/j.1748-0361.2007.00122.x.

Smokowski, P. R., Chapman, M. V., & Bacallao, M. L. (2006). Acculturation risk and protective factors and mental health symptoms in immigrant Latino adolescents. *Child Psychiatry and Human Development, 40*(4), 589–608. doi:10.1007/s10578-009-0146-9.

Snethen, G., & Van Puymbroeck, M. (2008). Girls and physical aggression: Causes, trends, and intervention guided by social learning theory. *Aggression and Violent Behavior, 13*(5), 346–354. doi:10.1016/j.avb.2008.05.003.

Snyder, F., Flay, B., Vuchinich, S., Acock, A., Washburn, I., Beets, M., et al. (2010). Impact of the *Positive Action* program on school-level indicators of academic achievement, absenteeism, and disciplinary outcomes: A matched-pair, cluster randomized, controlled trial. *Journal of Research on Educational Effectiveness, 3*(1), 26–55. doi:10.1080/19345740903353436.

Society for Research in Child Development. (2009). *Report of healthy development: A summit on young children's mental health. Partnering with communication scientists, collaborating across disciplines and leveraging impact to promote children's mental health.* Washington, DC: Author.

Solomon, B. G., Klein, S. A., & Polityilo, B. C. (2012). The effect of performance feedback on teachers' treatment integrity: A meta-analysis of the single-case. *Psychology in the Schools, 41*(2), 160–175. doi:10.1002/pits.21598.

Solorzano-Moreno, T. (2012). *The effectiveness of implementing a violence prevention curriculum: Second Step within preschools.* Unpublished master's thesis, California State University, Northridge, CA.

Song, S. J., Ziegler, R., Arsenault, L., Fried, L. E., & Hacker, K. (2011). Asian student depression in American high schools: Differences in risk factors. *The Journal of School Nursing, 27*(6), 455–462. doi:10.1177/1059840511418670.

Soole, D. W., Mazerolle, L., & Rombouts, S. (2008). School-based drug prevention programs: A review of what works. *Australian and New Zealand Journal of Criminology, 41*(2), 259–286. doi:10.1375/acri.41.2.259.

Spaulding, S. A., Irvin, L. K., Horner, R. H., May, S. L., Emeldi, M., Tobin, T. J., et al. (2010). Schoolwide social-behavioral climate, student problem behavior, and related administrative decisions: Empirical patterns from 1,510 schools nationwide. *Journal of Positive Behavior Interventions, 12*(2), 69–85. doi:10.1177/1098300708329011.

Spence, S., Burns, J., Boucher, S., Glover, S., Graetz, B., Kay, D., et al. (2005). The *beyondblue* Schools Research Initiative: Conceptual framework and intervention. *Australasian Psychiatry, 13*(2), 159–164. doi:10.1111/j.1440-1665.2005.02180.x.

Spence, S. H., Najman, J. M., Bor, W., O'Callaghan, M. J., & Williams, G. M. (2002). Maternal anxiety and depression, poverty and marital relationship factors during early childhood as predictors of anxiety and depressive symptoms in adolescence. *Journal of Child Psychology and Psychiatry, 43*(4), 457–469. doi:10.1111/1469-7610.00037.

Spence, S. H., Sheffield, J. K., & Donovan, C. L. (2003). Preventing adolescent depression: An evaluation of the Problem Solving for Life Program. *Journal of Counseling and Clinical Psychology, 71*(1), 3–13. doi:10.1037/0022-006X.71.1.3.

Spielvogle, H. N. (2011). *Understanding and addressing barriers: Engaging adolescents in mental health services.* Unpublished doctoral dissertation, University of Toronto, Toronto, Canada.

Spiro, J. (2009). *Leading change handbook: Concepts and tools.* Retrieved from http://www.wallacefoundation.org/

Spoth, R., Greenberg, M., & Turrisi, R. (2008). Preventive interventions addressing underage drinking: State of the evidence and steps toward public health impact. *Pediatrics, 121,* S311–S336. doi:10.1542/peds.2007-2243E.

Spoth, R., Greenberg, M., & Turrisi, R. (2009). Overview of preventive intervention addressing underage drinking: State of the evidence and steps toward public health impact. *Alcohol Research & Health, 32,* 53–66. Retrieved from http://pubs.niaaa.nih.gov

Spoth, R., Randall, G. K., Shin, C., & Redmond, C. (2005). Randomized study of combined universal family and school preventive interventions: Patterns of long-term effects on initiation, regular use, and weekly drunkenness. *Psychology of Addictive Behaviors, 19*(4), 372–381. doi:10.1037/0893-164X.19.4.372.

Spoth, R., Redmond, C., Haggerty, K., & Ward, T. (1995). A controlled parenting skills outcome study examining individual difference and attendance effects. *Journal of Marriage and the Family, 57*(2), 449–464. doi:10.2307/353698.

St. Pierre, T. L. (2004). Tales of refusal, adoption, and maintenance: Evidence-based substance abuse prevention via school-extension collaborations. *American Journal of Evaluation, 25*(4), 479–491. doi:10.1177/109821400402500405.

Stagman, S., & Cooper, J. L. (2010). *Children's mental health: What every policymaker should know.* New York: National Center for Children in Poverty.

Starcevic, V., & Berle, D. (2006). Cognitive specificity of anxiety disorders: A review of selected key constructs. *Depression and Anxiety, 23*(2), 51–61. doi:10.1002/da.20145.

Staubli, S., & Killias, M. (2011). Long-term outcomes of passive bullying during childhood: Suicide attempts, victimization and offending. *European Journal of Criminology, 8*(5), 377–385. doi:10.1177/1477370811415761.

Steiker, L. K. (2008). Making drug and alcohol prevention relevant: Adapting evidence-based curricula to unique adolescent cultures. *Family & Community Health, 31*(1S), S52–S60. doi:10.1097/01.FCH.0000304018.13255.f6.

Steiker, L. K., Castro, F. G., Kumpfer, K., Marsiglia, F. F., Coard, S., & Hopson, L. M. (2008). A dialogue regarding cultural adaptation of interventions. *Journal of Social Work Practice in the Addiction, 8*(1), 154–162. doi:10.1080/15332560802112094.

Steinberg, K. S., Bringle, R. G., & Williams, M. J. (2010). *Service-learning research primer.* Scotts Valley, CA: National Service-Learning Clearinghouse.

Steinberg, L. (2008). A social neuroscience perspective on adolescent risk-taking. *Developmental Review, 28*, 78–106. doi:10.1016/j.dr.2007.08.002.

Stephan, S. (2012, March 26). *Common elements of evidence-based mental health practice in schools* (Webinar). Center for School Mental Health and IDEA Partnership.

Sterling-Turner, H., & Watson, T. (2002). An analog investigation of the relationship between treatment acceptability and treatment integrity. *Journal of Behavioral Education, 11*, 39–50. doi:10.1023/A:1014333305011.

Sternberg, R. (2002). Effecting organizational change: A "Mineralogical" theory of organizational modifiability. *Consulting Psychology Journal, 54*(3), 147–156. doi:10.1037/1061-4087.54.3.147.

Stigler, M. H., Neusel, E., & Perry, C. L. (2011). School-based programs to prevent and reduce alcohol use among youth. *Alcohol Research and Health, 34*(2), 157–162. Retrieved from http://www.niaaa.nih.gov

Stillwell, R. (2009). *Public school graduates and dropouts from the common core of data: School year 2006–2007: First look* (NCES 2010-313). Washington, DC: National Center for Education Statistics, Institute of Education Sciences.

Stipek, D. J. (1996). Motivation and instruction. In D. C. Berliner & R. C. Calfee (Eds.), *Handbook of educational psychology.* New York: Simon & Schuster/Macmillan.

Stjernberg, T., & Philips, A. (1993). Organizational innovations in a long-term perspective: Legitimacy and souls-of-fire as critical factors of change and viability. *Human Relations, 46*(10), 1193–1219. doi:10.1177/001872679304601003.

Stoppel, C., Albrecht, A., Pape, H. C., & Stork, O. (2006). Genes and neurons: Molecular insights to fear and anxiety. *Genes, Brain, and Behavior, 5*(Suppl. 2), 34–47. doi:10.1111/j.1601-183X.2006.00229.x.

Strein, W., & Koehler, J. (2008). Best practices in developing prevention strategies for school psychology practice. In A. Thomas & A. J. Grimes (Eds.), *Best practices in school psychology V* (Vol. 4, pp. 1309–1322). Bethesda, MD: National Association of School Psychologists.

Substance Abuse and Mental Health Services Administration. (2011). *Identifying mental health and substance use problems of children and adolescents: A guide for child-serving organizations* (HHS Publication No. SMA 12-4670). Rockville, MD: Author.

Substance Abuse and Mental Health Services Administration. (2012). *Results from the 2011 national survey on drug use and health: national findings* (NSDUH Series H-42, HHS Publication No. (SMA) 11-4667). Rockville, MD: Author.

Sugai, G., & Horner, R. H. (2006). A promising approach for expanding and sustaining the school-wide positive behavior support. *School Psychology Review, 35*(2), 245–259. Retrieved from http://www.nasponline.org

Sullivan, T. N., Helms, S. W., Kliewer, W., & Goodman, K. L. (2010). Associations between sadness and anger regulation coping, emotional expression, and physical and relational aggression among urban adolescents. *Social Development, 19*(1), 30–51. doi:10.1111/j.1467-9507.2008.00531.x.

Sullivan, A. L., Long, L., & Kucera, M. (2011). A survey of school psychologists' preparation, participation, and perceptions related to positive behavior interventions and supports. *Psychology in the Schools, 48*(10), 971–985. doi:10.1102/pits.20605.

Sussman, S., Burton, D., Dent, C. W., Stacy, A. W., & Flay, B. R. (1991). Use of focus groups in developing an adolescent tobacco use cessation program: Collective norm effects. *Journal of Applied Social Psychology, 21*, 1772–1782. doi:10.1111/j.1559-1816.1991.tb00503.x.

Sussman, S., Dent, C. W., & Stacy, A. W. (2002). Project Towards No Drug Abuse: A review of the findings and future directions. *American Journal of Health Behavior, 26*(5), 354–365. doi:10.5993/AJHB.26.5.4.

Sussman, S., Dent, C. W., Stacy, A. W., Hodgson, C., Burton, D., & Flay, B. R. (1993). Project Towards No Tobacco Use: Implementation, process and posttest knowledge evaluation. *Health Education Research: Theory and Practice, 8*, 109–123. doi:10.1093/her/8.1.109.

Sussman, S., Dent, C. W., Stacy, A. W., Sun, P., Craig, S., Simon, T. R., et al. (1993). Project Towards No Tobacco Use: 1-year behavior outcomes. *American Journal of Public Health, 83*(9), 1245–1250. doi:10.2105/AJPH.83.9.1245.

Sussman, S., Rohrbach, L. A., Patel, R., & Holiday, K. A. (2003). A look at an interactive classroom-based drug abuse prevention program: Interactive contents and suggestions for research. *Journal of Drug Education, 33*(4), 355–368. doi:10.2190/H04H-KGQN-HW9X-6R60.

Suveg, C., Zeman, J., Flannery-Schroeder, E., & Cassano, M. (2005). Emotion socialization in families of children with an anxiety disorder. *Journal of Abnormal Child Psychology, 33*(2), 145–155. doi:10.1007/s10802-005-1823-1.

Swahn, M. H. (2012). Cross-national perspectives on early adolescence: Implications and strategies for public health prevention and interventions. *Journal of Early Adolescence, 32*(1), 20–25. doi:10.1177/0272431611432866.

Swartz, K. L. (2011). *Adolescent Depression Awareness Program (ADAP)*. Retrieved from http://www.mhainde.org/edADAP.asp

Swearer, S. M., Espelage, D. L., Love, K. B., & Kingsbury, W. (2008). School-wide approaches to intervention for school aggression and bullying. In B. Doll & A. Cummings (Eds.), *Transforming school mental health services: Population-based approaches to promoting the competency and wellness of children* (pp. 189–212). Thousand Oaks, CA: Corwin Press.

Sweeney, C., Goldner, J., & Richards, M. (2011). Exposure to community violence and daily feeling states among urban African American youth. *Journal of Prevention & Intervention in the Community, 39*(2), 114–131. doi:10.1080/10852352.2011.556560.

Swendsen, J., Burstrin, M., Case, B., Conway, K. P., Dierker, L., He, J., et al. (2012). Use and abuse of alcohol and illicit drugs in US adolescents: Results of the National Comorbidity Survey-Adolescent Supplement. *Archives of General Psychiatry, 69*(4), 390–398. doi:10.1001/archgenpsychiatry.2011.1503.

Swesey, M. (2008). *Evidence based practices and multicultural mental health* [White paper]. Retrieved from http://www.nami.org

Tableman, B., & Herron, A. (2004). School climate and learning. *Best Practice Briefs, 31*, 1–10. Retrieved from http://outreach.msu.edu

Tackett, J. L. (2010). Toward an externalizing spectrum in DSM-V: Incorporating developmental concerns. *Child Development Perspectives, 4*(3), 161–167. doi:10.1111/j.1750-8606.2010.00138.x.

Taub, J. (2001). Evaluation of the Second Step Violence Prevention Program at a rural elementary school. *School Psychology Review, 31*, 186-200. Retrieved from http://www.nasponline.org.

Taub, J. (2002). Evaluation of the *Second Step* violence prevention program at a rural elementary school. *School Psychology Review, 31*(2), 186–200. Retrieved from http://www.nasponline.org/

Taylor, L., & Parsons, J. (2011). Improving student engagement. *Current Issues in Education, 14*(1). Retrieved from http://cie.asu.edu/

Terzian, M., Moore, K. A., Williams-Taylor, L., & Nguyen, H. (2009). *Online resources for identifying evidence-based, out-of-school time programs: A user's guide*. Research-to-Results Brief (Publication #2009-36). Washington, DC: Child Trends. Retrieved from http://www.childtrends.org

The Collaborative for Academic, Social, and Emotional Learning (CASEL). (2003). *Safe and sound: An educational leader's guide to evidence-based social and emotional learning (SEL) programs*. Chicago: Author.

The Evidence-Based Intervention Work Group. (2005). Theories of change and adoption of innovations: The evolving evidence-based intervention and practice movement in school psychology. *Psychology in the Schools, 42*(5), 475–494. doi:10.1002/pits.20086.

The Multisite Violence Prevention Project. (2009). The ecological effects of universal and selective violence prevention programs for middle school students: A randomized trial. *Journal of Consulting and Clinical Psychology, 77*(3), 526–542. doi:10.1037a0014395.

The President's New Freedom Commission on Mental Health. (2003). *Achieving the promise: Transforming mental health care in America. Final report* (DHHS Publication No. SMA 03-3832). Washington, DC: U.S. Government Printing Office.

The Workgroup on Adapting Latino Services. (2008). *Adaptation guidelines for serving Latino children and families affected by trauma* (1st ed.). San Diego, CA: Chadwick Center for Children and Families.

Thomas, S. G., & Gravert, E. R. (2011). *Systematically adapting social and emotional curriculum and program content: A closer look at the Second Step early learning programs.* Specialist thesis. California State University, Sacramento, CA.

Thompson, V. L., Cavazos-Rehg, P. A., Jupka, K., Caito, N., Gratzke, J., Tate, K. Y., et al. (2008). Evidential preferences: Cultural appropriateness strategies in health communications. *Health Education Research, 23*(3), 549–559. doi:10.1093/her/cym029.

Thompson, R., Tabone, J. K., Litrownik, A. J., Briggs, E. C., Hussey, J. M., English, D. J., et al. (2011). Early adolescent risk behavior outcomes of childhood externalizing behavioral trajectories. *Journal of Early Adolescence, 31*(2), 234–257. doi:10.1177/0272431609361203.

Thurlow, M. L., Sinclari, M. F., & Johnson, D. R. (2002). Students with disabilities who drop out of school—Implications for policy and practice. *Issue Brief: Examining Current Challenges in Secondary Education and Transition, 1*(2). Minneapolis: MNL National Center on Secondary Education and Transition.

Tilleczek, K., & Ferguson, B. (2007). *Transitions and pathways from elementary to secondary school: A review of selected literature.* Toronto, Canada: Ontario Ministry of Education.

Tilly, W. D. (2008). The evolution of school psychology to science-based practice: Problem solving and the three-tiered model. In A. Thomas & A. J. Grimes (Eds.), *Best practices in school psychology V* (Vol. 1, pp. 17–36). Bethesda, MD: National Association of School Psychologists.

Tobin, T. J., & Vincent, C. G. (2010). *Culturally competent school-wide positive behavior support: From theory to evaluation data.* 7th International Conference on Positive Behavior Support, St. Louis, MO.

Tobin, T. J., & Vincent, C. G. (2011). *How can the SWPBS framework promote racially proportionate behavioral outcomes?* Paper presented at the Washington PBIS Conference, Washington, DC. Retrieved from http://www.pbisnetwork.org/?attachment_id=1168

Tobler, A. L., Komro, K. A., Dabroski, A., Aveyard, P., & Markham, W. A. (2011). Preventing the link between SES and high-risk behaviors: "value-added" education, drug use and delinquency in high-risk, urban schools. *Prevention Science, 12*(2), 211–221. doi:10.1007/s11121-011-0206-9.

Tobler, N. S., Roona, M. R., Ochshorn, P., Marshall, D. G., Streke, A. V., & Stackpole, K. M. (2000). School-based adolescent drug prevention programs: 1998 meta-analysis. *The Journal of Primary Prevention, 20*(4), 275–336. doi:10.1023/A:1021314704811.

Tobler, N. S., & Stratton, H. H. (1997). Effectiveness of school-based prevention programs: A meta-analysis of the research. *The Journal of Primary Prevention, 18*(1), 71–128. doi:10.1023/A:1024630205999.

Todd, A. W., Horner, R. H., Anderson, K., & Spriggs, M. (2002). Teaching recess: Low-cost efforts producing effective results. *Journal of Positive Behavior Interventions, 4*(1), 46–52. doi:10.1177/109830070200400108.

Tolman, D. L., Impett, E. A., Tracy, A. J., & Michael, A. (2006). Looking good, sounding good: Femininity ideology and adolescent girls' mental health. *Psychology of Women Quarterly, 30*(1), 85–95. doi:10.1111/j.1471-6402.2006.00265.x.

Tran, A. G., & Lee, R. M. (2010). Perceived ethnic-racial socialization, ethnic identity, and social competence among Asian American late adolescents. *Cultural Diversity and Ethnic Minority Psychology, 16*(2), 169–178. doi:10.1037/a0016400.

Tremblay, R. E., Mâsse, L. C., Pagani, L., & Vitaro, F. P. (1996). From childhood physical aggression to adolescent maladjustment: The Montreal Prevention Experiment. In R. D. Peters & R. J. McMahon (Eds.), *Preventing childhood disorders, substance abuse, and delinquency* (pp. 268–298). Thousand Oaks, CA: Sage.

Trickett, E. J., & Rowe, H. L. (2012). Emerging ecological approaches to prevention, health promotion, and public health in the school context: Next steps from a community psychology perspective. *Journal of Educational and Psychological Consultation, 22*, 125–140. doi:10.108 0/10474412.2011.649651.

Trumbull, E., & Rothstein-Fisch, C. (2011). The intersection of culture and achievement motivation. *The School Community Journal, 21*(2), 25–53. Retrieved from http://www.families-schools.org/CJindex.htm

Tseng, V. (2012). Sharing child and youth development knowledge: The uses of research in policy and practice. *Social Policy Report, 26*(2), 1–16. Retrieved from http://www.nationalcac.org

Tucker, P., Liao, Y., Giles, W. H., & Liburd, L. (2006). The REACH 2010 logic model: An illustration of expected performance. *Preventing Chronic Disease, 3*(1), A21. Retrieved from http://www.cdc.gov

Tudge, J., Mokrova, I., Hatfield, B., & Karnik, R. (2009). Uses and misuses of Bronfenbrenner's bioecological theory of human development. *Journal of Family Theory & Review, 1*(4), 198–210. doi:10.1111/j.1756-2589.2009.00026.x.

Turner, W. L. (2000). Cultural considerations in family-based primary prevention programs in drug abuse. *The Journal of Primary Prevention, 21*(2), 285–303. doi:10.1023/A:1007091405097.

Tyrer, P. (2001). The case for cothymia: Mixed anxiety and depression as a single diagnosis. *The British Journal of Psychiatry, 179*, 191–193. doi:10.1192/bjp.179.3.191.

U.S. Department of Education. (2011). *Public school graduates and dropouts from the common core of data: School year 2008–09.* Retrieved from http://nces.ed.gov/pubs2011/graduates/tables.asp

U.S. Department of Health and Human Services. (2008/2010). *An evaluation protocol for systematically evaluating efforts to improve racial and ethnic minority health, reduce health disparities, and effect systems approaches to racial and ethnic minority health problems.* Rockville, MD: Office of Minority Health.

U.S. Department of Health and Human Services. (2010). *Head start impact study.* Final report. Washington, DC: U.S. Department of Health and Human Services.

U.S. Department of Health, Human Services (U.S. DHHS). (1999). *Mental health: A report of the surgeon general.* Rockville, MD: U.S. Department of Health and Human Services, National Institute of Mental Health.

Unger, J. B., Chou, C. P., Palmer, P. H., Ritt-Olson, A., Gallaher, P., Cen, S., et al. (2004). Project FLAVOR: 1-year outcomes of a multicultural, school-based smoking prevention curriculum for adolescents. *American Journal of Public Health, 94*(2), 263–265. doi:10.2105/AJPH.94.2.263.

Utley, C. A., Kozleski, E., Smith, A., & Draper, I. L. (2002). Positive behavior support: A proactive strategy for minimizing behavior problems in urban multicultural youth. *Journal of Positive Behavior Interventions, 4*(4), 196–207. doi:10.1177/10983007020040040301.

Vaillancourt, T., Trinh, V., McDougall, P., Duku, E., Cuningham, L., Cunningham, C., et al. (2010). Optimizing population screening of bullying in school-aged children. *Journal of School Violence, 9*(3), 233–250. doi:10.1080/15388220.2010.483182.

Valente, T. W. (1996). Social network thresholds in the diffusion of innovations. *Social Networks, 18*(1), 69–89. doi:10.1016/0378-8733(95)00256-1.

Van de Ven, A., & Sun, K. (2011). Breakdowns in implementing models of organizational change. *Academy of Management Perspectives, 25*(3), 58–74. Retrieved from http://amp.aom.org

Van den Hoofdakker, B., Van der Veen-Mulders, L., Sytema, S., Emmelkamp, P. M., Minderaa, R. B., & Nsuta, M. H. (2007). Effectiveness of behavioral parent training for children with ADHD in routine clinical practice: A randomized controlled study. *Journal of the American Academy of Child and Adolescent Psychiatry, 46*(10), 1263–1271. doi:10.1097/chi.0b013e3181354bc2.

Van Duyn, M. A. S., McCrae, T., Wingrove, B. K., Henderson, K. M., Boyd, J. K., Kagawa-Singer, M., et al. (2007). Adapting evidence-based strategies to increase physical activity among African Americans, Hispanics, Hmong, and Native Hawaiians: A social marketing approach. *Preventing Chronic Disease, 4*(4). Retrieved from http://www.cdc.gov

Van Marter, D. F., Dyment, S. J., Evers, K. E., Johnson, J. L., & Prochaska, J. M. (2007). Effectiveness of a transtheoretical model-based effect system for bullying prevention among elementary school students. *Education Research, 49*(4), 397–414. doi:10.1363/4302311.

Van Oort, F. V., Greaves-Lord, K., Ormel, J., Verhulst, F. C., & Huizink, A. C. (2011). Risk indicators of anxiety throughout adolescence: The TRAILS study. *Depression and Anxiety, 28*(6), 485–494. doi:10.1002/da.20818.

Van Oort, F. V. A., Greaves-Lord, K., Verhulst, F. C., Ormel, J., & Huizink, A. C. (2009). The developmental course of anxiety symptoms during adolescence: The TRAILS study. *Journal of Child Psychology and Psychiatry, 50*(10), 1209–1217. doi:10.1111/j.1469-7610.2009.02092.x.

van Schoiack-Edstrom, L., Frey, K. S., & Beland, K. (2002). Changing adolescents' attitudes about relational and physical aggression: An early evaluation of a school-based intervention. *School Psychology Review, 31*(2), 201–216. Retrieved from http//www.nasponline.org/publications

Van Voorhis, F. L. (2011). Adding families to the homework equation: A longitudinal study of mathematics achievement. *Education and Urban Society, 43*(3), 313–338. doi:10.1177/0013124510380236.

Vazsonyi, A. T., & Belliston, L. M. (2006). The cultural and developmental significance of parenting processes in adolescent anxiety and depression symptoms. *Journal of Youth and Adolescence, 35*(4), 491–505. doi:10.1007/s10964-006-9064-3.

Vincent, C. G., & Tobin, T. J. (2011). *Minority students and support intensity: Discipline and intervention data.* Paper presented at the 8th International Conference on Positive Behavior Support, Denver, CO.

Vitiello, B. (2010). The importance of the discourse on the method. *Child and Adolescent Psychiatry and Mental Health, 4*(2), 2. doi:10.1186/1753-2000-4-2.

Vogel, I. (2012). *Review of the use of 'Theory of Change' in international development: Review report.* UK Department for International Development. Retrieved from http://www.dfid.gov.uk

Volkow, N. D. (2009). *Tobacco addiction. Research report series* (NIH Publication #09-4342). Rockville, MD: U.S. Department of Health and Human Services. Retrieved from http://drugabuse.gov/PDF/TobaccoRRS_v16.pdf

Vollmer, T. R., Sloman, K. N., & Pipkin, C. (2008). Practical implications of data reliability and treatment integrity monitoring. *Behavior Analysis Practitioner, 1*(2), 4–11. Retrieved from http://www.abainternational.org

Volpe, R. J., Briesch, A. M., & Chafouleas, S. M. (2010). Linking screening for emotional and behavioral problems to problem-solving efforts: An adaptive model of behavioral assessment. *Assessment for Effective Intervention, 35*(4), 240–244. doi:10.1177/1534508410377194.

Volpe, R. J., & Gadow, K. D. (2010). Creating abbreviated rating scales to monitor classroom inattention-overactivity, aggression, and peer conflict: Reliability validity, and treatment sensitivity. *School Psychology Review, 39*(3), 350–363. Retrieved from http://www.nasponline.org

Vreeman, R., & Carroll, A. (2007). A systematic review of school-based interventions to prevent bullying. *Archives of Pediatrics & Adolescent Medicine, 161*(1), 78–88. doi:10.1001/archpedi.161.1.78.

Waasdorp, T. E., Bradshaw, C. P., & Leaf, P. J. (2012). The impact of schoolwide positive behavioral interventions and supports on bullying and peer rejection: A randomized controlled effectiveness trial. *Archives of Pediatrics & Adolescent Medicine, 166*(2), 149–156. doi:10.1001/archpediatrics.2011.755.

Waddell, C., & Godderis, R. (2005). Rethinking evidence-based practice for children's mental health. *Evidence-Based Mental Health, 8*, 60–62. doi:10.1136/ebmh.8.3.60.

Waddell, C., Hua, J. M., Garland, O. M., Peters, R. D., & McEwan, K. (2007). Preventing mental disorders in children: A systematic review to inform policy-making. *Canadian Journal of Public Health, 98*(3), 166–173. Retrieved from http://journal.cpha.ca

Wag, J., Nansel, T. R., & Iannotti, R. J. (2011). Cyber and traditional bullying: Differential association with depression. *Journal of Adolescent Health, 48*(4), 415–417. doi:10.1016/j.jadohealth.2010.07.012.

Wagenaar, A. C., Gehan, J. P., Jones-Webb, R., Toomey, T. L., Forster, J. L., Wolfson, M., et al. (1999). Communities mobilizing for change on alcohol: Lessons and results from a 15-community randomized trial. *Journal of Community Psychology, 27*(3), 315–326. doi:10.1002/(SICI)1520-6629(199905)27:3<315::AID-JCOP6>3.0.CO;2-1.

Walker, H. M. (2008a, September 6). *Critical issues in the use of randomized clinical trials and control groups within applied settings: Rationale, challenges and benefits.* Paper presented at the 2008 ABA International Education Conference, Reston, VA.

Walker, E. (2008b). Meta-analysis: It's strengths and limitations. *Cleveland Clinic Journal of Medicine, 75*(6), 431–439. doi:10.3949/ccjm.75.6.431.

Walker, H. M., Kavanagh, K. A., Stiller, B., Golly, A., Severson, H. H., & Feil, E. G. (1998). First step to success: An early intervention approach for preventing school antisocial behavior. *Journal of Emotional and Behavioral Disorders, 6*, 66–81. doi:10.1177/106342669800600201.

Walker, H. M., Nishioka, V. M., Zeller, R., Severson, H. H., & Feil, E. G. (2000). Causal factors and potential solutions for the persistent underidentification of students having emotional or behavioral disorders in the context of schooling. *Assessment for Effective Intervention, 26*(1), 29–39. doi:10.1177/073724770002600105.

Walker, H., Stiller, B., Golly, A., Kavanagh, K., Severson, H., & Feil, E. (1997). *First step to success: Helping young children overcome antisocial behavior* (an early intervention program for grades K-3). Longmont, CO: Sopris.

Walsemann, K. M., Bell, B. A., & Maitra, D. (2011). The intersection of school racial composition and student race/ethnicity on adolescent depressive and somatic symptoms. *Social Science & Medicine, 72*(11), 1873–1883. doi:10.1016/j.socscimed.2011.03.033.

Walton, J. W., Johnson, S. B., & Algina, J. (1999). Mother and child perceptions of child anxiety: Effects of race, health status, and stress. *Journal of Pediatric Psychology, 24*(1), 29–39. doi:10.1093/jpepsy/24.1.29.

Wang, M., & Holcombe, R. (2010). Adolescents' perceptions of school environment, engagement, and academic achievement in middle schools. *American Educational Research Journal, 47*(3), 633–662. doi:10.3102/0002831209361209.

Wang, J., Iannotti, R. J., & Nansel, T. R. (2009). School bullying among US adolescents: Physical, verbal, relational, and cyber. *Journal of Adolescent Health, 45*(4), 368–375. doi:10.1016/j.jadohealth.2009.03.021.

Wang, Y., Tussing, L., Odoms-Young, A., Braunschweig, C., Flay, B., Hedeker, D., et al. (2006). Obesity prevention in low socioeconomic status urban African-American adolescents: Study design and preliminary finding of the HEALTH-KIDS study. *European Journal of Clinical Nutrition, 60*, 92–103. doi:10.1038/sj.ejcn.1602272.

Watkins, R., Meiers, M. W., & Visser, Y. L. (2012). *A guide to assessing needs: Essential tools for collecting information, making decisions, and achieving development results.* Washington, DC: The World Bank. Retrieved from http://ryanrwatkins.com

Watson, D. L., & Emory, C. (2010). From rhetoric to reality: The problematic nature and assessment of children and young people's social and emotional learning. *British Educational Research Journal, 36*(5), 767–786. doi:10.1080/01411920903159424.

Weare, K., & Nind, M. (2011). Mental health promotion and problem prevention in schools: What does the evidence say? *Health Promotion International, 26*(Suppl. 1), 129–169. doi:10.1093/heapro/dar075.

Webb, M. S., Rodriguez-Esquivel, D., & Baker, E. A. (2010). Smoking cessation interventions among Hispanics in the United States: A systematic review and mini meta-analysis. *American Journal of Health Promotion, 25*(2), 109–118. doi:10.4278/ajhp.090123-LIT-25.

Webster-Stratton, C. (1982). Teaching mothers through videotape modeling to change their children's behavior. *Journal of Pediatric Psychology, 7*(3), 279–294. doi:10.1093/jpepsy/7.3.279.

Webster-Stratton, C. (1990). *The teachers and children's videotape series: Dina Dinosaur's social skills and problem-solving curriculum.* Seattle: University of Washington Press.

Webster-Stratton, C. (1994). Advancing videotape parent training: A comparison study. *Journal of Consulting and Clinical Psychology, 62*(3), 583–593. doi:10.1037/0022-006X.62.3.583.

Webster-Stratton, C. (2000). *The Incredible Years training series.* Juvenile Justice Bulletin NCJ173422. Washington, DC: Office of Juvenile Justice and Delinquency Prevention.

Webster-Stratton, C. (2007). Tailoring the Incredible Years parent programs according to children's developmental needs and family risk factors. In J. M. Briesmeister & C. E. Schaefer (Eds.), *Handbook of parent training: Helping parents prevent and solve problem behaviors* (3rd ed., pp. 305–344). Hoboken, NJ: Wiley.

Webster-Stratton, C. (2009). Affirming diversity: Multi-cultural collaboration to deliver the Incredible Years parent programs. *International Journal of Child Health and Human Development, 2*(1), 17–32. Retrieved from https://www.novapublishers.com

Webster-Stratton, C., & Herman, K. C. (2010). Disseminating incredible years series early-intervention programs: Integrating and sustaining services between school and home. *Psychology in the Schools, 47*(1), 36–54. doi:10.1002/pits.20450.

Webster-Stratton, C., & Reid, M. J. (2008). Adapting the Incredible Years child dinosaur social, emotional, and problem-solving intervention to address comorbid diagnoses. *Journal of Children's Services, 3*(3), 17–30. doi:10.1108/17466660200800016.

Webster-Stratton, C., Reid, J., & Hammond, M. (2001). Preventing conduct problems, promoting social competence: A parent and teacher training partnership in Head Start. *Journal of Clinical Child Psychology, 30*(3), 283–302. doi:10.1207/S15374424JCCP3003_2.

Webster-Stratton, C., Reid, M. J., & Stoolmiller, M. (2008). Preventing conduct problems and improving school readiness: Evaluation of the Incredible Years teacher and child training programs in high-risk schools. *Journal of Child Psychology and Psychiatry, 49*(5), 471–488. doi:10.1111/j.1469-7610.2007.01861.x.

Webster-Stratton, C., Reinke, W. M., Herman, K. C., & Newcomer, L. L. (2011). The Incredible Years teacher classroom, management training: The methods and principles that support fidelity of training delivery. *School Psychology Review, 40*(4), 509–529. Retrieved from http://www.nasponline.org/

Wehipeihana, N., Davidson, E. J., McKegg, K., & Shanker, V. (2010). What does it take to do evaluation in communities and cultural contexts other than our own? *Journal of MultiDisciplinary Evaluation, 6*(13), 182–192. Retrieved from http://survey.ate.wmich.edu

Weiner, B. J. (2009). A theory of organizational readiness for change. *Implementation Science, 4*, 67. doi:10.1186/1748-5908-4-67.

Weinreich, N. K. (2011). *Hands-on social marketing: A step-by-step guide to designing change for good* (2nd ed., pp. 1–24). Thousand Oaks, CA: Sage.

Weisburd, D., Lum, C. M., & Petrosino, A. (2001). Does research design affect study outcomes in criminal justice? *Annals of the American Academy of Political and Social Science, 578*, 50–70. doi:10.1177/000271620157800104.

Weiss, H. B., Bouffard, S. M., Bridglall, B. L., & Gordon, E. W. (2009). Reframing family involvement in education: Supporting families to support educational equity. *Equity matters: Research Review No. 5.* NYL Teachers College, Columbia University. Retrieved from http://www.equitycampaign.org

Weiss, J. W., Cen, S., Mouttapa, M., Johnson, A. C., & Unger, J. (2011). Longitudinal effects of hostility, depression, and bullying on adolescent smoking initiation. *Journal of Adolescent Health, 48*(6), 591–596. doi:10.1016/j.jadohealth.2010.09.012.

Weiss, A. R., & Siddall, A. J. (2012). *Schools at the hub: Community partnerships in the Boston Public Schools.* Brookline, MA: Mendelsohn, Gittleman & Associates, LLC.

Weiss, H. B., & Stephen, N. C. (2010). From periphery to center: A new vision and strategy for family, school, and community partnerships. In S. L. Christenson & A. L. Reschly (Eds.), *Handbook of school-family partnerships* (pp. 448–472). New York: Routledge.

Weissberg, R. P., Kumpfer, K. L., & Seligman, M. E. P. (2003). Prevention that works for children and youth: An introduction. *American Psychologist, 58*(6/7), 425–432. doi:10.1037/0003-066X.58.6-7.425.

Weissberg, R. P., & O'Brien, M. U. (2004). What works in school-based social and emotional learning programs for positive youth development. *The Annals of the American Academy of Political Science and Social Science, 591*(1), 86–97. doi:10.1177/0002716203260093.

Weissman, M. M., Wickramaratne, P., Nomura, Y., Warner, V., Pilowsky, D., & Verdeli, H. (2006). Offspring of depressed parents: 20 years later. *The American Journal of Psychiatry, 163*, 1001–1008. doi:10.1176/appi.ajp.163.6.1001.

Weist, M. D. (2003a). Challenges and opportunities in moving toward a public health approach in school mental health. *Journal of School Psychology, 41*(1), 77–82. doi:10.1016/S0022-4405(02)00146-2.

Weist, M. D. (2003b). Commentary: Promoting paradigmatic change in child and adolescent mental health and schools. *School Psychology Review, 32*(3), 336–341. Retrieved from http://www.nasponline.org/

Weist, M. D., Rubin, M., Moore, E., Adelsheim, S., & Wrobel, G. (2007). Mental health screening in schools. *Journal of School Health, 77*(2), 53–57. doi:10.1111/j.1746-1561.2007.00167.x.

Weist, M. D., Stiegler, K., Stephan, S., Cox, J., & Vaughan, C. (2010). School mental health and prevention science in the Baltimore City schools. *Psychology in the Schools, 47*(1), 89–100. doi:10.1002/pits.20453.

Weisz, J. (2006, September 11). *Evidence-based practice in child & adolescent mental health: Recent news and my ESP on EBP*. Portland, Oregon: Children's Array of Psychiatric Programs.

Weisz, J. R., Chorpita, B. F., Palinkas, L., Schoenwald, S. K., Miranda, J., Bearman, S. K. (2012). Research Network on Youth Mental Health. Testing standard and modular designs for psychotherapy treatment for depression, anxiety, and conduct problems in youth: A randomized effectiveness trial. *Archives of General Psychiatry, 69*(3), 274–282. doi: 10.1001/archgenpsychiatry.2011.147.

Wenz-Gross, M., & Upshur, C. (2012). Implementing a primary prevention social skills intervention in urban schools: Factors associated with quantity and fidelity. *Early Education & Development, 23*(4), 427–450. doi:10.1080/10409289.2011.589043.

West, A. E., & Newman, D. (2007). Childhood behavioral inhibition and the experience of social anxiety in American Indian adolescents. *Cultural Diversity and Ethnic Minority Psychology, 13*(3), 197–206. doi:10.1037/1099-9809.13.3.197.

Westhues, A., Nelson, G., & MacLeod, J. (2003). The long-term impact of preschool prevention programs: Looking to the future. *Prevention & Treatment, 6*(1), Article 36. doi:10.1037/1522-3736.6.1.636r.

Whitcomb, S. (2009). *Strong Start: Impact of direct teaching of a social-emotional learning curriculum and infusion of skills on emotion knowledge of first grade students*. Doctoral dissertation, University of Oregon.

White, L. K., McDermott, J. M., Degnan, K. A., Henderson, H. A., & Fox, N. A. (2011). Behavioral inhibition and anxiety: The moderating roles of inhibitory control and attention shifting. *Journal of Abnormal Child Psychology, 39*(5), 735–747. doi:10.1007/s10802-011-9490-x.

Whittaker, R., Dorey, E., Parag, V., Rodgers, A., & Salmon, P. (2010). A theory-based video messaging mobile phone intervention for smoking cessation: Randomized controlled trial. *Journal of Medical Internet Research, 13*(1), e10. doi:10.2196/jmir.1553.

Whitted, K. S. (2011). Understanding how social and emotional skills deficits contribute to school failure. *Preventing School Failure, 55*(1), 10–16. doi:10.1080/10459880903286755.

Wildenger, L. K., & McIntyre, L. L. (2012). Investigating the relation between kindergarten preparation and child socio-behavioral school outcomes. *Early Childhood Education, 40*, 169–176. doi:10.1007/10643-012-0509-x.

Wille, N., Bettge, S., Ravens-Sieberer, U., & BELLA Study Group. (2008). Risk and protective factors for children's and adolescents' mental health: Results of the Bella study. *European Child & Adolescent Psychiatry, 17*(Suppl. 1), 133–147. doi:10.1007/s00787-008-1015-y.

Williams, S. L. (2008). Anxiety disorders. In J. E. Maddux & B. A. Winstead (Eds.), *Psychopathology: Foundations for a contemporary understanding* (2nd ed., pp. 151–169). New York: Routledge.

Williams, J. M., & Greenleaf, A. T. (2012). Ecological psychology: Potential contributions to social justice and advocacy in school settings. *Journal of Educational and Psychological Consultations, 22*, 141–157. doi:10.1080/10474412.2011.649653.

Williams, K. R., & Guerra, N. G. (2007). Prevalence and predictors of Internet bullying. *Journal of Adolescent Health, 41*(6), S14–S21. doi:10.1016/j.jadohealth.2007.08.018.

Williams-Taylor, L. (2010). *The journey to evidence-based programming: Changing the face of social services.* Boynton Beach, FL: Children's Services Council of Palm Beach County.

Wilson, S. J., & Lipsey, M. J. (2007). School-based interventions for aggressive and disruptive behavior: Update of a meta-analysis. *American Journal of Preventive Medicine, 33*(2S), S130–S145. doi:10.1016/j.amepre.2007.04.011.

Windle, M., Spear, L., Fuligni, A. J., Angold, A., Brown, J. D., Pine, D., et al. (2008). Transitions into underage and problem drinking: Developmental processes and mechanisms between 10 and 15 years of age. *Pediatrics, 121*(Suppl. 4), S273–S289. doi:10.1542/peds.2007-2243C.

Winsper, C., Lereya, T., Zanarini, M., & Wolke, D. (2012). Involvement in bullying and suicide-related behavior at 11 years: A prospective birth cohort study. *Journal of the American Academy of Child and Adolescent Psychiatry, 51*(3), 271–282. doi:10.1016/j.jaac.2012.01.001.

Winstead, B. A., & Sanchez-Hucles, J. (2008). The role of gender, race, and class in psychopathology. In J. E. Maddux & B. A. Winstead (Eds.), *Psychopathology: Foundations for a contemporary understanding* (2nd ed., pp. 39–65). New York: Routledge.

Winters, K. C., Fawkes, T., Fahnhorst, T., Botzet, A., & August, G. (2007). A synthesis review of exemplary drug abuse prevention programs in the United States. *Journal of Substance Abuse Treatment, 32*, 371–380. doi:10.1016/j.jsat.2006.10.002.

Witkiewitz, K., King, K., McMahon, R. J., Wu, J., Luk, J., Bierman, K. L., et al. (2013). Evidence for a multi-dimensional latent structural model of externalizing disorders. *Journal of Abnormal Child Psychology, 41*(2), 223–237. doi:10.1007/s10802-012-9674-z.

Wolfe, V. V., Dozois, D. J., Fisman, S., & DePace, J. (2008). Preventing depression among adolescent girls: Pathways toward effective and sustainable programs. *Cognitive and Behavioral Practice, 15*(1), 36–46. doi:10.1016/j.cbpra.2007.01.001.

Wood, J. J., Chiu, A. W., Hwang, W., Jacobs, J., & Ifekwunigwe, M. (2008). Adapting cognitive-behavioral therapy for Mexican American students with anxiety disorders: Recommendations for school psychologists. *School Psychology Quarterly, 23*(4), 515–532. doi:10.1037/1045-3830.23.4.515.

Woods-Groves, S., & Hendrickson, J. M. (2012). The role of assessment in informing our decision-making processes. *Assessment for Effective Intervention, 38*(1), 3–5. doi:10.1177/1534508412456200.

World Health Organization (2011). Good practice appraisal tool for obesity prevention programmes, projects, initiative and interventions. Copenhagen, Denmark: Author. Retrieved from http://www.euro.who.int.

Wurtlele, S. K., Marrs, S. R., & Miller-Perrin, C. L. (1987). Practice makes perfect: The role of participant modeling in sexual abuse prevention programs. *Journal of Consulting and Clinical Psychology, 55*(4), 599–602. doi:10.1037/0022-006X.55.4.599.

Xu, L., Qu, X. P., Mao, C. J., Ma, H. Y., Liu, T. J., Hu, H. Q., et al. (2011). Evaluation on the effects of an education program regarding the sedentary behavior among school-aged children using Transtheoretical Model. *Chinese Journal of Epidemiology, 32*(2), 142–145. doi:10.3760/cma.j.issn.0254-6450.2011.02.009.

Yarcheski, A., & Mahon, N. E. (2000). A causal model of depression in early adolescence. *Western Journal of Nursing Research, 22*(8), 879–894. doi:10.1177/01939450022044854.

Yazzie-Mintz, E. (2009). *Charting the path from engagement to achievement: A report on the 2009 high school survey of student engagement.* Bloomington, IN: Center for Evaluation and Educational Policy.

Ybarra, M. L., Diener-West, M., & Leaf, P. J. (2007). Examining the overlap in Internet harassment and school bullying: Implications for school intervention. *Journal of Adolescent Health, 41*(6), S42–S50. doi:10.1016/j.jadohealth.2007.09.004.

Yesil-Dagli, U. (2011). Center-based childcare use by Hispanic families: Reasons and predictors. *Children and Youth Services Review, 33*(7), 1298–1308. doi:10.1016/j.childyouth.2011.03.004.

Ysseldyke, J., & Geenen, K. (1996). Integrating the special education and compensatory education systems into the school reform process: A national perspective. *School Psychology Review, 25*(4), 418–430. Retrieved from http://www.nasponline.org

Ysseldyke, J., Lekwa, A. J., Klingbeil, D. A., & Cormier, D. C. (2012). Assessment of ecological factors as an integral part of academic and mental health consultation. *Journal of Educational and Psychological Consultation, 22*, 21–43. doi:10.1080/10474412.2011.649641.

Ysseldyke, J. E., & McLeod, S. (2006). Using technology tools to monitor response to intervention. In S. R. Jimerson, M. K. Burns, & A. M. VanDerHeyden (Eds.), *Handbook of response to intervention* (pp. 396–407). New York: Springer.

Yue, W. (2008). Resistance, the echo of change. *International Journal of Business and Management, 3*(2), 84–89. Retrieved from www.ccsenet.org.

Zayas, L. H. (2010). Seeking models and methods for cultural adaptation of interventions: Commentary on the special section. *Cognitive and Behavioral Practice, 17*, 198–202. doi:10.1016/j.cbpra.2010.01.006.

Zimmerman, J. A. (2008). Working the system: Building capacity for school change. *Journal of Scholarship & Practice, 5*(1), 9–14. Retrieved from http://www.aasa.org

Zimmerman, M. A., Ramirez-Valles, J., Washienko, K. M., Walter, B., & Dyer, S. (1996). The development of a measure of enculturation for Native American youth. *American Journal of Community Psychology, 24*(2), 295–310. doi:10.1007/BF02510403.

About the Author

Gayle L. Macklem, MA, NCSP, LEP, is a nationally certified school psychologist and a Massachusetts-licensed educational psychologist. She has served in the field of education for more than 30 years. She is a former president of the Massachusetts School Psychologists Association (MSPA); she serves as the Technology Chairperson of the state association. She is an instructor in the School Psychology Specialist and Doctoral Training Programs at the Massachusetts School of Professional Psychology in Newton. She writes curricula and writes on topics of interest to educators. She is a frequent presenter at regional and national conferences. Ms. Macklem is the author of Springer's *Evidence-Based School Mental Health Services: Affect Education, Emotion Regulation Training, and Cognitive Behavioral Therapy* (2011); *Practitioner's Guide to Emotion Regulation in School-Aged Children* (2008); and *Bullying and Teasing: Social Power in Children's Groups* (2003).

G.L. Macklem, *Preventive Mental Health at School: Evidence-Based Services for Students,* 369
DOI 10.1007/978-1-4614-8609-1, © Springer Science+Business Media New York 2014

Index

G.L. Macklem, *Preventive Mental Health at School: Evidence-Based Services for Students,*   371
DOI 10.1007/978-1-4614-8609-1, © Springer Science+Business Media New York 2014

Made in the USA
Lexington, KY
01 February 2017